Counseling Pregnancy, Politics, and Biomedicine
Empowering Discernment

Counseling Pregnancy, Politics, and Biomedicine
Empowering Discernment

Patricia Elyse Terrell, PhD, MTS

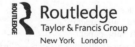

Routledge
Taylor & Francis Group
New York   London

First published by

The Haworth Pastoral Press®, an imprint of The Haworth Press, Inc., 10 Alice Street, Binghamton, NY 13904-1580.

This edition published 2012 by Routledge

Routledge
Taylor & Francis Group
711 Third Avenue
New York, NY 10017

Routledge
Taylor & Francis Group
2 Park Square, Milton Park
Abingdon, Oxon OX14 4RN

PUBLISHER'S NOTE
The development, preparation, and publication of this work has been undertaken with great care. However, the Publisher, employees, editors, and agents of The Haworth Press are not responsible for any errors contained herein or for consequences that may ensue from use of materials or information contained in this work. The Haworth Press is committed to the dissemination of ideas and information according to the highest standards of intellectual freedom and the free exchange of ideas. Statements made and opinions expressed in this publication do not necessarily reflect the views of the Publisher, Directors, management, or staff of The Haworth Press, Inc., or an endorsement by them.

Cover design by Kerry E. Mack.

Library of Congress Cataloging-in-Publication Data

Terrell, Patricia Elyse.
    Counseling pregnancy, politics, and biomedicine : empowering discernment / Patricia Elyse Terrell.
        p. cm.
    Includes bibliographical references and index.
    ISBN: 978-0-7890-3044-3 (hard : alk. paper)
    ISBN: 978-0-7890-3045-0 (soft : alk. paper)
    1. Human reproductive technology—Religious aspects—Christianity. 2. Human reproductive technology—Moral and ethical aspects. 3. Pastoral counseling. 4. Medical ethics. 5. Pregnancy—Religious aspects—Christianity. I. Title.

RG133.5.T47 2007
176—dc22

                                                                                        2006038680

This book is dedicated to Phillip, my only son,
whose optimism provided real inspiration.

John and Betty, my father and mother,
who provided a spirit of friendship
during the completion of this book.

ABOUT THE AUTHOR

Patricia Elyse Terrell, PhD, is an academic visitor to the Faculty of Theology at the University of Oxford in England. She was appointed an official Observer for the United Nations Educational, Scientific, and Cultural Organization's International Bioethics Committee (UNESCO IBC) and has participated in the negotiations, drafting, and delivery of international legal instruments with bioethic goals, including the European Convention on Biomedicine and Human Rights and the United Nations Declaration on the Universal Norms for Bioethics and Human Rights. Dr. Terrell has participated in the World Congress on Ethics in Medicine and made recommendations to the UNESCO IBC Committee for Ethics Education in Medical Schools.

CONTENTS

Acknowledgments

I am deeply grateful to the wonderful individuals and organizations who have contributed resources for this book. A special thank you to Derek Davis, James Wood Jr., and John Jonsson, J.M., Dawson Institute of Church-State Studies, Baylor University, for their commitment to liberty of conscience. University of Oxford scholars provided cutting-edge research data in genetics, law, philosophy, genetic medicine, and theology, especially John Hedley Brooke, Robert Morgan, the late Arthur Peacocke, Nicholas Proudfoot, Christopher Rowland, Richard Swinburne, David Vaux, Keith Ward, Margaret Yee, among the fine students who offered their insights. I offer my thanks to Denise McDonough for preparing the illustrations for this publication.

Many thanks to the international secretariats who generously included me in their legislative proceedings on modern reproductive medicine and genetics, including Carlos de Sola, Director for Bioethics and Family Law at the Council of Europe and the International Bioethics Committee, United Nations Educational, Scientific, and Cultural Organization's International Bioethics Committee (UNESCO IBC). Outstanding scholars from recognized universities around the globe broadened the perspective of this writing, contributing rich diversity, especially Alexander McCall Smith and Michel Revel. Papal legates Monsignor Michael Courtney, the Very Reverend Maurice Dooley, and Monsignor Jean-Marie Mpendawatu equipped me with diplomatic skills to show tranquility, gentleness, and strength in the face of difficult issues.

Finally, I would like to express my love and gratitude to my son, Phillip, and to John and Betty Terrell who encouraged and inspired my dedication to equipping, empowering, and protecting the health of mothers and children.

This book is offered in thanksgiving to the One Holy God, Creator, Redeemer, and Sustainer-Trinity living in Unity. Amen.

Counseling Pregnancy, Politics, and Biomedicine
© 2007 by The Haworth Press, Inc. All rights reserved.
doi:10.1300/5697_a

In the beginning was the Word, and the Word was with God, and the Word was God.

And the Word became flesh and lived among us, and we have seen his glory as the Father's true son full of grace and truth.

John 1:1-2, 14

Introduction

The Goals of the Book

The Christian church is a community of people dedicated to helping one another on a journey toward God's Promise. It represents God's activity in a pluralistic world in which religion and science coexist and, in many cases, religion has little to say about the scientific inventions of man. Genetics has moved from science to medicine, and genetic diagnosis has become a regularly prescribed technique in predicting risky pregnancies and other reproductive situations. As a science, genetics is constantly being revised, and this means that there is a constant need for ethical clarification and revision. Fortunately, ethical theories developed across centuries and provide a few constants in the formula, but pastors, ministers, priests, and health group leaders must be prepared to help communicants who come to them for guidance and reflection.

The church has an obligation to bring its contemporary ethical position into balance with the *qualities of life* it values for Christian living. This assists those who stand in the avalanche of disorganized news and magazine articles, which seem to confuse more than inform. Many church professionals and members think that *ethics* means drafting and imposing laws that protect patients from peculiar therapies. The church has an obligation to research the regulations, the ins and outs of writing health guidelines, laws, and to explore other avenues for protecting and informing its community about good health practices.

The effectiveness of communicating any Christian position depends on developing substantive issues with a user-friendly, instruc-

Counseling Pregnancy, Politics, and Biomedicine
© 2007 by The Haworth Press, Inc. All rights reserved.
doi:10.1300/5697_01

tive framework. Therefore, this book has adopted a format that is: (1) appropriate for teaching and informing a household of Christian believers, beginning with its leaders, and (2) suitable for people of conscience who are called to inspire lawmakers to write legal protections in the area of genetic diagnosis.

The ideas and conceptualizations presented in this book offer ministers and Christians a way to sharpen and transform discernment abilities in the faith and in practical matters, through the following features:

- It presents a complete discussion on humankind created in the image of God *(imago Dei),* the goals of the Christian faith, and how these images intersect a *living* religion with *live science.*
- It offers a broad-based orientation to each field with lay language and places important aspects, issues, and terminology in its particular context.
- Each subject is developed and made relevant through its history, normative practices, and internal competing systems.
- The new terminology that has evolved in theology, ethics, law, and medicine as a result of genetic therapy is explained and defined.
- The boundaries, positions, and recommendations by the church are clarified.
- Information is communicated in lay terminology to assist clergy in discussing genetic therapy intelligently (i.e., sharing information).
- It teaches and equips others to be self-directing (c.f., counseling suggestions) and to make personal decisions (i.e., discernment) based on solid ethical theories, not memorized prescriptive formulas for *XYZ-type illness,* because circumstances alter cases.
- People are equipped to take personal, proactive positions in health care-even participation in the public forum.
- The application of the information is demonstrated through examples provided in the last two chapters of the book—one for women and one for the unborn baby.

The book simplifies science and the law, so that laypersons can be active too. It suggests important issues that need to be addressed by elected officials and lawmakers, such as:

- Writing laws that provide educational opportunities for *all* people to learn about the benefits and risks of genetic medicine, especially women of childbearing age, who may wish to participate in their own health care.
- The allocation of funds needed to train and provide counselors and information centers for patients using genetic diagnosis (distributive justice).
- Delineation of a minimum standard of practice for medical practitioners and researchers, with the appropriate penalties for failing to meet the obligations.
- Emphasizing the need for laws providing just and equitable access to genetic diagnosis services, clinics, and technology.

One reason why congressmen and women have not adequately represented their constituencies in regulating genetics is because they are not educated to do so. Representatives have to hire scientific experts to translate genetic language (jargon), interpret molecular technology, and recommend the appropriate actions. As a result, science has become *self-regulating*. Scientific experts do not have a duty to represent anyone and have, notoriously, pursued their own interests. Private firms have *no* legal restrictions—even when using human subjects. In the wake of the separation of church and state as well as some ferocious divides between science and theology, many lawmakers have fallen into thinking that health matters are just plumber–plumbing routines. Nonetheless, the fact that medical science is complex does not change the responsibility of the church to follow through.

On more than one occasion, politicians have asked religious professionals to explain why these *biological* issues mattered to the body of Christ. If the clergy cannot articulate it now, they will be able to after reading *Counseling Pregnancy, Politics, and Biomedicine: Empowering Discernment*. One of the longest-standing reasons behind the church's involvement in the politics of human health came from the tradition that human beings were created in God's image, *imago Dei*. The mote surrounding *imago Dei* was partially a result of the high degree of academic specialization. Scholars excluded data from fields beyond their own subject, but honest research needed to investigate the whole picture. Being made in the image of God is explicable in concrete terms that cut to the core of the Christian faith, which is very anthropological. Thanks to science, there are now vivid and wonderful technical descriptions that help explain and integrate theological information and goals.

There are several important reasons why being created in the image of God means so much. *Imago Dei* refers to the entire human race. The research in this book cuts to the very essence of human origin, even before creation, to explore the *divine–human relationship* (where we came from and where we are going)—including, but not limited to, God's Promise for the heirs of the Christian faith.

The discussion about Christianity needs to follow one cohesive doctrine. Since the life of Christ is the focal point for *all* Christian denominations, Jesus' life is the common denominator for church community. The *universal* Church is not dependent on the variety of tenets around which a myriad of denominations have organized their communities. Jesus was the Archetypical *Imago Dei*. The Christian faith was founded on Jesus' example, and biblical narratives depict life with ideas and activities that we see through history.

In a health-related text, it is especially important that the relationship of God-in-Christ, as *imago Dei*, be explained with realism. Hence, the chapter on theology explains the natural, physiological properties of humankind, so that one understands in which ways human genetic health can directly influence the God–human relationship. This defends why reproductive health and science is the business of the church and its theology.

In addition to locating a solid fulcrum for human health in theology, ethics, and law, a fair and balanced viewpoint has to consider its ethical priorities from a medical perspective. The truth is that public policy makers will only listen to a church opinion when it can be qualified and substantiated in material terms. The general environment of genetics has become so broad that, in order to understand it, one has to have an in-depth acquaintance with the many faces of experimental medicine. To achieve this challenge, the book looks at medical philosophies, techniques, and the rationale behind human experimentation.

The primary disciplines impacting the present discussion are theology, ethics, law, and medical experimentation. The terminology and the subject matter are defined in a format that teaches. It does not prescribe terms or conclusions. A historical framework for experimental medicine is employed to place it within its own context, explaining the various branches that have emerged within the subject, while showing how and why experimentation has paved a way for molecular and genetic medicine. Examples of workable, contemporary therapies in genetics are provided as well as those that are not yet viable. Adopting lay language in place of the professional terminology assists the reader.

After Part One presents four chapters containing information, it is time for practical lessons. Part Two consists of two chapters that demonstrate how the information may be applied in specific situations. Chapter 5 enters the environment of expectant mothers, with its myths, discomforts, quandaries, and hard decisions. Four contemporary dilemmas are raised. One targets human dignity and ethical behavior, encouraging an education that meets the demands of an age of biotechnology. Moving to issues related to medicine, suggestions are made on how the environment can be improved to respect and protect women from situations that manipulate them and force codependency or moral compromise. Applying law and politics opens the fiery debate in America over abortion, turning to the U.S. Constitution and its legal history. With pertinent issues raised in several fields, it is time to hear how experts in other jurisdictions dealt with some of the legal challenges.

Chapter 6 dares to examine the moral status of the embryo. It considers the fetus in light of human connectivity as well as utilitarian biotechnology. Arguments about the definitions of a fetus and fetal stem cell research are grounded in tangible logic, even when the research inherently contradicts established values. Then it raises the issues that beg for the appropriate policy and legal restraints.

In summary, the overall aim of this book is to organize all the basic definitions and theses from theology, ethics, law, and medical science that assist people in making holistic health care decisions and encouraging community members to respect and trust them. Hopefully, when physicians and researchers listen to clergy who have studied these concepts, it will demonstrate a thoughtful interest and open doors for discussions about all that ministers have to say—on many subjects. Life has a primary value that moves beyond pregenetic ethics into a mature, realistic approach to values and admits that sentience is part of the cure.

A wide variety of resources has been used to develop the text, explain the issues, and rectify gaps, including books, articles, seminars, symposia, laboratory experiments, government legislative sessions, as well as interfaith, ecumenical dialogues among various church communities. This Christian writing was intended to edify the marvels and accomplishments achieved by theologians, ethicists, lawyers, and medical scientists—since each one has contributed to the pool of knowledge that serves life and health. In addition, the writing recognizes that Christ's ministry heals and protects the vulnerable, the weak, the disabled, and other members of society who experience marginalization—and in the course of healing and defending others Jesus challenged existing political and religious norms to accomplish his goals. This serves as an example, making it our duty to protect the rights of those who have no one else to defend them.

A FORMULA THAT LISTENS AND TEACHES: PLACING DEFINITIONS AND THESES INTO NARRATIVE FORMAT

How does one research the Christian church's position on genetic diagnosis and conduct an investigation supportive of legislation? There is an enormous amount of information that impacts bioethics, and this investigation of reproduction and its genetic counterparts includes translating professional jargon and technical terminology into more readable language. On the one hand, the research takes a macro approach, so the task far surpasses simply writing basic lists to define the most frequently used terms. That has certainly been done in various books and articles. Many of the terms, descriptions, and theses contained herein are presented in story form to help the readers locate their own impressions and preferences—this creates flexibility and an adaptable instrument. Although ethics was originally a branch of religious studies, bioethicists now emerge from several disciplines that have declared independence from religion and theology—legal ethics, social morality, industrial ethics and the psychology of relationships, genomic ethics for the financial business of genetic discoveries, and medical ethics, which itself harbors even more specialized subjects, such as divisions of biological ethics and genetic ethics.

Over the centuries, several different ethical approaches reached heights of popularity and preference. As one ponders reproductive applications, there are prevailing accents from one or more of the antecedent ethical styles. An Englishman or a biochemist may favor *utilitarian ethics;* a German or a physician might prefer *Kantian* ethics; an American or a sociologist may lean into *feminist or womanist* ethics, etc. Again, each theory helping to clarify the reasons behind good health stewardship merits a description. Humankind has invented several independent ethical formulas on how to express the *best* and *highest* care to one another; that is why there is a chapter devoted to reviewing ethical theories.

In addition to studying values from within each field, this investigation also had to integrate multiple, interdisciplinary relationships. Interdisciplinary encounters included interfacing science and theology, politics and religion, law and theology, science and medicine, and law and science—to name a few. Simplifying the subject matter preserves the instructional nature of the work, so the categories will be general headings such as theology, ethics, law, and medical experimentation.

Each subject will identify its own influences and subdivisions. The theories may or may not be interdependent—usually not. Some scholars believe ideologies and methodologies have an emergent pattern, and other experts, such as phenomenologists, consider each different attitude as a unique phenomenon that impacts a particular culture. The present assessments try not to prejudge one theory or the other, though there are points of convergence with obvious prejudices. The subtopics make a difference since, for example, one country uses common law and relies on legislation more than another nation that uses Napoleonic law; one generation of doctors prefers a more traditional approach, whereas another uses state-of-the-art molecular medical practices; there are religious teachers who teach "essential dogmas," while some theologians gravitate toward explanations from particular schools, such as those from stemming from the Alexandrian or Antiochene schools. The mixed backgrounds of a country's citizens will color its attitudes. In America's melting pot, there are a plethora of opinions in bioethics, stemming from its potpourri of heritages. Thusly, multiple categories are compared and contrasted to provide a place where readers can locate a fulcrum that suits their values as they apply to this subject.

It is a major challenge to interpret and articulate a realistic view of the Christian church as a community whose faith is in One Lord, Christ Jesus, when there are multifactional Christian communities. At the end of the day, the theological chapter intentionally leaves the door open to the different ways people understand the God-human relationship so as not to offend the mission of the church or the conscience of individual believers—and this does not detract from the cohesiveness of a community centered on the example of Jesus, the God–Human. Understanding the influences of reproductive medicine in late modernity through the lens of informed theology about the divine–human relationship is a primary concern for theologians and church professionals, since they are called to reflect on the long-term social–psychological effects for the church community and the surrounding environment. The church has a passionate desire for each person to have an opportunity to reach his or her full potential. *Freedom of conscience* figures into this because it empowers free moral agents to make conscientious decisions and provides a constitutional bill of inalienable rights. The author respects every person's unique identity and liberty of conscience. This book desires to furnish knowledge pursuant to the equitable access of fair, moral health practices, without discouraging the treasures in store for humankind through genetic discoveries.

WHAT TO EXPECT UNDER EACH HEADING

Part I

Chapter 1—Humankind Created in the Image of God,
Imago Dei: *The Passon and Politics of Human Biology*

Chapter 1 takes a look at humanity in the image of God, *imago Dei*. Jewish and Christian scriptures present a compelling and practical understanding of human potential by narrating examples of people's lifestyles—some are righteous and some are not. Biological function plays a significant role in the practice of faith. But, before launching into an informed theology about *imago Dei,* it has to navigate some obvious dichotomies. First of all, a theological approach to medically assisted reproduction involves a discussion on scientifically related information, which asks that science, *per se,* be introduced into theology. Connections come from resources provided by individuals accomplished in both science and theology, such as the late Arthur Peacocke, Keith Ward, John Hedley Brooke, John Polkinghorne, Margaret Yee, Ian Barbour, among others.

Secondly, God's single message has many expressions as seen in Christian denominationalism, so it is helpful to focus the reader on the core of Christian thought—Jesus Christ himself and the character traits that he expressed. This way, Christianity appears as a single Christian community rather than several associations. It respects and briefly discusses the different worldviews that arise from people who adhere to either the Semitic or the Hellenist traditions. Some refer to the Antiochene or Alexandrian schools as the two most influential teachings. Kallistos Ware and George Maloney contributed insights that helped organize this topic.

The *imago Dei* chapter develops an informed theology that explains why a healthy human *body* is of tremendous concern to God. This is important because classical theology divided the human and heavenly, as did the "divine clockmaker" idea in which God watches his creatures from afar. This chapter explains why God is not aloof and detached. It presents, rather, a case for divine–human interdependencies. *Imago Dei* refers to all of humanity, and God having a relationship with the entire species. Therefore the discussion is not isolated to Christian believers, but it considers all of humankind, which possesses some common heritable properties and others that are more specific.

Jesus was born into the human community as the Exemplar par excellence of the God-human relationship. He was created in the image of God, and so was humankind. The chapter proceeds step-by-step in the unveiling of *imago Dei* using a definitive biblical verse or theological concept that can be systematically unraveled and interpreted. The idea is to steer the reader through an uninterrupted course of awareness about the human-divine relationship. The trail begins with the Jewish community in the Old Testament who proffered the genes that made-up Jesus' genome. Jesus came to the Jews to instruct each person, by example, on how to live faith that fulfilled God's law. Biblical commentaries from Old Testament scholars such as Samuel Driver, Franz Delitzsche, John Skinner, M. Rosenbaum, and Arthur Silbermann are interfaced with modern scientific explanations and imagery, such as cosmology, physics, human anatomy, and biochemistry, in analyzing the Creator *before* creation, the concept of *Logos,* and *imago Dei.*

Verses from the New Testament describe Christ as the Word made flesh. These speak of Jesus' birth and life in its expression of both human and divine qualitites that created a library for future generations—that comprise *the* church. Skilled theologians compare modern scientific discoveries with theological propositions. Among these erudite contributors stand John Jonsson, Keith Ward, Nancey Murphy, John Habgood, and many, many others. This study requires scientific information about DNA, embryology, biochemistry, and neurophysiology from writers such as Susan Greenfield, who explained the anatomical wonders of the human brain and neurological pathways in a very comprehensible manner. In examining the texts, one discovers that God responds to those who were, and are, devoted to pursuing the course of faith in astonishing ways. Reflections on Jürgen Moltmann, Tim Bradshaw's thoughts on Wolfgang Pannenberg, Morwena Ludlow's research on Karl Rahner, as well as Keith Ward's volumes on comparative theology are used to gather insights about *Theobiogenesis*—what happened when God put His signature on Jesus' life. Human consciousness changes and human capacities are enlarged so that people encounter eternity in life *and* death. Richard Swinburne, Christopher Rowland, and John Jonnson offered major insights about the road to Resurrection and why this became popular among Christian believers. Mixing divine qualities with human potential poses a startling, immensely powerful, and intimate relationship between divine and human natures. The natural outplay of this discovery logically leads to the conclusion that the church has a legitimate interest in human health, biomedical discussions, and, therefore, genetic diagnosis.

*Chapter 2—Ethics: Has Morality Become a Maze
or a Prism?*

Over the ages, religious leaders from many cultures believed that certain civilizations achieved prominent positions because the god or gods of that particular tribe or culture was the most powerful god in the *council of gods*. Chiefs, kings, philosophers, and prophets have pondered ways to impress, worship, and empower their god(s). Human strength, an army's victory, intellect, and civic diligence were all components of how human beings went about life in the *right* way. *Being right* and *being ethical* have similar meanings, but the rationale and motivations to those goals differed according to time and culture.

Civilizations all over the world have contributed to ethics scholarship and what it means to *do* or *be* right and good. Henry Sidgwick's *History of Ethics* offered concrete starting points for defining ethics, morality, and rationale, and he contributed much to the overall shape of this discussion. Theories and examples chosen for health care ethics gravitate toward points emphasizing respect for the whole person— body, mind, and soul. Since the Hippocratic Oath, medicine has had its own branch of ethics—its standard of practice.

Christians need to develop their own ethical rationale about health care and genetic diagnosis that conforms to the directions Christ gave in his teachings, not simply an echo of the reasoning developed and passed on by medical scientists. In Chapter 2, basic Christian values as well as philosophers on medical ethics are considered, such as Tom Beauchamp, Oliver O'Donovan, Bernard Mayo, Robert Veatch, and Baruch Brody. To understand which moral positions best suit genetic diagnosis, the discussion surveys all the ethical systems that inform human rights and justice—classical ethics from Greek poetry and philosophers, religious ethics, natural law, Kantian, Utilitarian, principle-based medical ethics, womanist ethics, as well as Mesoethics.

The presentation of ethical theories for the purposes of assisting the discernment of reproductive and genetic health will be kept intact, while made succinct. The author connects the ethical theories to the medical venue by developing the stories and theories about the ethical stewardship of the human body. Greek poetry told of people who took care of their bodies to impress the gods. Although the Greek philosophers were a few steps ahead of Jesus' revelation that he, in fact, had a human nature tied to his heavenly origin, the ideas coalesced concerning the God–human dynamic. Natural law, Kant, and the British empiricists, all have particular philosophies that contribute to medical ethics, and Christian ethics as well. Thinkers from different times and places made coherent and useful contributions for discerning issues. This chapter locates the most helpful definitions and contributions for understanding our subject matter.

For example, Socrates, Plato, and Aristotle favored virtuous attributes and studied ways to teach these so as to raise the standards of the ancient Greek civilization. Christian texts also came out of Greece and featured a special brand of virtues, some of which Paul and the Evangelists associated with Holy behavior. This chapter reviews several contemporary publications on Christian ethics, such as Joseph Fletcher's *Situation Ethics,* and publications by Alaisdair MacIntyre, Keith Ward, James Gustafson, Stephen Pope, Stanley Hauerwas, John Jonsson, and Daniel McGee, as well as Lisa Cahill's review of the Paul Ramsey–Richard McCormick debate.

Aristotle also gave vision to natural law, which was later corralled in the writings of Thomas Aquinas and was largely developed during the Middle Ages by philosophers from Christian, Jewish, and Islamic backgrounds. Walter Kaufman and Forrest Baird described the era of Aquinas and other medieval philosophers as each reflected upon God's Being and His desires for human behavior. Clerics during this period began to develop ideas about how divine communications occurred in human consciousness and conscience.

Alternatively, Immanuel Kant abandoned the religious frame of reference although not the Ultimate vision, as he preferred a more objective and less intuitive emphasis. In time, secular ethics became popular and were given expression by Jeremy Bentham and John S. Mill. Each, in his own British way, defined utilitarianism. Since utilitarianism was growing side-by-side with an increase in scientific investigations, the chapter visits the history of science from David Lindberg, as well as John Hedley Brooke's inspired history of religion and science. How one behaves in a particular setting at a given time in history influences the type of moral behavior that can be expected.

Standing on the ground floor of medical ethics involves principle-based ethics, womanist ethics, and perspectives from Mesoethics that deliver the reader to the ethical and legal platforms where human rights issues come into play. Womanist ethics are important because the new medical technology focuses heavily on reproduction, which involves women's bodies. Ethical principles are steeped in issues regarding freedom of conscience, which drew authors such as James E. Wood, Jr., Derek Davis, C. A. Pierce, and Michael Baylor, to name a few. Scholarship about women's ethics was limited, so the author created a new, original womanist ethic to specifically correlate challenges that women face with making decisions about reproduction and genetic therapy. In many cases, pregnant women do not have sufficient education and are particularly vulnerable to discrimination. Thoughts and writings from Lois Daly and Carol Gilligan provided background and ideas. Equal rights, equal opportunity, health management organizations (HMOs), and forms of socialized medicine merged together and issued a wake-up call for Mesoethics to dive into the heart of justice, civil liberties, and human rights issues—all part of balancing health care resources. This chapter considers *rights* and *justice* concepts proposed by famous political theorists such as John Rawls, Arthur Sade, Robert Nozick, Andrew Williams, T.M. Scanlon, and G.A. Cohen. Considering these views, it seems that patient-centered medicine and socioeconomic medicine may not be heading in the same direction. It is important that this Christian position be familiar with society's moral attitudes—law needs to come from society and be received by that society in order to be effective. How does political thought nurture respect for personhood, liberty of conscience, and human rights?

The chapter provides a myriad of values that may be useful in evaluating assisted reproductive practices. More than one ethical form may apply to the reader's formation of values, and he or she may notice a particular absence in cohesions that could indicate a need for generating new solutions. It is all part of the discernment process that leads to good ethical choices.

Chapter 3—What Politics? Which Legal System?

The purpose of this chapter is to offer a study in comparative law, looking at religious law, civil law, common law, human rights law, international law, and the twists and turns that these took, which compounded attempts to regulate reproductive biotechnology and therapies. Considering legal systems is in keeping with the proper expression of guidelines and standards that frame Christian values about genetic diagnoses. In order to set forth principles in society and make them legally binding, one has to understand the legal and political system; and one has to know the boundaries that separate church motives from public secular purposes by understanding what is involved in suitable legal and political vehicles.

For example, this writing uses a Christian value system, which invokes *religious law*. Religious law was the foundation for many of the statutes appearing in the civilized world, yet it differs from the *civil law* that was set forth in the Greek and Roman periods from which religious canons germinated. Civil law has much to do with present-day international human rights law as well as the *common law* that is practiced in many Western and American societies. The American Congress has to consider common law as well as constitutional provisions (c.f., bill of rights and human rights law). Most of the existing legislation on genetics comes from nations using civil law as well as international human rights law. All the legal formats have developed intersections over the years. If the desire is to express religious values so that they are fair to people of *all* faith traditions and of the *no-faith* background, then the delivery system and the language have to be amicable to *public* law systems. One has to consider the legal vessels, rather than merely presume that it is possible to take laws from foreign (i.e., different) law systems and cut-and-paste into one that, in reality, is inherently different.

Here is an examination of the law systems, antecedents, changing attitudes, and recent influences that are directly associated with issues from genetic screening. Each legal category begins with a definition, and then places the law system in a familiar context, communicating the principles and terminology in common language—teaching as it proceeds.

The study begins with religious law because it has the most ancient background and was widely practiced, even though the religious cults differed over the generations. Zeroing in on the Christian tradition places the researcher in Rome with religious texts that were written by a Roman citizen, Paul of Tarsus. Robert Morgan considered the Roman environment as he elaborated on Paul's epistle to the *Romans*. He gave a clear impression of how Roman law impacted Christian thought. Mircea Eliade offers some broader religious impressions, and Geoffrey Sawer provides insights into legal structures and divisions. There was much to say about *rights* from Christian perspectives vis-à-vis their modern equivalents. Can attitudes from 2000 years ago be interpreted into modern human rights? Were religious law and civil codes woven together by Justinian? Some of the former priestly traditions, such as long robes and decorum, have shifted into the secular courtroom, according to Harold Berman. Berman's erudite observations are complimented by the professional writings from Derek Davis and James Wood, Jr., at the J.M. Dawson Institute of Church-State Studies, Baylor University.

The comparative law experts, David Sawyer and Geoffrey René, explain the journey of civil law and common law. James E. Wood, Jr., contributed insights about the diversity caused by Eastern and Western cultures. Politics often lacked virtue, but power also corrupted religious leadership, and these struggles for power cast dark, lingering shadows that eventually erected a wall of separation between those who governed the church and those manning government posts. Experts in religious matters lacked expertise in state affairs, and professional politicians were not qualified to make decisions for the churches. Jean-Jacques Rousseau, Diderot, and others strove for completely new social orders. Derek Davis reflected on whether or not *neutrality* between religion and politics was even possible in the judicial setting.

After a discussion on the three primary law systems, the chapter begins to reconstruct law to fit biomedicine. Roger Dworkin reviewed the bioethical cases that have already been disputed in court—controversy arose over experimentation, wrongful birth, wrongful life, embryo experiments, etc. Bernard Dickens evaluates reproductive sciences in terms of law, ethics, and justice. Sheila Jasonoff takes a look at science at the [legal] bar.

The goals of science have to be weighed next to the vision that society has created for its short- and long-term health organization. Bertha Knoppers and Andrea Bonniksen examined the dichotomy already present between private and public pursuits. The chapter brings the reader to an understanding of how the legal system operates, its swarthy influences, and the power of money in minimalizing the regulation of science and medicine. These important considerations help set the tone for what ethics may have become in view of money, power, and technology—dilemmas in trying to get protections surrounding genetic research have emerged into radical *laissez faire* policies. Chapter 5 and Chapter 6 cannot ignore the signals that these issues raise for women and embryos, nor can society allow itself to be sold for a pittance.

Concerns about the direction of modern reproductive medicine have been legislated at the international level. The process of evaluating bioethics and genetics requires patience. Considering international rights has advantages for Americans, because the laws center on pluralism, the stuff of modern America. The international laws could assist in establishing universal standards with just, uniform, regulatory offices, so that offenders could not hop frontiers to pursue business interests that offend human values. The discussion presents some interesting examples.

Chapter 4—Medical Experimentation and Reproduction

Chapter 2 gave a face to each different ethical approach, Chapter 3 defined the legal and political systems that are involved in legislating social morals, and this chapter surveys different medical philosophies that are important to the tenor of experimental medicine. The categories are divided into: (1) defining health and background on traditional medicine; (2) the philosophy of holocaust medicine (the way *not* to go); (3) molecular medicine; and (4) palliative care as an alternative to modern technology, as therapy.

An exploration of medical history and experimentation illustrates the growing acceptance of experimental research and therapy. Insights into medical history by E.H. Ackernecht are heightened by what Michel Foucault revealed in the *Birth of the Clinic*. John Brooke, Geoffrey Cantor, William May, and Alan Johnson help the reader to integrate medicine with religion, tradition, and covenants. Henrik Wulff, Stig Andur Petersen, and Raben Rosenberg carry medical philosophy to the gate of the medical revolution—as told by Robert B. Baker, Arthur Caplan, Linda L. Emanuel, and Stephan Latham. F. Campagnari explains society's desire for biotechnology.

Civilization reached an enlightened medical pinnacle by the mid-twentieth century, and then it crashed. Examining medical experimentation during the German Holocaust is a *must* when evaluating the high stakes of ideological goals. The scientific expectations revolved around racial purity and all too familiar aspects of genetic manipulation—mixed with social engineering. The emerging medical techniques and premeditated manipulation of circumstances lead to atrocities that bioethicists want to eliminate forever. Yehuda Bauer, William Brennan, Donald Diedrich, and Robert Lifton are but a few of the scholars who detailed World War II episodes that set up the myriad of tragic narratives, as shared by Eli Wiesel. Human experimentation has existed in other societies, but not to the extent that occurred in World War II. George Annas and Michael Grodin brought to life the Nuremberg Code that was implemented after the Nazi Doctors' trial, as have John Jonsson's writings about post-Holocaust studies. Out of the Nuremberg Doctors' Trials came postwar legal instruments that focused on the protection of human life-proclaiming that every person is entitled to respect because he or she is *human*. Professor E. BenGershôm campaigned for medical students to be educated about the responsibilities that accompany the heroic aspects of medicine.

The third section blazes the trail into postwar scientific achievements that came about due to the advancements in molecular medicine and a very different approach to medical practices. The history behind genetics traveled from Charles Darwin's theories to Gregor Mendel's experiments and beyond. This chapter offers the details behind the double helix and DNA as explained by James Watson, Lubert Stryer, and other scientists. From Oxford University, lessons from John Knowland unravel the *jargon* while Nicholas Proudfoot and David Vaux set up laboratory experiments on cloning bacteria and cancer cells. The research continues to explore the animal experiments that led up to human applications in an attempt to discern the *actual* level of progress that is being achieved. Can the embryology of animals be transferred to human applications? The answer, at present, is no.

Genetic screening can give confidence to expectant mothers. The details of the screening processes (i.e., PID, PND) are explained, as well as the goals that each method is striving to accomplish. This section also evaluates the identification and treatment of particular heritable diseases. Alternative methodologies are also discussed, because each contributes to major medical breakthroughs and provides *hope* for patients. The ethical implications of genetic treatments are reviewed by James Childress, Allen Verney, Richard Devine, Eric Juengst, LeRoy Walters, and many other qualified scholars in the bioethical field. The *best interests of the patient* means reconciling the goals of science and medicine, so that the health of the patient is the final frontier.

The philosophy of genetic medicine is also challenged. The floor is given to professionals who, among others, support DNA's "lariat" hypothesis, a less-circulated theory, and skeletal development observations that illustrate system interdependency, diverting from genetics only propositions. Peter Cook's theory about *genetic processes* indicates that there are still many unanswered questions. Steven J. Goss is another academic physician who stands apart from the crowd, as he explains how cells differentiate into specific tissues and organs as well as the myriad of genetic matrixes that are possible and which cannot be predicted. Tim Horder challenges genetic primacy with his research on limb development patterns. Kay Davis is a very fine scientist, and her experiments have increased her confidence that patients with Duchenne muscular dystrophy (DMD) will be treated successfully in the future. These are all thoughtful assessments, backed by controlled experiments, and they are all worthy of consideration, in addition to being quite interesting. Knowing that physicians and scientists are receiving different training from one another enhances the prospects for developing a broad variety of treatments and creating new opportunities to advance human health. This chapter is designed to equip the reader with details about most of the genetic therapies that have been developed, or to look at a particular treatment's stage of development. The information is specific enough to assist people in making qualified decisions for themselves—with counseling from professional molecular therapists or assisted by licensed medical experts.

Not all people wish to tread the road of high technology. Some patients and families prefer to follow the natural course of life and death rather than become involved in genetic solutions. It is important to know that palliative care systems offer an alternative. Robert Twycross is the foremost authority on the subject of palliative care. Palliative therapy makes life, suffering, and death a family experience. It is about relationships. William May speaks of a quality of life that takes the spotlight off of the quantity of life. The discussion emphasizes that death is not failure—life becomes very precious when it is measured. Nancey Murphy raises important dimensions about Ultimate reality, as does David Jones in his discourse on death—from the viewpoint of a religious professional. Palliative care allows a patient and his or her family to opt out of high-technology therapy. People need not be intimidated into genetic engineering if they prefer to take a different route.

Part II

Chapter 5—Issues Faced by the Expectant Mother

Motherhood has been honored from age to age. Women conceive, carry, and deliver babies. Mothers usually have the responsibility of raising children. Over the years, women have also received education that prepares them for numerous other professions. Providing a woman with the tools to make health care decisions, especially for pregnancy, does not seem inconsistent with her other social roles.

In the ordinary course of reflection, an expectant mother will: (1) evaluate the benefits and risks of having genetic screening; (2) want to learn about medical alternatives, corrective therapy, abortion, or make special medical and educational plans for the infant and family if her suspicion of a heritable illness is confirmed; (3) ask for details and get opinions from professional counselors, consult family members, and take encouragement from clergy; and (4) weigh the information and advice in order to make an informed decision. This seems to be a reasonable approach to decision making; so, what, if anything, is wrong with this picture?

The previously mentioned formula contains presumptions, which are not universal. This exercise acts similar to a case study. It provides an opportunity to consider real-life hypothetical questions, with ways to answer them using the information from previous chapters. The reader has a chance to see the information from Chapter 1 through Chapter 4 in action—to discern and prioritize decisions and dig deeper to see if alternatives exist. It will increase one's ability to make moral decisions across the board. Based on the above scenario, consider the following: (1) a woman's self-determination may be challenged; (2) she needs to be educated in order to make informed decisions and would benefit from a clinical setting that provides a more homelike environment, one that communicates kindness and sympathy rather than brass and steel; (3) a woman may have serious quandaries about abortion, and reviewing abortion-related legal cases explains how others thought, and fought, through the struggle; and (4) there are circumstances that ask for legislative protections to safeguard pregnant women involved in genetic therapy. This *practice* involves real issues.

Issue (1) is couched in an old debate: David Thomasma and Edmund Pellegrino defend medical paternalism as the only responsible way to treat expectant mothers, while Robert Veatch et al. stand firmly with autonomy. Many believe paternalism is damaging to a woman's character, as a female class of persons. The chapter on expectant women employs a *womanist ethic,* referring to studies from Carol Gilligan and Lois Daly; Christian writer Richard Niebuhr offers substance, as do positions articulated by the erudite scholar Albert Schweitzer.

Next, issue (2) makes it ethically incumbent upon the trained medical professional to share knowledge with patients and provide counseling, so that decisions are made based on concrete, positive resources. Specific examples are provided about technical information, statistical data, and social adjustments that will be encountered. Several ethicists would like to see women equipped for decision making, such as Joel Feinberg, Arthur Caplan, Thomas Murray, and Jeffrey Botkin. Others tread more cautiously—as becomes apparent in discussions offered by Sisela Bok, Ronald Cole-Turner, and Brent Waters. Issues regarding conduct during genetic screening, teaching, and counseling environments, and how to respond sympathetically are raised. John Fletcher and *Personal Origins* place genetic screening into a broader perspective. There are several areas in a person's life and family that are impacted by serious illnesses.

One of the most serious challenges to troubled pregnancies is abortion, issue (3), and it has to be addressed. This section takes a roll call of lawsuits involving abortion—challenges that made it to the Supreme Court-in order to examine what turns abortion into a social outcry. There is a case-by-case review of how society adjusted to abortion, its legalization, and the different measures of persuasion and rationale used by opposing parties. The content allows the reader to step into the ring, so that she can make up her own mind about the ethics of interrupting a pregnancy—and own the decision.

The arguments *for* and *against* the regulation of genetic practices form the last segment, issue (4). The primary responsibility rests on the health care providers and the research environment, rather than the individual. Resources such as Baruch Brody and Eric Meslin, formerly on President Clinton's Advisory Committee on Bioethics, are consulted. In the final analysis, recommendations from medical law experts are provided. Secular presentations by Bertha Knoppers and Oliver Guillod correspond well with the overall tenor of Christian thought-what is best for *all* of our *neighbors,* people who are created in the image of God, *imago Dei.* While the chapter provides a work-study, it also intends to confer real legislative-oriented solutions.

Chapter 6—The Moral Status of the Embryo

In contrast to the ethics concerning expectant women, this chapter stretches the reader past the outer, visible world and into the microscopic and symbolic realm embracing the meaning of human life in its basic original conception and development. This is the epitome of ethical reflection, because it challenges a person's sense of worth with scientific data about statistical probabilities.

The history of *in utero* experimentation begins with Michael Harrison's animal research. What he learned from the experiments would, one day, be used to save human babies, and he designed his experiments so that the methodology and results were applicable to human fetuses (i.e., he used pregnant ewes that had a size similar to human mother, etc.). Professor Steinbock weighed the alternatives for a woman with an endangered pregnancy. In her analysis, she considered the potential suffering of the fetus and conflicts with the mother's well-being. One section ponders the many attributes that form a person's life—the fetus's physiology as well as its potential character. The medical therapy is for the patients themselves. Snapshots on value considerations were derived from Patricia Baird, Alexander McCall Smith, Michel Revel, Robert Solomon, Joseph Schenker, George Boer, and others. These represent the more stellar scholars, and much of the scholarship is very contemporary.

Experimentation on human fetuses, not for the patient's own benefit, but for the benefit of society, raises additional, major ethical issues. There are very few publications about the ethics of fetal experimentation, also known as stem cell research. Most articles are technical, found in medical journals, and are primarily theories for the treatments that may eventually arise as a result of the experimentation. Writings and years of experience about issues arising early in human reproduction by George Annas, Arthur Caplan, S. Elias, etc., are consulted. Public debates at academic symposia and during legislative assemblies are the most frequent references—especially recent scholarship presented by UNESCO bioethics committee members M. McCall-Smith and M. Revel. The level of technology that science would like to achieve in medical therapy is astounding and sincere, but so are the reasons for postponing research on human fetuses. Genomics, monetary, and utilitarian motives drive much of the development and forestall legislation. The chapter weighs fetal stem cell research with several uncontrovertibly accepted ethical practices.

The final pages of the chapter and, therefore, of the book, open an analysis on the political, legislative alternatives that could be called from existing statutes to redirect the crowd back to ethical rationale. Legal and medical experts from the International Society of Family Law, Robert Lee, B. Dickens, Bertha Knoppers, and Lawrence Wardle, to name a few, look at issues that parlay *rights* into statutory considerations. UNESCO weighs the sources of embryos, consent issues, privacy, confidentiality, and more—as it makes recommendations on moral guidelines that governments can justly implement concerning fetal experimentation. The exercise in applied ethics that this chapter creates is also intended as a lens on the reality that our generation is facing—real issues in fetal stem cell research. The conclusion of Chapter 6 reflects an accurate appraisal of values that the Christian church supports, as well as the hope it represents for those who are marginalized by society—upholding the church's responsibility to carry out God's promises to care for the weak, vulnerable, and those who have no one else to defend them.

Humanitarian efforts assist the goals and ideals of Christian church. At the same time, the community of faith has a far greater heritage than many understand, and identifying humankind with *that* image is one goal worth pursuing! The chapter about *imago Dei,* Chapter 1, explains the most profound reality that humankind has ever known, as well as the justification for the church's interest and activity in biomedical ethics—specifically, genetic diagnosis.

PART I:
INFORMATION
TO EQUIP DECISIONS

Chapter 1

Humankind Created in the Image of God, *Imago Dei:* The Passion and Politics of Human Biology

INTRODUCTION

Wisdom, knowledge, education, and discernment are at the heart of a pastoral response to a potentially difficult pregnancy. The goal of the following chapters is to equip the reader with the best and most relevant information on procreative strategies and to empower confident health care decision-making for the minister, the mother, her family members, and the significant others in that family's community.

Pregnancy is an intimate topic. Inside the human mother is a growing embryo, which will probably look like its parents and inherit family characteristics. A pregnant woman is someone's daughter, sister, aunt, wife, and friend. She lives and works in a community; therefore her decisions during gestation impact other individuals. One day, that child could live and play in the same neighborhood. If there are health problems, the community will be supporting the special educational or medical needs of the child—supplying professional expertise, emotional support, or even financial assistance. Our society has become more sensitive to persons with special needs and recognizes that everyone possesses different abilities. On the other hand, innovations in medical technology spark concerns for any mother whose family has a history of genetic illness, birth defects, or even, for example, a hear-

Counseling Pregnancy, Politics, and Biomedicine
© 2007 by The Haworth Press, Inc. All rights reserved.
doi:10.1300/5697_02

ing impairment, and she will question whether or not to continue her pregnancy. No one is closer to the embryo in her body than a mother. She doesn't want to end a baby's life or confound it with years of suffering. Our individualistic, competitive, fast-paced, technology-driven, and culturally dominated society tends to lose touch with the individual. Those making decisions about difficult pregnancies can be guided by ministers, priests, and pastors who are well enough informed to equip and empower a balanced understanding, which enables a clear conscience.

This chapter develops, step-by-step, a Christian theological foundation to explain the empirical and implied values God has endowed to every human life. God, Christology, and ethics were inseparably united prior to creation. God's creative process inherently packaged God's ethical nature into the spark of life and fashioned humankind in God's image, *imago Dei*. The chapter presents Jesus as the Archetype because Jesus exemplified the workings of Christ and the Ethic. It is this Christological combination that expresses the fullness of God in Jesus' life and actions. Jesus came to know God as his Father: "my testimony is valid because I know where I have come from and where I am going."[1] This means Jesus came from God because he was integral in the Godhead prior to his earthly birth and intends to re-unite within the Godhead in his Resurrected Life. All this is explained in the pages to come.

Jesus' *in utero* divine–human nature initiated ensoulment—it was not completed instantaneously. The human reproductive process gives birth to a helpless infant whose body and soul is nurtured by loved ones. God intended to communicate a message by showing humanity the lifestyle that most pleased God. For those who followed Jesus' example, it would restore the brokenness that occurred as a result of human disobedience. To create the highest identity with humankind, Jesus developed in the way that all people do—biologically, psychologically, and theologically. His example is understood gradually by studying his lifestyle in Christian traditions and texts. They describe the shaping of the human soul as it grows into the God–human relationship in order to be raised to God's Ultimate goal for each living person, even little ones who are only "ideas."

Jesus, as fully human and fully God, immediately initiates a conversation between nature and the transcendent. The interplay of God and humanity becomes more relevant for today's readers if it explores religious awareness in real terms, such as human consciousness, the story inside DNA, and the neurological system that fuels our emotions. Scientific discovery provides beacons for theology, but mixing the disciplines often raises eyebrows. Therefore, a few conciliatory comments will be helpful.

NAVIGATING DICHOTOMIES: RELIGION, SCIENCE, AND A CHRISTOCENTRIC FAITH

Introducing Science into Theology

Humanity was created in the image of God—with a physiology. Therefore, it is important that this investigation begin by locating a positive fulcrum for science within the theological discussion. In common, religion and science use human experience to discover and disclose truth, but their tests are different.[2] Werner Heisenberg dismissed the idea that science could be neutral and objective, because scientists bring their own bias into any evaluation, which affects how truth is measured. In fact, Arthur Peacocke insists scientists and theologians be self-critical, because they both explore worlds that can only be partially and imperfectly understood. Collaborating with other disciplines is wise and advantageous.[3] Science makes knowledge possible about worlds that cannot otherwise be seen or known (e.g., cell biology, chemistry, or God). Using accessible language, metaphors, and models leads to coherent, fruitful, comprehensive, and cogent ideas. Scientists collect, try, and retest their conclusions. Likewise, theologians gather past and present experiences into its interpretive community to be examined and restated, often in a liturgical context. The liturgy is repeated and frequently invites an active and emotional response. Cross-disciplinary probes invite mutual respect between science and theology—theology creating the space for a view of the natural world and science recognizing that there is at least one Reality that is not totally, scientifically discernable.[4]

Many scholars agree Christianity is the most anthropological of all religions; hence, being "created in the image of God" (Lat., *imago Dei*) becomes a common proposition between nature and religion. Indeed, most Christian denominations will agree that Jesus Christ had both a divine and a human nature in order to reveal *imago Dei* to all people. God became human, opening the possibility for a partially natural interpretation about God's activity in the world, and it was around this message that congregations united in sharing the message of Christ— God's Promise.[5]

Locating God's Single Message Among Its Many Expressions

Finding a common stance for the Christian Church on any subject may appear challenging due to its mosaic of denominations. Indeed, there are six billion unique individuals in this world, who bring very different experiences and religious ideas into daily life.

The earliest assemblies of Christians believed that following Jesus' behavior was central to the faith, but very early in Christianity, the establishment of schools brought to light the fact that there were two very different, culturally driven worldviews about Christ's life— the Semitic and the Hellenist. George Maloney and Kallistos Ware explain that Semitic [Jewish] Christians believe in a dynamic, existential transformation of the whole person. Hellenist Christians, such as Clement of Alexandria, Origin, and Evagrius, favor the belief that God conveys a special light or knowledge (Gk., *Gnosis*) to those with a privileged relationship—one was called to know God. The Hellenists with a Platonist background could not conceive of the Most High intermingling with God's creation. They believed in a division between the material world and the spiritual world. The poorer souls with nothing else to offer but their own selves tended to see themselves as servants, vessels, or hosts for God's activity on earth; in this view, God was incarnational.[6] God worked through human biology.

Today's biblical commentators inevitably prefer one belief over the other. Despite scholars' interpretive differences, the mainstream churches have essentially the same religion. Christianity embodies the same rudimentary principles of faith in one and the same God, revealed in Jesus Christ.

Discovering the Meaning Behind Being Created in the Image of God

If society is ever to hold a sincere respect for humanity, it will need to rediscover the divinity entrusted to it. Ancient authorities have pondered the secrets of life with great curiosity, as have modern scholars, who have literally formed a myriad of academic disciplines in search of understanding what it means to be human. Each tightly focused discipline provides a piece of the puzzle explaining the God–human relationship; yet, together and only together do they form a whole picture. This book defines and gives context to bioethical knowledge from different disciplines to equip well-informed decisions about difficult pregnancies, and this chapter unfolds avenues to human wholeness by interpreting biblical verses (e.g., God's wisdom.). It systematically builds the whole picture subject by subject. The study will open the ancient scrolls and examine what can be learned about the Christology within the Creator—God *before* creation. This exposé will also look at God's creating activity because it dynamically reveals the Christocentricity and energy that lives within the things that God has made. Citations from ancient authorities, Old and New Testaments, Patristics (early Church councils), and medieval philosophy will be joined with scientific theories and illustrations to explore God's concrete involvement in Jesus' life and its implications for our lives today—and Ultimate aims. The scholarship presented is the cumulative result of centuries of significant reflection.

THE CHRISTOLOGICAL AND ETHICAL ORIGINS INHERITED BY HUMANITY

Thesis: Christology is One with God. "Prior" to time and creation, the primitive Ethic was also one with God and Christology. The Ethic flowed through the spark of life into creation. God trusted humanity to bear the image of God—*imago Dei.* Eternity was God, Christ, the Ethic, and Wisdom—from whence humanity came forth.[7]

First Things About the Creator of the Universe

The only way to illuminate the importance of being human is to explain how God's own Ethic passed into the stream of human life so that people could aspire to reach their full potential. For this to be true, God had to precede all universes, being all in all. Hence, the Creator made what exists from God's own Self. Christ and the Ethic were human entitlements in God's legacy. This section gives evidence of God and Christ as a unified entity who existed prior to everything that was created—and from whom the tangible things of this world were brought into existence (Jn. 1:3).

Across the ages, biblical scholars, theologians, and philosophers have contributed volumes on the divine origin of the universe. The Jewish Old Testament creation episodes are found in the Hebrew Bible.

Genesis 1:1 reads:

בְּרֵאשִׁית בָּרָא אֱלֹהִים אֵת הַשָּׁמַיִם וְאֵת הָאָרֶץ: ¹

The translation is: "In the beginning, God created the heavens and the earth." The idea of a *beginning* inferred that God preexisted his creating activity (cf., Job 38:4-7), and there was only one way we all got here. The psalmist spelled it out: " . . . in holy splendor; *before* the Daystar, like the dew, I have begotten you" (Ps 110:3).

What does the first verse of the Jewish Bible reveal about the Creator? Genesis 1:1 named the Creator *Eloheim. El* (אֵל) signified God, and *heim* (חִים) denoted a plural ending. Jewish scholars insisted God was only *One* and not a plurality. For Samuel Driver, the plural ending qualified Christian Trinitarianism (i.e., God as Father, Son, and Holy Spirit)—calling it an Ecclesiastical Court. To resolve any confusion about the Oneness of God, John Skinner, Samuel Driver, and A. von Dillman agreed that *Eloheim* referred to a living synthesis of the powers and forces within God. Some biblical texts named God *Eloheim,* and, in other Bible verses, the Jews called God *Yahweh,* which originally may have been a verb describing God's simultaneous Being and Activity. Both Genesis 1:1 and the *imago Dei* texts of Genesis 1:26-27 referred to God as *Eloheim.* God was Himself *before* the beginning.

These citations, as well as the rest of the creation narratives (Genesis 1-11), are viewed as a composite work, and scholars have cited many sources, including the *Elohist* and *Yahwistic* documents, the Priestly Code, and the Pentateuch.[9] The Genesis verses do not offer any information as to whether the primitive heavens and earth were created in a few thousand or over millions of years. Only God was present at creation, and one is not likely to find him sitting at his table mixing cinnamon and spices or crafting creation by carving tools and a painting mallet, since those too would be created articles.

Aristotle and early philosophers understood the Creator to be "the great thought thinking itself" and conceptualized God as the *Logos* (i.e., the Creative Word). That culture used masculine nouns/pronouns for generalized references. It was Philo who gave currency to the all-pervasive, intelligent *mind* of God theory. Greek stoics spoke of the *Logos* as the One who generated souls. *Logos* was also a divine fire, permeating the universe. This electrified mind of God strangely resembled the florescent lighting used in brain imaging of later years. Many early Greco-Roman legends personified *Logos* as wisdom incarnate.

From within the Hellenistic environment, John's gospel resounded with God's Creative Authority: "In the beginning was the *Logos* (Gk., λόγος, Eng., Word), and the *Logos* was with God and the *Logos* was God." The early Christian community, originally consisting of Jews, reconciled energy for creative, formative power, the mystical source of divine wisdom as well as a divine light that produces holiness, the Ethic.

The Orthodox Church's official position on creation became *creatio ex Nihilo,* creation out of Nothing, because God was incomprehensible to the natural mind. No one could describe exactly what God was, only what He was not. In the fourth century, all references to God were curbed *via Negativa,* and the Nothing of *Creatio ex Nihilo* respectfully referred to God—it was never intended to be a void. Now, many contemporary theologians tend toward *creatio continuum,* God's continual creativity.

God was present at the beginning, and all that was created came through the Creator, including the human soul. Nonetheless, religious authorities saw the Creator and his creation as distinctly separate. Consistent with *creatio ex Nihilo,* Gregory of Nyssa denied any natural kinship between a human soul and God, since the Eternal was limitless and the human soul was bound to a linear journey. However, Gregory wrote many hymns about divine–human Union, and he used his own experience as he taught others about the unity of Christ's "energies" in humanity. He was describing the inexpressible *Nihilo* as a real event in the life of the faithful, sometimes described as divine darkness or holy light. In a Hellenistic culture subsumed by neo-Platonian idealism, the beauty of the natural environment only gave hints of the true heavenly Perfection. Of course, all the doctrines of the early Church, including *ex Nihilo,* were Capital "T" Truth, but, in more recent conversations with biblical scholars who are also scientists, there are new and realistic explanations that are also theologically sound.[10]

Within the context of science, one cannot refute theological discourses and various creation hypotheses *prior* to creation. If *Nihilo* is removed from its original culture, it renders a false picture because "nothing" cannot give rise to existence, especially conscious life. Physical propositions actually support the existence of God's mysterious all-pervasive firmament. Christology preexisted creation.

The Creative Process: Christology and Ethics Flow into the Natural World

God has to do with *being,* which, by its very nature, cannot *not be.* Keith Ward claims Being has a necessary nature, but the Being is not the universe because the universe is dependent and contingent, and God is completely free. As philosophers and theologians before him, Ward considers the mind of God to have birthed the universe and all therein, including human life. In Ward's congenial style, he insisted that the mind of God is not nothing.[11] Simply stated, God created humankind in His own image, arguably from God's own Self since God preexisted all else. God passed his Christology and Ethic to his creation, mindful of varying levels of stewardship. The higher responsibility to creation rested upon humans because they were endowed with a greater social consciousness.[12]

Astronomers, cosmologists, and physicists have postulated as to how the universe came into being. In many cases, theologians who were also qualified scientists found that their propositions agreed with biblical texts on creation—there was room for exploding stars and a Quantum God between Genesis 1:1 and Genesis 1:2. Friedmann, LeMaitre, Robertson, and Walker described the beginning of time, space, and matter as coming from a cosmic explosion—the Hot Big Bang theory.[13] Russell Stannard's anthropic principles explained that gases exploded planets into existence, blue hot, then cooling to sub-freezing temperatures (befitting cryopreservation) until the planets found a place to orbit the sun—this warmed the earth enough to sustain life. Stannard's theory was scientifically cohesive with more recent interstellar investigations that simulated the magnetic gathering of planetoids into orbits around the sun.[14] God was free to create or not to create, but, having begun creation, nature's proliferation of life depended on the right balance of carbons, air, and warmth in order to produce life (see Figures 1.1-1.5).

Quantum mechanics (QM) explained the "nothing" in nano-terminology, saying space has always been occupied with energy-emitting

FIGURE 1.1. God is All-in-All before creation. Nothing exists.

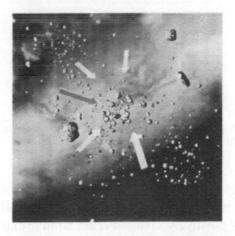

FIGURE 1.2. Friction: Big Bang explosion looses stars, surrounded by whirling dust (chaos). *Source*: Photo © Alan Boss. Used with permission.

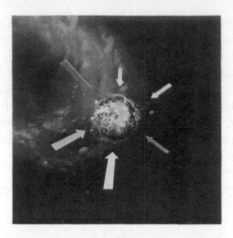

FIGURE 1.3. Dust sticks together, forming masses; gravity draws gases and forms clouds. *Source*: Photo © Alan Boss. Used with permission.

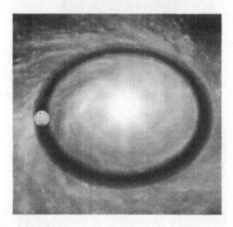

FIGURE 1.4. Core planet formed at center of clouds carves a ring in gases. *Source*: Photo © Derek Richardson. Used with permission.

waves and particles. Like planets orbiting the sun, electrons circle a nucleus without touching. Electrons that are negatively charged and a nucleus that is positively charged react countermagnetically. QM waves and particles travel invisibly across the electromagnetic spectrum, unsupported. Physicist Niels H.D. Bohr concluded that physical

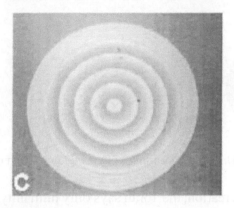

FIGURE 1.5. Target pattern radio wave CDH-BZ reaction. *Source:* Chad T. Hamik and Oliver Steinbock, Excitation waves in reaction–diffusion media with non-monotonic dispersion relations. *New Journal of Physics* 5(2003): 58.1- 58.12. © Institute of Physics. Used with permission.

particles are forever changing and unpredictable, freely spinning and reversing direction spontaneously—there are no fixed values, hence the Copenhagen Principle of Indeterminacy and Heisenberg's Uncertainty Principle overturned Einstein's idea that there could be an explanation for everything.[15]

In light of these discussions and the grand drama of creation, there is more and more evidence that God ordered the universe to accommodate human life. Philosophers saw the creative cycle generated from the mind of God. Pierre Teillard de Chardin described God's brilliant and mystical cosmological order in which landscapes unfolded, cell-by-cell, the way embryos grow. David Atkins, a scientist and self-described atheist, lauded the symmetry and grace evidenced in the natural world in which we live with awe.[16] We observe, behold, and explain. J. Kempler once said, "it was as if thinking God's thoughts after him." Does humankind, *imago Dei,* share God's consciousness?

God Fashioned Humankind in God's Image, **Imago Dei**

As biblical literature suggests and scientific hypotheses confirms, the environment became compatible with and home to many differing life forms and species (see Figure 1.6).

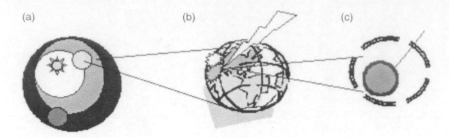

FIGURE 1.6. (a) Universe (b) Earth (c) First single-cell, with nucleus (model).

Of all God's creation, the Torah says only humanity was fashioned in God's image:

Gen. 1:26:

²⁶ וַיֹּאמֶר אֱלֹהִים נַעֲשֶׂה אָדָם בְּצַלְמֵנוּ

כִּדְמוּתֵנוּ וְיִרְדּוּ בִדְגַת הַיָּם וּבְעוֹף הַשָּׁמַיִם וּבַבְּהֵמָה וּבְכָל־הָאָרֶץ

וּבְכָל־הָרֶמֶשׂ הָרֹמֵשׂ עַל־הָאָרֶץ:

Gen 1:27:

²⁷ וַיִּבְרָא אֱלֹהִים ׀ אֶת־הָאָדָם

בְּצַלְמוֹ בְּצֶלֶם אֱלֹהִים בָּרָא אֹתוֹ זָכָר וּנְקֵבָה בָּרָא אֹתָם:

The New Revised Standard Version (NRSV) translation reads:

Then God [Eloheim] said, let *us* make humankind in *our* image, according to *our* likeness, and let them have dominion over the fish of the sea, and over the birds of the air, and over the cattle, and over the wild animals of the earth, and over every creeping thing that creeps on the earth. (Gen. 1:26)

So God [Eloheim] created humankind in His image, in the image of God he created them; male and female he created them. (Gen. 1:27)[17]

The text has an interesting change of words: "God *made*" in 1:26 and "God *created*" in 1:27. Delitzsche thought *imago Dei* was "made," originally, from that which already existed—God's Self? Comparatively, "creating" signifies uniqueness. Some hold that *imago Dei* was "made" like God, without gender. Then God created gender, male and female. Adam and Eve were pure, fashioned in God's likeness. They did not lose their innocence until later (Gen. 9:6). Jewish commentaries highlighted God's desire to "make" humanity *for* God's own pleasure.[18] Was the image of God only for the Jews?

Jewish Christians shared the "beginning" with Israel—God's chosen people. They also shared that which was *before* creation—*Eloheim*, God. There was sufficient unity of thought about God's Eternal State and His creating activity to achieve a level of continuity from the Old to the New Testament. The first eleven chapters of Genesis were readily accepted as Scripture in the primitive church; its authority was certain.

The Johannine gospel sounded like Genesis 1:1, but, rather than using *Eloheim*, John named God, *Logos*, which means the Word. In John 1:1-4, the Prologue introduces the idea that Otherness was inside *and* outside of time, at the point of beginning. John 1:1-4 reads:

> Ἐν ἀρχῇ ἦν ὁ λόγος, καὶ ὁ λόγος ἦν πρὸς τὸν θεόν, καὶ θεὸς ἦν ὁ λόγος.ᵃ 2 οὗτος ἦν ἐν ἀρχῇ πρὸς τὸν θεόν.ᵇ 3 πάντα δι' αὐτοῦ ἐγένετο, καὶ χωρὶς αὐτοῦ ἐγένετο οὐδὲ ἕν.ᶜ ὃ γέγονενᵈ 4 ἐν¹ αὐτῷ ζωὴ ἦν², καὶ ἡ ζωὴ ἦν τὸ φῶς τῶν ἀνθρώπων·

He reveals *Logos* as the source of "light and life" for humanity, connecting Eternity with time:

> In the beginning was the Word *[Logos]*, and the Word was with God, and the Word was God. He [the *Logos* of Christ] was in the beginning with God. All things came into being through him, and without him not one thing came into being. What was come into being was life, and the life was the light of all people.[20]

In addition, the Johannine Prologue (Jn. 1:1-4) bridged some of the Jewish and Hellenistic cultural differences since John was a Jew writing in the midst of the Greek world. Ruth Edwards clarified the Hellenist identity of *Logos* was a rational utterance, a word directed by reason. Indeed, the universal sense of *Logos* carried the Aristotelian air of "the great thought thinking itself," which communicated rational principles for governing all things—a panpsychism. For the Jews, *Logos* was God's *dabar* (Heb., דְּבַר; Eng., Word), representing God's creative power (cf., Ps. 33:6, 9) and God's reliable revelation of Truth and Law.[21] As such, it conformed to Jewish solidarity in which God dwelt within the community. Consequently, Word (λόγος) was meaningful to Jews and Gentiles; in the Divine sense, it represented Mosaic Law (cf., Prophetic inspiration) and Greek wisdom (cf., embodied Light). The connection suggests that Jewish Law was an internal Knowing, inspired wisdom, not simply a set of positive regulations that one had to obey like a checklist.[22]

The Johannine *Logos* spoke positively of the order, structure, and beauty of the universe. As his text continued, it confirmed that the source of "life and light," God Incarnate, had come into the temporal world. God's gracious presence empowered "life" (η ζωη) with a fresh start and a clear conscience. The "Light" (τὸ φῶς) brought an intellectual awakening and the literal physical restoration of sight to the blind. *Logos* was the embodiment of true law, righteousness, and Christology's preexistent force of life and light, which contained God's Ethic. In John 1:14, the evangelist introduces the reader to the "Word made Flesh" (η σὰρξ) prior to actually naming Jesus:

> 14 Καὶ ὁ λόγος σὰρξ ἐγένετο καὶ ἐσκήνωσεν ἐν ἡμῖν,
> καὶ ἐθεασάμεθα τὴν δόξαν αὐτοῦ, δόξαν ὡς μονογενοῦς
> παρὰ πατρός, πλήρης χάριτος καὶ ἀληθείας.[m]

The word was personified in the flesh:

> The Word became flesh and lived among us, and we have seen his glory, the glory as of a Father's only son, full of grace and truth.[24]

The gospel writers knew the importance of legitimizing Christ in a Jewish sense. John likened the Word to Moses (verse 1:17), whom the Jews: (1) knew as a man and (2) recognized as a messenger of God, a Prophet, and Deliverer. Matthew presented the genealogy of Jesus to demonstrate the integrity of his Jewish heritage.

God sent Moses and several other prophets and messengers, who were rejected. Then God sent his human Son, Jesus. Chris Rowland and many other scholars focus on the "sending," as described in John 1:17-18:

> The law was indeed given through Moses; grace and truth came through Jesus Christ. No one has ever seen God. It is God the

only son that is close to the Father's heart, who has made him known.[25]

Jesus was sent, in the flesh, to make God known. Jesus' instrument was himself—his person and body. According to this text, Jesus enjoyed a nascent memory of the Creator–Father. It connected Jesus' human brain with Jesus' Father *via* consciousness. Jesus' mind acted through the same biological means as all people. He made choices and acted upon them in a physical way, but he was preexistent in Christology:

> He is the image of the invisible God, the firstborn of all creation; for in him all things in heaven and on earth were created, things visible and invisible, whether thrones or dominions or rulers or powers—all things have been created through him and for him. He himself is before all things, and in him all things hold together . . . through him God was pleased to reconcile to Himself all things, whether on earth or in heaven, by making peace through the blood of his cross.[26]

Jesus was *in* the beginning. The *Logos* of Jesus was co-Eternal with the Father. He was *not becoming* "likeness" or virtue.[27]

The gospels proclaimed Jesus' life, death, and resurrection. Living and dying were part of human nature, but Jesus' resurrection was God's own signature of approval. After Jesus and his apostles left their legacy to the early church, its leaders struggled for a proper teaching on embodied divinity. A close relationship between Jesus and God offended Jewish Christians, who were strongly influenced by solidarity, that is God *in community,* and not in the individual sense. Those influenced by Greek dualism struggled with the idea that God would intermingle with corruptible bodily materials and even more so by a God who would suffer and die. The early Christians were slow to interpret the events surrounding Jesus' humanity.[28] Classical theologians described God as Eternal, immutable, changeless, and totally without temporal and spatial relations in the created cosmos and adopted the doctrine of *impassability*—affirming that God could not suffer.[29] Augustine's *City of God* (Book 11) declared that God did not exist in time at all. He created time, but God did not exist in it, not then, and not now. It hedged on self-negation because Augustine also believed that every possible universe existed within the "mind of God."[30] Wrestling to resolve the Cross, others said Jesus was "sent" to humanity as a divine *agent* (1 Cor. 8:6; cf., Col. 1:16—"all things come [εκ] from God through [διά] Christ").[31] Despite apostolic testimony to the contrary, many churchmen would not reckon Jesus with his humanity. Impassability was a paradox for Christianity. It disassociated the Redeemer from creation, voided the purpose behind the Cross, and challenged the morality of the Resurrection—all of which are foundational principles for the Christian faith.

Perplexed by the incongruity of these earlier doctrines in light of the Crucifixion, contemporary scholars were convinced that God was affected by his creation. Barth recognized that "Christ was antecedently in himself for us," and again, "Jesus was God brought forth from God," but Barth stopped short of any panhuman manifestation of divine energy. David Brown proposed three centers of consciousness that were indivisible, cooperative, omnipotent, and omniscient. Brown believed Jesus was conscious of the Holy Spirit and that he also drew ideas from the *Torah* (Law) and Wisdom oral traditions. In this way, Jesus was personal and historical as well as a product of the Jewish community and culture. Rudolf Bultmann demythologized Christ in order to locate God in human history, but he did admit that Jesus preexisted as a divine being and was presented as the Son of God.[32] For John Habgood, Jesus' connection with the Holy took place *within* the created order, and he was definitely identified with the entire human race.[33] Presumably, God knew all things as they really were and was aware of good and evil; yet, God surrendered the perfect life (*kenosis,* Phil 2:4-9) and, instead, became part of the earthly drama, voluntarily facing the shame of the Cross. John Polkinghorne walked the fine line between incarnational theology and the Otherness of God by saying God placed a simple Eternity *in* a created nature, *cum tempore,* not *in tempore.* This way, God could realize new forms of value that would not have otherwise been realized or expressed in nature.[34]

God expressed his desire to be in relationship with humankind when he willingly and intimately entered into the humanity of Jesus—creatively energizing Jesus' natural person so he could respond to humankind with love for the glory of God.

JESUS: THE INCARNATE WORD
WITH HUMAN ATTRIBUTES

Thesis: Jesus is the Archetype of humankind, *imago Dei,* conceived by Mary and shaped by his faith, relationships, environment, his five senses, and human experience. He resisted iniquity and was ennobled by God to reveal the divine nature in humanity as he lived the Jewish story. God endowed human beings with a far greater potential than we have thus far believed possible.

God, Christology, and Ethics existed in a simple and perfect unity before all things. When God formed creation, it was "The" parental catalytic act. Christology and all its attributes entered creation. The universe was intelligently ordered as planets and stars fell into place on spiraling radio waves, which we now know since these same forces send signals and sounds to antennas around the world. God's genius was so incredible that even the stars hosted myriads of cells with infinite varieties of species and, at the right time, each received its distinct *genus* and some were filled with the sacred mystery of life's breath and became conscious beings.[35] Thusly, the *Logos* and the mind of God generated and filled the depths of space as well as entered into the finite, palpable, biological realm.

Now, it is time to identify certain aspects of Jesus' humanness as a matter of visualizing the transmission of God's Energy, with its attributes, beginning with the microscopic level—DNA (deoxyribonucleic acid). Of course, there were no specifics about DNA in Scripture, and neither were there any specific descriptions about the color of Jesus' hair or face. There were, however, early Jewish traditions about God as the One who bestows life's breath, and Christian texts say God fathered Jesus with Mary, Jesus' human mother. Present in Mary's body as well as that of Jesus, but obscured from sight was the nanoworld of DNA. From the earliest fossils to the birth of Jesus and beyond, it appeared that every cell contained life and energy that came from somewhere beyond the horizon.

Jesus' Embryonic Genesis

Jesus' conception was of God and Mary because his divinity universally bequeathed his life to all humankind—it was a simple yet profound message:

She [Mary] gave birth to her firstborn son, wrapped him in bands of cloth, and laid him in a manger, because there was no place for them in the inn.[36]

Bethlehem was home to Jesus' ancient Jewish relatives and so it was that he came to be born there. Bethlehem was Hebrew for "house [beth] of bread (Lehema)," for it had been a shrine to the god of bread, Le-Hema. Bethlehem signified the anthropological survival of Eloheim's covenant community and its stalwart struggles were on the lips of the prophets. It was King David's native land; now it was the birthplace of Jesus.

The gospels of Matthew and Luke listed Jesus' biological genealogy. Luke explained that God and Mary conceived Jesus. Mary contributed her biological history and, after being "overshadowed by the Holy Spirit," Jesus gestated in Mary's womb.[37] In the ancient world, universal greatness was expected of one born by a virgin. All Pharaohs had virgin births.[38] Historians and theologians have researched Jesus' humanity for more than two thousand Christmases, but scholars struggle to explain the presence of the Infinite within the finite figure of Jesus. Although it looms humbly in the shadows of God's ineffable energy, DNA does define human traits—across eons.

It would be difficult to say exactly how Mary's reproductive DNA information-bites were configured after her conception of God's Son. Jesus was one with God in Christology, and Jesus was conceived, uniquely, by God and Mary. In fact, God's own Christology imbued those of natural parentage with the potential to become children of God.[39] The DNA code originated at the beginning of time, and the DNA information was inherited by Jesus through his Jewish ancestors, unhindered by the boundaries of life and death, because every parent since Adam and Eve had contributed to the DNA pool, recombining the DNA at each new fertilization. God intended to palpably reveal himself in Jesus.[40] Across the millennia, environmental, emotional, and cultural variations have altered DNA biochemistry and provided rich diversity.[41] Of Mary's DNA introns, 97 percent were common to all living creatures, but it was the remaining 3 percent, the exons, which expressed Mary's unique anatomical features, and this was also true of Jesus' personal traits because exons provide the key to individual identity. Jesus was flesh of Mary's flesh and blood of her blood; hence Jesus shared DNA with the human species.[42] When the virgin conceived God's baby, many were skeptical about the physiology, but such a birth was packed with symbolism in that culture. It signified kingship; *Maria Theotokos* made Mary the throne of God and even a woman pregnant with the Holy Spirit growing inside of her. His virgin birth did not preclude his humanness. Jesus was born and, like all babies, he began in primitive reproductive cells, went through the process of meiosis, and developed as an embryo (see Figures 1.7-1.9). Were Jesus' nuclear substance available for testing, it would match the DNA of his ancestors. Body samples could be tested for dietary substances that suited Jewish eating laws and the historical environment.[43] For example, Jesus' ancestors ate quail and bread,

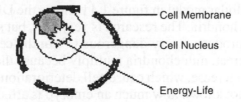

FIGURE 1.7. Prokaryote cell, asexual reproduction, "round" nuclear DNA.

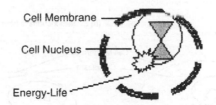

FIGURE 1.8. Eukaryote cell, heterosexual, "antiparallel" nuclear DNA.

FIGURE 1.9. Cell "arousal": Spark/mutation may have differentiated male and female.

called *manna,* while living in the Sinai desert; scientists might therefore try to identify ions/elements from that particular geography. Later, Jesus was called *Bread of Life,* a symbolic macro for Israel. Being of God and Mary, the Eternity of *Logos* coexisted with Jesus' *sui generis* DNA. DNA was *not* "the Source," but it was in service to Jesus.[44]

Woven into this chapter are examples of differing levels of energy waves and signals that create and communicate within the solar system and the natural world. Radio waves crossed through the cosmos during the discussion of Christology. Here are examples of energy emissions that build human bodies—from the inner working of molecules, *intracellular,* to signaling that causes tissue/organ generation, *intercellular.*

This intracellular model in figure 1.11 shows the DNA nucleus instructing mitochondria. The research is very new, but scientists know mitochondria produce a very dangerous O^2. In the cells of older females who overeat, mitochondria multiply because the DNA sends a signal. Toxins increase, which cause cell deterioration and the effects of aging. It is not known how much an embryo is affected by the toxins when a woman of a mature age conceives. Figure 1.10 shows intercellular signaling.

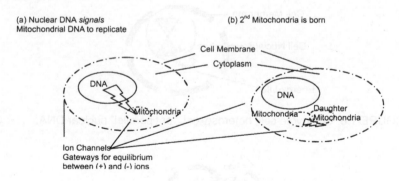

(a) Nuclear DNA *signals* Mitochondrial DNA to replicate

(b) 2nd Mitochondria is born

Cell Membrane

Cytoplasm

DNA

Mitochondria

DNA

Mitochondria

Daughter Mitochondria

Ion Channels
Gateways for equilibrium
between (+) and (-) ions

FIGURE 1.10. Inside the cell, mitochondria are sending signals.

When baby Jesus was an embryo, his cells instructed amino acids to form tissue, build organs, and orchestrate all the complex functions within his human architecture. This symphony of signals position and polarize the embryo in the womb while instructing the differentiation

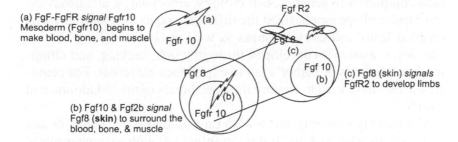

(a) FgF-FgFR *signal* Fgfr10
Mesoderm (Fgfr10) begins to
make blood, bone, and muscle

(b) Fgf10 & Fgf2b *signal*
Fgf8 (**skin**) to surround the
blood, bone, & muscle

(c) Fgf8 (skin) *signals*
FgfR2 to develop limbs

FIGURE 1.11a,b,c. Fibroblast growth factor (Fgf) *signaling* differentiation of body parts: An example of cells "signaling" whole systems can be seen during mitosis when embryonic DNA signals multiplication, polarization, and differentiation: cells organize for particular functions. Cells will generate particular "limbs" at the proper location.

of his heart and lungs, etc. Figure 1.11 demonstrates the order in which the "signals" encode. When FgfR (fibroblast growth factors) signals Fgf10, blood, bone, and muscle are manufactured (Figure 1.11a). After Fgf10 joins FgfR2b, an epidermis (Fgf8) is made to encase the blood, etc., and generate the neurological system (Figure 1.11b). Fgf8 bonds FgfR2, and limbs begin to protrude (Figure 1.11c). The dance of the fibroblasts (Fgfr) is illustrated below.

At the molecular level, fibroblast growth factors (Fgf) efficiently differentiated the parts that made up Jesus' whole person. In gestation, his cells were internally consistent, coherent, and collaborative. Jesus had human biology (Gk., *bios* is life).

God's Son was a carefully packaged genesis of past, present, and future. Jesus' physical humanness distinguished the second and third persons of the Godhead. Like normal people, Jesus still had to mature before he could complete the work that his Father sent him to do. The *Bread of Life* came to fill the *House of Bread*.[45] Of course, no one's story is chemically bound—it was Jesus' life that grew into the story of redemption.[46]

Jesus and Sentience: Religious Teachings, Socialization, and Neurological Systems

Jesus responded to God and humanity in his natural body, with his emotional chemistry, gradual affections, and the metaphysical dimensions of his life. Sociobiologist E.O. Wilson tried to reduce human complexity to genetics, cell biology, embryology, and behavior, but Stephen Pope emphasized the different stages of reciprocity that enabled Jesus' self-consciousness as well as God's "calling" on his life. Jesus' awareness developed through touch, sucking, and climbing into Mother's or Father's lap to experience closeness. For centuries, artists have tried to capture the deep bonds of the "Madonna and Child."[47]

Community solidarity and Jewish Law guided Jesus' behavior and educated his relationships. Today, an infant left with a stranger might fear separation from its parents, fear strangers, or trust its caregivers, but the Jewish community fostered the security of extended relationships. Mosaic Law tried to counter alienation, but maintaining personal honor was also part of the culture, and self-justification often worked through vindication, which marginalized others. As a child, Jesus' unusual conception may have affected the way his own family treated him. Not much is known about Jesus' earlier years, but kinship was a *de facto* part of Jewish life. It cultivated a self-love that blossomed into satisfying and stable emotions, which touched and ministered to several social levels: family, disciples, synagogue leaders, tax collectors, lepers, seafarers, farmers, and Roman authorities.[48]

Jewish religious teachings molded Jesus' worldview, attitudes, and emotional patterns because he learned the Jewish law, prophets, and wisdom sayings.[49] Jesus encountered the moods and poetry of the Psalms in his day-to-day life, which strummed the full range of his sentiments. Table 1.1 shows the emotional interaction between Israel and God using the Egyptian Hallel (Pss. 113-118), Gordon Mursell described the rainbow of emotions in the Jewish world: lament turned

TABLE 1.1. God toward Israel and Israel toward God.

Psalm	God toward Israel	Israel toward God
113	God showed *compassion*	Israel exhibited *heartfelt gratitude* Israel *hoped* with *expectation*
114	God responded by *empowering Faith*	Israel was *freed*
115	*God gives* Israel *holy fear*	Israel offers *praise and thanksgiving*
116		Israel's *dependency* on God Israel *waits* for piety
117		Israel *celebrates* God
118	God gives *victory* over enemies	Israel's leader shares God's *glory*

to boldness, anger met intimacy, intimacy stooped to mourning, and weeping erupted into praise. Unwavering legalism was displaced with an inner desire to please God.

In Psalm 113, the psalmist offers tearful appreciation because God showed mercy for the lowly and needy. Psalm 114 tells of a God who had power over all creation, and, in his tenderness, God confounded natural laws to free Israel from Egypt. Israel trusted that God would redeem families (Ps. 115). Amid the spiral of praise, the Psalmist pleads for Israel to stand in fear of God by being faithful to the Law. The petitioner in Psalm 116 appeals to God alone for a desperately needed healing. Psalm 117 heralded a doxology. The crescendo (Ps. 118) gives military victory to the righteous and the right to enter the temple. God inhabits praise in active sentience, not in logical gratitude.[50]

The harp of the human soul played an emotional tune, and only God knew the lyrics. Hasdi Cresda knew *Torah* was the human recipe for growing into the image of God: bodily, intellectually, morally, and theologically. He quotes the Deuteronomist: "So Israel, what does the Lord your God require of you? Only to fear the Lord your God, to walk in all his ways, to love him, to serve him with all thy heart and with all your soul."[51]

In the midst of self-sacrifice and human tragedy, God's wisdom appeared through redemptive processes. The *Torah* was filled with rough characters and nasty situations stemming from volatile moods, which were a very normal and natural outgrowth of humanity, but needed taming (recovery). Personal genetic makeup, hormonal secretions, environment, and negative interactions with others affected emotions. They were often driven by basic self-interest, honor, and pride. People in biblical narratives express pain, anger, and rage, which were provoked either psychologically or physically. Before the person had time to think, his adrenal glands released hormones, blood flow increased to the muscles, neurons transmitted signals to the brain's hypothalamus, neuronal circuitry released blood-born chemical agents that charged a muscular response—someone was struck down!

Jesus was humanly capable of all these reactions. He walked, talked, prayed, worked, ate, slept, and wept. He expressed emotion, conflict, discrimination, effort, desire, motives, moods, and appetites—exercising every one of his five senses. Like all people, his nervous system transferred signals from axons to dendrites, penetrated cell membranes, and excited hormones that even modified genetic expression. These affected Jesus' spontaneous thoughts, sensations, reaction, and reason. Jesus also had to be a risk taker, challenging religious authority about certain Sabbath rules when these interfered with God's higher motivations.[52] He learned to forgive as a reconciling and healing power. It was a great deal more than "mind over matter" or "will power." Jesus' promise to God necessitated a thorough biological transformation.

Arthur Peacocke explained the bottom-up and top-down workings of biological and natural systems, but he emphasized the importance of the "total-system-as-a-whole" influence.[53] The biological ladder shown in Figure 1.12 gives a simple illustration of complex human neurology as it triggers emotions that inform mental experiences.[54]

In the course of Jesus' life, teachings from Jewish law produced a healthy set of habits and emotions. Jesus' assimilation came *via* neuromuscular pathways, biochemistry, as well as tradition and liturgy. Jesus was manifest in Christology, and he was born a biologically natural *Homo sapien*. He had to be righteous before God and the Jews. For this reason, Jesus had to strive for unwavering, unconditional kindness in and through his natural relationships while experiencing the natural, deep, abiding feelings that drove human compassion.[55] During Jesus'

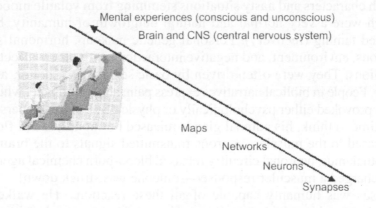

FIGURE 1.12. Hierarchy of communication between the nervous system and the brain, a two-way stream.

upbringing, the history of the Jewish people was imprinted on Jesus' genes, in his body, and mind—and in his behavior, which his mother seemed to understood better than anyone.[56]

Religious Commitment, Divine Response, and Forms of Participation

Jesus was trained in obedience and weighted in love so he could teach his community what his human story meant for every person— God's new covenant had come.[57] He had a special *logic* (cf., λογος) and mysterious intelligence about the ordered knowledge of the earth, natural life, and God. Jesus' behavior bespoke God's steadfast love because Jesus set aside his own needs for the benefit of the other—revealing an emotional maturity of a distinct nature.[58] It was chesed (Heb.) love, unique to God (cf., Gk., *agape,* ἀγαπε). Some-times, God deposited his delight into the Soul, and the person felt joy and passion that penetrated both the heart and the loins (i.e., Heb, *kelayot wale'b*; cf., Greek, *eros,* ερως). Friends felt *ahabah* toward one another (cf., Gk., phileo, πιλω).[59] Jesus lived in the love of God.

At the age of 30, Jesus went to the Jordan River to be baptized. Baptism was a ritual cleansing, not unlike some temple observances (cf., *miqveh*). Jesus made a public commitment to God through this purification rite and, thereby, transferred it to humanity.[60] When God sent the Holy Spirit, He anointed Jesus' mission and proclaimed: "This is my son, the Beloved, with whom I am well pleased."[61] Paradig-matically, the Holy Spirit descended on humanity and made anoint-ing possible for all God's faithful. Jesus entered a volitional covenant with God on behalf of humankind that was witnessed by John.[62] It ushered in Jesus' second birth. The first birth was by Mary.[63]

Many scholars disputed whether Jesus was sentiently tied to God or simply had a conscious connection. According to John Cornwall, consciousness was received directly from God and not *via* the senses. According to Margaret Boden, human thought processes, *qualia,* were inexplicable. John Searle placed intelligence in the high brain and sensitivity in a separate, lower-brain function (cf. animal reflex).[64] Therefore, some well-meaning theologians tried to protect Jesus' holy estate by pretending that Jesus could not experience human feelings.

René Descartes considered consciousness nonspatial, effectually leaving Jesus' relationship with God a nonembodied mystery.

Realistically, Jesus was a human being who had a special relationship with God. Jesus' sentience and intelligence worked together. According to Bernard Ballentine and Anthony Dickenson's research, cognition *emoted* preferences. Stephen Rose said whether one's decisions were objective or subjective, they had social and biological influences. [65] The five senses contributed to the complexity of meaning, as did experience and a symphony of neurological functions, including electric gestalts and the central nervous system (CNS). Consequences from any action involved chemistry, culture, environment, age, time, and location. High sensitivity and genius go hand-in-hand for artists, poets, musicians, and brilliant minds of all kinds.

Indeed, Jesus' loyalty to God permeated his entire being—as it danced with his increasing awareness of his divinity. Jesus Christ developed a character strangely reminiscent of God—moral and compassionate, with a sacrificial lifestyle.[66] His commitment to a holy life showed others the way to live in order to reach toward the Penultimate Promise.[67] Christ's genius, discernment, and life grew through prayer.

Today, prayer and mediation can be monitored using electrode sensors and brain-imaging technology. In a contemplative state, neuronal "rest" occurs in the Amygdala, the lower-right lobe, and there is only a tiny gestalt near the central tip of the visual cortex (Figures 1.13-1.15).[68]

Prayer and contemplation require the entire body to be calm and focused in order to clear the mind of invading thoughts, so God may dwell with the person in peace.

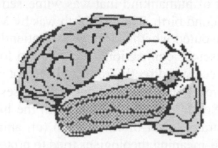

FIGURE 1.13. Brain: Meditation in lower region, "resting."

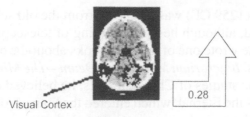

Visual Cortex

0.28

FIGURE 1.14. Brain: Meditation top view, "arousal"; visual cortex region.

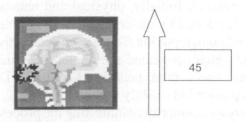

45

FIGURE 1.15. Meditation in back of head, "arousal"; visual cortex region.

Jesus' faith matured and was challenged by his own human nature as well as events in everyday life in first-century Palestine. Light, touch, hearing, smell, and taste translated into sight, silence, feelings of joy, and grief. These were mediated through his human architecture, memory, and prayer. Jesus' mind interpreted God's will for his life, and he himself mediated the human correspondence with heaven.[69]

God and Human Consciousness

Across generations, thinking about the Creator initiated a system of beliefs about the universe—myths about cosmogenesis and biogenesis. God entered history, so Israel and generations to come would experience God in nature and through conscious reflection. The Church Fathers said God's *Essence* was uniquely God's and could not be known, but God's activity on earth came through His *Energies*. By the Middle Ages, theologians, philosophers, and intellectuals examined theology using religious and scientific lenses. They wished to gaze into the ways in which God made his will known to people. Hence, metaphysics achieved credibility in spite of the Church's apophatic dogmas.

Bonaventure (1259 CE) was a scholar from the old school of tonsured clerics and, although he knew nothing of telescopic or microscopic worlds, he wrote one of the first books about the development of consciousness, *Itinerarium Mentum ad Deum—The Mind's Journey to God*. From his studies of Christian texts, he believed each person had a memory of the Eternal, which entered the brain through the soul and, over time, developed and trained the mind toward reunion with the Creator—using intelligence, reason, understanding, imagination, and moral discernment. Initially, physical and natural powers (cf., Greek, *anima*) developed by observing the environment, appreciating goodness, and contemplating God. Devotional activities attracted God's energies, which permeated the human soul and chiseled the love of God onto one's mind, heart, and soul (cf., Dt. 10:12; Mk. 12:30). Contemplation led to Holy ascent.[70]

Guilt was a strong counterforce inhibiting the process of achieving divine unity because it interfered with concentration and one's true self-image. Bonaventure believed human guilt originated when Adam first disobeyed God in the Garden of Eden. Human culpability for Adam's sin continued until Jesus painfully conquered death in his own body. His suffering was a definitive part of the journey (cf., *kenosis; Def.*, emptying, suffering love). For Luther, guilt was mediated by one's conscience, which rejected or restored moral turpitude.[71] Today, Mary Midgley would argue that parents, family members, and others make derogatory or flattering comments that create false self-images. A person spends a lifetime peeling away the opinions of others.[72] Self-forgiveness tamed the guilt and relieved the stress. Bonaventure believed that following Jesus' life style would reduce anxiety and clear one's mind. Having stilled the mind, the pathway was open for God's enrichment of the human Soul. Jesus totally gave of himself to accomplish God's work, constantly battling human nature (i.e., hormones, biochemistry, etc.).

God was wise beyond human understanding, and Jesus himself interpreted the examples of righteousness told in ancestral tales. Choices made of one's free will was certainly necessary for moral responsibility rather than merely acting on someone else's decision, but it was a matter of discerning God's way, or not.[73] He thoroughly examined the teachings and weighed the implications for his own life and the consequences for others. He did not blindly accept the construct handed to him. Christian, Sephardic, and Muslim philosophers believed faith was a metaphysical transaction. Being conscious meant "someone was there"—the *genius* (spirit, in Latin). In effect, the faithful desired God's participation in making choices for the best result.[74] Constancy in prayer and sound ethical teachings illuminated the mind toward right judgments. How does one recognize the spirit?

Scholars and scientists, such as Isaac Newton, concluded that God's existence was spatial and, therefore, physical. Physicists wondered if fiery particles entered the brain to initiate and transmit messages. Antoni Van Leeuwenhoek (1632-1723) found a liquid in nerve cells that he associated with mental activity and the epiphenomenal (e.g., the animal spirit of man). Luigi Galvani (1737-1798) deduced that electric currents conducted impulses along neuro pathways.[75]

Those bright ideas came together in the twentieth century in the form of brain imaging, in which phosphorescent lighting cast images of the brain and neurocircuitry onto a screen. For example, it shows up in persons who read books and, as their thoughts increase, little fiery balls, electrogestalts, multiply on the screen (in the cortex interpretive complex).

An electroencephalogram (EEG) mapped the gestalts, but marking the epicenters was not possible since they were multiple, divergent, and lacked synchronization; therefore, one could not pinpoint a physical or mental deficiency. In addition, moods and behavior fluctuate with levels of serotonin, acetylcholine, norepinephrine, histamine, and dopamine. This amine fountain varies.[76]

There is a remarkable contrast between a brain responding to human stimulus and a brain engaged in prayer or meditation. Conscious thought generates myriads of gestalts (Figure 1.16) and a mind submitted to prayer or mediation "rests."

Donald McKay and Nancey Murphy developed a chart for mental causation.[77] Comments about electric gestalts were added to enhance the visual integration of the concepts. The McKay–Murphy graph began by assessing an idea with relevant data and experience (R). Electric gestalts begin to multiply. Figure 1.17 illustrates first, second, and third choices (C, O). The fiery area increases as possibilities

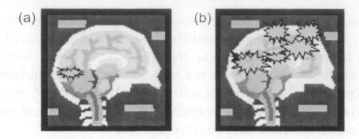

FIGURE 1.16. Brain image, (a) low concentration/small gestalt; (b) hyper-stimulation/arousals. An electroencephalogram (EEG) mapped the gestalts.

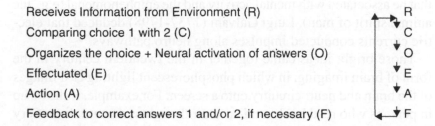

Receives Information from Environment (R)

Comparing choice 1 with 2 (C)

Organizes the choice + Neural activation of answers (O)

Effectuated (E)

Action (A)

Feedback to correct answers 1 and/or 2, if necessary (F)

FIGURE 1.17. Rational processes (from Murphy's paper, adapting McKay's Figure 6).

are compared (E). The person chooses the action (A), and then re-evaluates it (F).

In a second graph, McKay opened a gate for input—perhaps a commentary from another person, a surprise sound, or an inspiration from God. Adding the metaorganizer illustrated in Figure 1.18 and a metaevaluator made room for any number of higher-level supervisory systems. Priorities were constantly revised because they were affected by new information as well as natural brain mechanisms, such as biochemistry and brain surface electricity fluctuations. Humans are discursive thinkers—in continuum.

According to these metaorganizing systems, people have the ability to apply reason over and above natural instincts. They fit snugly into the maturation process and facilitate sound ethical decisions that are essential to pleasing God.

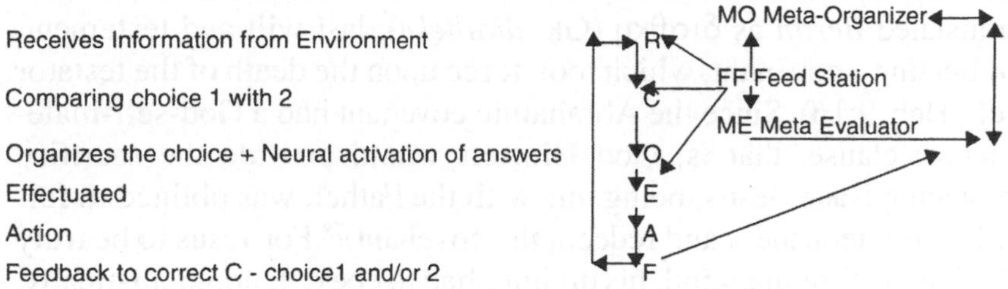

Receives Information from Environment

Comparing choice 1 with 2

Organizes the choice + Neural activation of answers

Effectuated

Action

Feedback to correct C - choice1 and/or 2

R
C
O
E
A
F

MO Meta-Organizer

FF Feed Station

ME Meta Evaluator

FIGURE 1.18. Meta-conceptualization.

THEOBIOGENESIS: GOD'S TRANSFORMATION OF HUMAN BIOLOGY

Thesis: God's penultimate moral nature empowered Jesus to make a fully informed choice about accepting death on the Cross. God enhanced his psychosomatic understanding of the humiliation, pain, and ultimate joy of the Cross. The Father also reassured Jesus about Resurrection by sending Moses and Elijah to speak to him. Originally, resurrection was of Jewish eschatology. Human nature was created for the divine metamorphosis, so all righteousness might be fulfilled according to God's Word.

The Creator's energy flowed through physics and molecules. Clearly, *Eloheim* entered history and participated in several covenants with people from diverse locations and cultures. God repeatedly ennobled those who honored these covenants. In the Hebrew *Torah, Tanakh,* the agreement between Israel and God, was known as a *Berith* (Gk., συν θηκη, *suntheke*). Noah received pairs of animals and a promise for the restoration of humankind and the environment. Abraham received a land grant and promise for progeny (in God's Self-maledictory covenant). The Priestly covenants celebrated God and made provisions for peace among the tribes. The Mosaic covenant harmonized God's relationship with His chosen ones by delivering them from slavery and providing for their needs in the desolate wilderness, and David was promised an Eternal Kingdom. For generations, God lovingly taught Israel through hardship, endurance, hope, and faithfulness, but Israel had become numb and blind to God's word.

In the covenant with Jesus, the Creator's intention became clear when God created a life for himself and named that life Jesus (i.e., the

Savior) and Immanuel (i.e., God with us). Interestingly, the *Septuagint* translated *Berith* as διαθκη (Gk. *diatheke*), last will and testament, indicating a covenant, which took force upon the death of the testator (cf., Heb. 9:16). Since the Abrahamic covenant had a God-self-maledictory clause, that is, God Himself would provide the sacrifice replacing Isaac, Jesus, being one with the Father, was obliged to fulfill all righteousness and redeem the covenant.[78] For Jesus to be truly the Savior of humankind, his divinity had to coexist, nondualistically, with his humanity.[79]

Theo-biogenesis made Jesus one mind with God, so he could be raised up (cf., Rahner). The natural deterrents to the goal percolated in Jesus' biochemistry, hormones, the lure to live alternative lifestyles, and temptations to deny the truth, but he chose to exemplify *Torah*. Jesus' obedience and faith crafted him into the Archetype for the Image of God—to the Jews as well as for those who would follow Christ's way.

Brilliant scholars such as Rudolph Bultmann, Wolfgang Pannenberg, Friedrich Schleiermacher, and Karl Rahner provided excellent discourses on the humanity of Jesus, but problems arose when the discussion moved to the divinity of Christ—the miracles and his Resurrection. Bultmann dismissed the miracles. Pannenberg, perhaps challenged by the dualism described by Barth and Bultmann, made a strong historical and scientific case, but after Hegel, Pannenberg's resurrection account collapsed into a hermeneutic (i.e., Jesus' own self-understanding). Schleiermacher carefully maintained a tension between the physical world and the Spirit, but the Spirit-matter dichotomy was left unresolved. Much indebted to Heidegger, Kant, and Aquinas, Karl Rahner explicated, in several volumes, that self-transcendence was built into humanity. He believed Jesus was a historical person, shaped by his culture, and incarnate of an omniscient God, which enabled Jesus to comprehend his own mission in light of an eschatological fulfillment.[80] God and Jesus had a relationship that could not be reduced to mere history, a personal inclination, or dualism, because Jesus was the macro of a truly good Jew, with an exemplary lifestyle for the sake of humanity.[81] Nonetheless, the Jesus message did not happen in a day, but across generations of human development.

God's Supreme Morality and the Transfiguration—Enosis

According to Jürgen Moltmann, Jesus' incarnation at birth provided a relationship between God and Jesus, but the nature of God was not absorbed into his humanity or memory. Jesus was limited to his conscious state, senses, and intuition.[82] The baptismal covenant proclaimed his commitment, but Jesus had to discipline his mind and body. Implied in the New Covenant was eschatological fulfillment—the blind would receive sight, the deaf would hear, the lame would walk, the poor would receive the good news, and the dead would be raised.[83] Jesus performed many miracles because he wanted to glorify God. Therefore, God led Jesus into a righteous judgment for the sake of righting humanity, but first, God wanted to equip Jesus with maximum human sensitivity because God wanted Jesus to fully understand the suffering and fulfillment associated with the profound decision that was required of him; therefore, God transfigured him:

2 καὶ
μετεμορφώθη ἔμπροσθεν αὐτῶν, καὶ ἔλαμψεν τὸ πρόσωπον αὐτοῦ ὡς ὁ ἥλιος, τὰ δὲ ἱμάτια αὐτοῦ ἐγένετο λευκὰ ὡς τὸ φῶς¹. 3 καὶ ἰδοὺ ὤφθη αὐτοῖς Μωϋσῆς καὶ Ἡλίας συλλαλοῦντες μετ' αὐτοῦ.[84]

In it, God demonstrated His own Perfect morality by transfiguring Jesus with the sentience to comprehend the humiliation, rejection, pain, and suffering that he would experience on the cross, as well as enlightening (Gk. φῶς) him with the full magnificence of what he was about to do (glorifying God's victory over death). Jesus' decision to go to the cross was fully informed and volitional.[85] John Jonsson equated *metamorphoomai* (μετεμορφώθη) to Jesus' "transvaluation"—within a physical event, not a dream, and it changed ordinary life into a manifestation of brilliance.[86] In it, αὐτοῦ signaled a divine event.

> And he was transfigured before them, and his face shone like the sun, and his clothes became dazzling white. Suddenly, there appeared to them Moses and Elijah, talking with him.[87]

When Jesus saw and spoke with Moses and Elijah, two prophets who were regenerated from the dead, it proved that the resurrection was genuine.[88] This was a physical resurgence of two very significant beings who were embodied, and the scriptures said they never experienced death so their bodies were not subject to decay.[89] It was real enough for Peter to decide to build shelters for the three.[90] Jesus received Moses and Elijah (i.e., the law and the prophets) into himself because they were no longer visible on the mount and no one has seen them since. In addition, Jesus' confidence was such that he was now able to countenance and defend his own testimony, as divine.[91]

... Μοϋσῆς καὶ Ἠλίας, οἱ ὀφθέντες ἐν δόξῃ ἔλεγον τὴν ἔξοδον αὐτοῦ, ἣν ἤμελλεν πληροῦεν ἐν Ἱερουσαλήμ.[92]

Moses and Elijah spoke to Jesus about his death at Jerusalem (Gk., εξοδον Eng., exodus).[93] Jesus was, thereby, integrated into Jewish eschatology. This varies from Rahner's understanding that Jesus had a natural Omniscient presence, but the concept was not contrary to Rahner's overall thesis.

> ... Moses and Elijah, talking to him. They appeared in glory and were speaking of his departure, which he was about to accomplish at Jerusalem.[94]

Jesus was "fully informed" (intellectually and sentiently) about the magnitude of his death and resurrection. His consent to go ahead with the redeeming work of the cross was unconditionally volitional and open to change any time along the way.

Jesus' transfiguration characterized *enosis* as a human phenomenon in which God intervened to equip and empower him according to God's own moral purposes. It was a condition precedent to Jesus' fulfillment of the covenant and entry into God's glory, and *enosis* fully engaged Jesus' mind and five senses. The transfiguration could be described as God's photon emissions, signals, moving throughout Jesus' body (Figure 1.19) and one can presume he had super-numerous electric gestalts (Figure 1.20) as he rationalized the activity (Figure 1.21) and prayed for perfect clarity in his life's purposes (Figure 1.22). *Phos* (Gk., φως) described *phos*phorescing, the energy that was overwhelming his life (cf., electro-energy signifiers). It appears science borrowed *phos* from the Greek. The communication between Moses, Elijah, and Jesus as well as God's commandment to "listen to him [Jesus]" spoke of *phonas* (Gk. φων−ας; Eng., hearing, listening, and knowing). *Phonas* implied there was audible sound riding on

Jesus' Enosis:

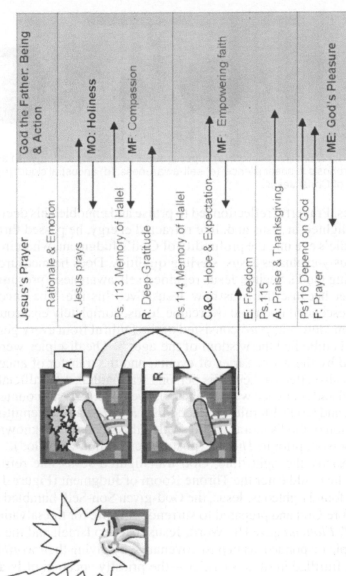

Jesus's Prayer | **God the Father: Being & Action**

Rationale & Emotion

A: Jesus prays — MO: Holiness

Ps. 113 Memory of Hallel

R: Deep Gratitude — MF: Compassion

Ps. 114 Memory of Hallel

C&O: Hope & Expectation

MF: Empowering faith

E: Freedom

Ps. 115

A: Praise & Thanksgiving

Ps116 Depend on God

F: Prayer — ME: God's Pleasure

FIGURE 1.19. Enosis memories.

FIGURE 1.20. Brain state: A = natural arousals; R = prayerful response.

FIGURE 1.21. Natural (rationale and emotion) and meta-system (Hillel Psalms and God: Father/Holy).

59

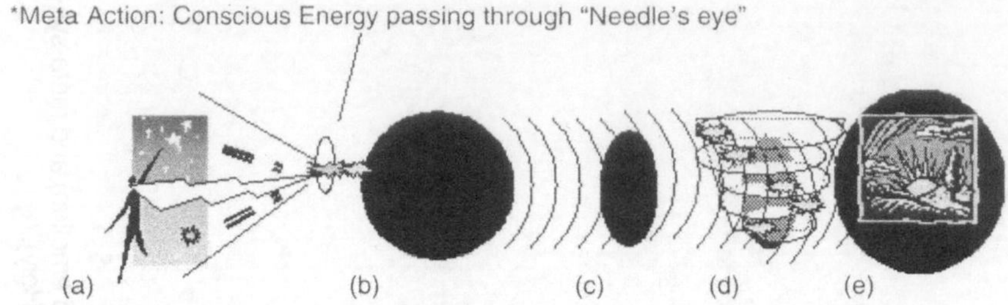

*Meta Action: Conscious Energy passing through "Needle's eye"

(a)   (b)   (c)   (d)   (e)

FIGURE 1.22. Enosis-in-action: (a) super-arousal of conscious energy; (b) energy metamorphosis to sheer silence; (c) self-awareness; (d) ancestral cloud; (e) Qua Persona of Christ Jesus.

airwaves. Prayerful reflection led to praise and ennobled his decision. God delighted in Jesus and, like refracted energy, he passed through the needle's eye into the profundity of God's Judgment, wherein God righteously evaluates Jesus' sterling qualities. Does he measure up? Following God's Seeing, Jesus regained self-awareness, presumably in prayer because that was how Jesus lived his life. The ancestral cloud descended upon and overcame Jesus, completely enshrouding him from view—its *phos* consisted of the faithful from every generation and embodied the wisdom of the ages.[95] The disciples were astonished by the whole series of events, and the transfer of ancestral wisdom also affected them. His persona was natural, not artificial, but his mind and sentience were enhanced, even poetic. Jesus countenanced joy, and God's Eternity sparked bliss. *Enosis* was the Penultimate expression of God's morality and seeded the greatest love known to a living person, prior to *Theosis* (postmortem Union with God).

At exactly the right time, God transfigured Jesus like refracted light so he could enter the Throne Room of Judgment (Figure 1.24). He was found righteous; Jesus, the God-given Son-Self, humbled himself before God and prepared to surrender his life for the salvation of others.[96] *Eloheim* gave His Word, Jesus, back to Israel, and the Jewish people responded, as in past covenants, by giving their *word* back to God, fulfilled in ritual sacrifice—the priestly vocation of Israel.

The Passion of Christ

Jesus discerned the Father's call for his life—to be Messiah. He was anointed by God to be the Archetype of humankind. Accordingly, he was tempted by the earthly passions that broke the divine–human relationship and, in full knowledge of human guilt and shame, he, universally, became sin—so he could put it to death and restore the divine–human relationship.[97] He placed the salvation needs of others above his own life, especially wary of the off-center and hypocritical device of religious authorities.[98] The template explaining Jesus' rich messianic and eschatological dimensions was in circulation, mostly from second temple Judaism—Isaiah's "Suffering Servant" passages, Daniel 12:2ff, Isaiah 26:7, 19, Hosea 6:2, Job 19:26 the Psalms of Solomon 3:1, Mishnah Sanhedrin 10:1, Testament of Judah, Wisdom of Solomon 3, Testament of Abraham 20 and 2 Maccabees 7:9.[99] The scriptures were troubling and prophesied great pain, rejection, and death to the Christ, but Jesus stood firm despite objections from the temple authorities.[100]

Jesus' activity sufficiently challenged the authority of Jewish leaders and they were concerned that religious toleration would cease if Rome heard of the dissention.[101] To counter repercussions, the Chief Priests persuaded Judas, Jesus' disciple, to hand him over to be tried for blasphemy by the Sanhedrin, but before the Roman governor— Jesus was accused of undermining Imperial authority, as a king-pretender. Who was really on trial? Was man trying God or was God testing human integrity? Jesus had several opportunities to remedy the intensity of suffering, but he endured for the sake of human redemption.[102] The betrayal of friends, the hatred of the crowds shouting against him, the mentality of those inflicting the punishments were tortuous, and the horror of the crucifixion appalled even the Romans.

The Cross changed the boundaries of God because when the nails pierced Jesus' body it caused him to become, irreversibly, one in suffering and death with every human being.[103] The suffering exceeded the limits of human capacity. Jesus was born in the flesh, lived, and became the crucified Christ.

> And they crucified him. . . . Then Jesus gave a loud cry and breathed his last.[104]

As he bled to death on the cross, Jesus' hanging, vertical position caused his lungs to fill up with water, and he drowned. The crucified bodies had to be removed in order to prevent the defilement of the feast commemorating the Jewish delivery from Egyptian slavery by Moses. Ironically, Jesus had just died so humankind could be delivered from the perversity of life. A soldier pierced Jesus' side with a spear to make sure he was dead; the spear must have torn his lung open because it drew blood and water.[105]

> . . . [Pilate] he granted the body to Joseph . . . [who] wrapped it in a linen cloth . . . and laid it in a tomb . . . [and] rolled a stone against the door of the tomb.[106]

No scholar denies the fact that Jesus was crucified and died. His heart and breathing ceased. Nonetheless, Jesus was united to God in Christology, as the son of Mary and God, through his holy lifestyle and, at Mt. Tabor; he was completely infused with Eternity. The interruption of love bespoke the preciousness of life contained in the eternal union.

Jesus Was Resurrected

All people die, and some die innocent deaths fighting for their beliefs, but no one has ever risen from death—except Jesus, the Son of God. Richard Swinburne evaluated the *prior* historical evidence as to the kind of life one would have to live so that God would consider raising that person from the dead. It is similar to Rahner's perfection of the whole person. Jesus practiced love, mercy, grace, repentance, and forgiveness of sin—he was an extraordinary Jew. Jesus offered holy and deeply moral teachings that revealed God's will. He identified with human suffering so even the undeserving could be forgiven, and his own sacrifice atoned for human failings. Christ led a perfect human life that taught about his own divinity and made it available to other generations and cultures through the church. Jesus' ethics and voluntary crucifixion were sufficient to bring him to life again— bearing God's indelible signature.

Mary Magdalene and the other Mary went to Jesus' tomb to anoint the body, but found it empty. Instead, in an illumination scene that was nearly identical with Jesus' transfiguration, they encountered angels and Jesus himself.

. . . ἄγγελος γὰρ κυρίου . . . ἦν δὲ ἡ εἰδέα αὐτοῦ ὡς ἀστραπὴ καὶ τὸ ἔνδυμα αὐτοῦ λευκὸν ὡς χιών. . . . καὶ ἰδοὺ Ἰησοῦς ὑπήντησεν αὐταῖς λέγων, Χαίρετε. αἱ δὲ προσελθοῦσαι ἐκράτησαν αὐτοῦ τοὺς πόδας καὶ προσεκύνησαν αὐτῷ.[107]

In the synoptic accounts, the angelic presence and αὐτοῦ signaled a theophany. The incandescence preceded Jesus' greeting, and the women *held* his body as they worshipped:

> . . . the angel of the Lord . . . His appearance was like lightening, and his clothing like white snow . . . Suddenly Jesus met them and said: "Greetings!" And they came to him took hold of his feet and worshipped him.[108]

In some cases, the respondents acted with ambiguity and delayed recognition.[109] Often, religious texts use poor vision to describe a lack of understanding. Mary mistook Jesus for the gardener. The disciples on the road to Emmaus did not know that it was Jesus speaking to them until he broke bread with them, and even Jesus' apostles did not recognize him on the beach.[110] The expectations of the disciples and others were decisively different from the actual events, and a severe psychological shock ensued.

In keeping with the integrity of Jesus' death and the sanctity of his Resurrection, the gospel reporters favored tangible evidence and played down mysticism. Luke portrayed orderly and material views; for example, Jesus was eating after he was resurrected (which dispelled angelmorphism). John, Luke, and Matthew pointed to an authentic witness using the soldier's testimony, the empty tomb, and the women. Although the women's testimony had no legal standing, it authenticated the reports because the accounts were *not* embellished, or it would have been omitted. The disciples were slow to respond to Jesus' resurrection. Eventually, they remembered Jesus' promise to return and believed. The Marys, Joanna, the apostles, and the disciples received Jesus' resurrection—with the same fruit that Jesus received from Elijah and Moses.

When Paul, the apostle, met the resurrected Jesus on the way to Damascus, he experienced an audible voice and a brilliant flash of light that rendered him blind (for three days). He continually retold the story about his theophany and used εγειρω *(egeiro)* to differentiate resurrection from a mere exaltation of spirit. Paul also documented resurrection appearances for other witnesses.[111]

Surviving literature of the early centuries gave wide currency to the resurrection, including Jewish sources such as Josephus (90 CE). Origin's *Contra Celsum* and the *Letter to Rheginos* brought Jewish sources together with the polemic against Jesus. He investigated 1 Kings 17:21f., 2 Kings 4:34, Moses, and myth, concluding that prophets intervened in the Old Testament resurrection narratives, but God acted directly in Jesus' resurrection. Followers were encouraged to live like people who already possessed the resurrection since the spread of Christianity was too great to be of mere human origin.[112]

Many Christian scholars believed Jesus was the trajectory of reconciliation. God's civilizing covenants bespoke God's perfect morality and the steadfast love Christ would exemplify in his life, death, and resurrection. Jesus accepted his own death without blame while satisfying Israel's covenantal obligations to God.[113] The New Testament was based on the faith of/in Christ, πιστου Χριστου, and the resurrection reinstated the hopes of humanity as inheritors of Eternal life.[114]

Conclusively, men and women in the first century received Jesus' resurrection, but the incandescence of God's energies have broken into natural settings in several centuries because the resurrection was intended for the faithful of every generation.[115] The writings of the Church patriarchs and doctors corroborated similar testimony, describing either a divine darkness, such as Moses at Mt. Sinai, or an illumination—an extraordinary implosion of intelligence coupled with supreme joy. St. Simeon spoke of a "non-material αὐτῶν, a non-metaphorical uncreated light which had no shape or form, by which he became that which he contemplated without losing identity," and he believed that this was available for everyone.[116] William James, a nineteenth-century psychiatrist, described his experience as a sudden extraordinary awareness:

> All at once . . . there came upon me a sense of exaltation of immense joyousness, accompanied or immediately followed by an intellectual illumination impossible to describe . . . I saw the universe is not composed of dead matter, but is on the contrary a living Presence; I became conscious in myself of Eternal life. It was not a conviction that I would have eternal life, but a con-

sciousness that I possessed eternal life then; I saw that all men are immortal. . . .[117]

Not unlike biblical accounts, modern enlightenment reports indicate thanksgiving, exuberance, joy, and a deep love of God—heaven on earth in the temporal structure of things, ideas, and history.[118] Orthodoxy refers to those blessed souls as *logoi* (cf., little *Logos'*), the faithful who were open to Christ's resurrection. Nonbelievers might have difficulty recognizing something with which they had no experience. Spontaneous enlightenment carries with it an eschatological intelligence, a special consortium of wisdom gathered from the faithful of every generation. In the natural, joy rises with the release of epinephrine into the brain, and energy flows through the limbic system when hormones and natural peptides respond in the pituitary and hypothalamus cortical regions, but tends to be momentary, fleeting. The small band of disciples knew the great joy of the resurrection and the sentient energy that Jesus spoke of flowing in those "rivers of living water." Inspired by the Holy Spirit, the Apostles wrote the New Testament collection, aware that *enosis*-salvation was intended for all who believe Jesus.

HUMAN WHOLENESS

Thesis: Christ entered human life with compassion for the marginalized, the weak, and those who were ill, loving the very image of God in each person—body and soul. Scripture calls humanity to be like Jesus and live in the world for God's glory.

The price of life is high, but the value of life in God goes beyond natural comprehension. It emerges through relationships with God, humankind, and the environment.[119] Gathering these unique qualities into a community leads to the quantum experience of human *wholeness* and, ultimately, a cosmic redemption in Christ.[120] The Resurrection of Christ extended human life beyond the material world. While the vastness of God's omnipotence (all powerful), omnipresence (unbounded by space and time), and omniscience (all knowing and wise) cannot be singularly contained in a one temporal human body, Christology and Ethics can flow into every person's being and activities. God lives in the midst of humankind. In *Torah,* God dwells in the midst of Israel's community. In Christianity, God's co-Eternal, indivisible Trinity became visible in Jesus' human life.

This chapter described the way God was evident in Jesus' *being*, his Christology and Ethic, while grounding him as a full-fledged member of the human species through Mary's heritage (i.e., genetic traits/ DNA). Jesus' portrait was cloaked in the Holy—born in Bethlehem and raised a Jew. He was tuned into his five senses and expressed emotion, but Jesus consciously contoured his response to the fulfillment of God's Word. God's Christology entered Jesus' flesh, and Christ worshipped God with his whole being.

The church, the gathered body of Christ, is directly concerned with the vitality and health of the community and provides a public conscience on behalf of those who need a voice—children, women, the disabled, the ill, the elderly, and minorities. It recognizes that every person is an important part of God's plan. Mary gave birth to the Messiah and, by his very existence, each new life brings a message from God to others. Therefore, the church has a responsibility to counsel and pray with individuals who face mental, physical, or emotional impairments—or must make difficult decisions about someone else's life and future. Counseling requires good information, and having that knowledge can assist in shaping specific prayers. The persons who must decide need to make an informed choice, so their conscience will be clear and everyone of sound mind is morally entitled to make a choice. God respected Jesus' right to make a fully informed decision— God enlightened him. Christ became the exemplar of compassion for society, attending to the physical needs of others as he ministered the divine *persona*. Frederick Houk Borsch, well-known ecclesiastical teacher and New Testament scholar, described the God–human relationship as anthropological, psychological, and, then, theological.[121] Borsch agreed that Jesus' *Imago Dei* provided a sound Christian perspective upon which the church and the people it serves can model present and future hopes and ethical determinations.

The church stands with the Universal Declaration of Human Rights in maintaining a vigil to protect human beings from exploitation by affirming respect for human dignity. To predetermine the life of another, without their consent, for any other reason than the certain elimination of a congenital illness, is a form of slavery. Every person has different abilities, so discrimination is not an option—everyone, every life, is valuable. To assign heritable traits, the stigma of "spelling mistakes" can marginalize whole groups of people who express their attributes differently (i.e., a deaf person has accelerated sight and a disabled veteran attains mastery of paraplegic sports). Sometimes, overcoming affliction provides the character and meaning that creates human wholeness and purpose. Protecting individual dignity honors the sacredness that was born *in* all creation. The church wishes to affirm genetic variation and the attributes of unique being—characterized by the genetic mutation.

When God surveyed his creation and declared, "it is very good," the definition for "good" rested in a Truth, an emerging Truth. "Good" has been interpreted subjectively, residing in the cultural community of its time, from age to age.[122] Life has value because others care. The people and their relatives who are born with particular afflictions form communities as a result of common heritable and degenerative illnesses, such as Trisome 21 or Duchenne Muscular Dystrophy. These same groups also serve as a healing vessel for those who develop a disability as a result of an accident or war—people who share similar nongenetic impairments. The L'Arche organization developed so Mongoloid individuals could live as adults, and many a visitor has been inspired by the lack of guile and guilt that characterizes these charming people, contributing to a healthy attitude about variations of mental awareness. Integrating disadvantaged persons into educational and other group activities, such as inspired by the Montessori kindergarten, creates an atmosphere of wholeness and inclusion in the community. Continued improvements in prosthesis have enabled many to live easier lives—reaching out to victims of wars, people with degenerative diseases, those who suffer from dermatological diseases, and those with varieties of cancer. National health services and health management companies provide wellness information and therapy groups to disadvantaged individuals and their families. All these communities facilitate a continual open exchange of information and support, which enables one to make a fully informed decision, and this honors the essence of being born into the human family. Any society that considers itself civilized holds human dignity in high regard, regardless of physical limitations. The Christian church desires wholeness for the entire human community toward the eradication of disease and rectification of organic, limbic, motor, or other limitations—where it is plausible.

Jesus was created in the image of God, *imago Dei*—just as we are—and *imago Dei,* as a fully physiological being, is the real reason for the church's legitimate interest in the legislative discussions on biogenesis. God is inextricable from personal consciousness, making liberty of conscience quintessential to being human; it is therefore a biological event—and a necessity. Derek Davis, liberty of conscience scholar, joins many scholars in the public defense of freedom of conscience as an inviolable right—central to human life and a living faith.

Humanity is entitled to strive for God's favor and to live into the Christology and Ethic bequeathed to creation. Living the way Jesus modeled, including making healthy, informed decisions with a clear conscience, opens the door for the Resurrection to initiate an enlightened existence, including heightened intellect and sensitivity, in which one participates in the Holy spectrum of omnipresence, omnipotence, and omniscience. In fact, some philosophy of regenerated/Resurrected life is common to most of the traditions, although it may be expressed in different terms. It is not surprising that humanitarians from differing religious and philosophical traditions reverence "life" as a universal value. In humanity, matter has become aware of itself; in Christianity, God has empowered creation with a voice that responds to God's immanent Presence—our stewardship is for a whole system of life in the cosmos. *Imago Dei* is the very expression of God's activity on earth, and the church is the vessel that nurtures those who live up to the Ethic instilled in each of us—by the way we live together (Figures 1.23 and 1.24).

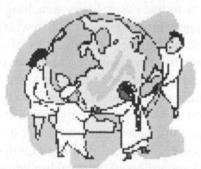

FIGURE 1.23. Summit of the mind: Ethical reverence for humankind.

FIGURE 1.24. Peace: Arriving at the place it all began.

The Truth is waiting in stillness . . . at the point of Origin . . .

Chapter 2

Ethics: Has Morality Become a Maze or a Prism?

INTRODUCTION: ENTERING THE RECONSTRUCTION ZONE

The purpose of this book is to equip and empower ethical decisions for difficult pregnancies by providing the information necessary to comprehend key aspects in such important decisions. In order to understand the potential of every person, God sent Jesus as a model and message. The previous chapter explained Christ's *being,* but this chapter will view its companion, ethical action, and the various formulas written for guiding moral behavior. The church is obliged to adhere to Christian principles and to engage in moral reflection about biomedicine on behalf of its community, but the church cannot begin by simply adopting existing medical ethics and going on from there, for that presumes something over Christ. This chapter looks at choosing the right or wrong *decision* and *action* by considering a variety of formulas for ethical thought, motivations, and conclusions. The scholarly contributions come from various cultural and geographical settings and contribute rational, social, and religious reasons for valuing every person. Each discussion is placed into a historical context while illuminating the value for which it became best known, delineating the major tenets that correspond best with Christian principles. The moral architecture covers classical ethical antecedents, principle-based ethics, womanist ethics, and the Mesoethics of rights and justice. The

Counseling Pregnancy, Politics, and Biomedicine
© 2007 by The Haworth Press, Inc. All rights reserved.
doi:10.1300/5697_03

womanist perspective is especially relevant since modern reproductive technologies and genetic diagnosis affect women and their bodies.

Taking systems of ethical thought on board generates the confidence necessary to buttress tough decisions and liberate the conscience for responsible action. Contributions came out of different centuries, from several countries, and from respectable experts whose ideas have received much attention. It will become evident that each decision has the capacity to send great ripples across the whole of society, but readers will only be able to choose from among those ethical patterns that resonate with their own understanding of what is *good*—or *right*.

Due to the myriad of values within a society of diverse people, it is very difficult to universalize social morals to one absolute *good* for all. Global migration, Westernization, pluralism, post-modernity, deconstructionist philosophies, and pragmatism have restructured traditional presuppositions about religious ethics, medicine, and moral philosophy. In the early days of democracy, society had common antecedents in race, nationality, and religious heritage, but pluralism brought a wide variety of cultures into the same community, irrespective of the country being discussed. For the sake of equity and justice, Michael Walzer accentuated the local and particular character of that group's idea of *good*.[1] The individualization of the "good" led to a new respect for autonomy, whereby each person deserved the right to choose her/his own values.[2] This dichotomy between justice and rights forced society to neutralize its values—referencing only "facts" so no one imposed and elevated their concept of good over another. Objectivity was packaged as the proper scientific method. Hence, the courts of law could only apply neutral, objective values—empirical evidence became the standard. Philosophical and religious evidence lost its footing to the technical emphasis. Michael Sandel surmised that this sequence of rationale yielded the procedural, rule-bound system of today's society.[3] Facts were sterilized, human sensitivity was sacrificed, and the ordering of appropriate categories of good was compromised.[4]

Sheila Jasonoff's evaluation of biomedical case law recognized that examining other people's experiences, including emotions, data, and technology, presented better choices in locating the best decisions.[5] Interpreting the information in light of one's culture and beliefs constituted one's *right*. For the Christian culture, it is important to locate the fulcrum of meaning and aptly apply its principles in reconciling standard values. As the reader will discover, right and good became distinguished very early in Greek history. Christian texts proceeded to richly express ethics, linguistics, and metaphor in light of its goals.

LOCATING A MEANINGFUL STARTING PLACE: DEFINITION AND GOALS

According to Oliver O'Donovan, the term *ethics* differs only slightly from *morality,* in that ethics are reflections on right living, and morality is the experience lived in one's life (the actual living); one is contemplating the good, and the other is doing it.[6] Aristotle's society highly esteemed those who lived a moral life. When someone achieved the ηθικα (ethic), the person was appointed to a high political position as an example to others. Good moral behavior was an end in itself. On the other side of the Mediterranean, Origin deduced ethics *(ithiki)* as the means by which one became holy. A person's conscience deciphered ethics and was the throne of morality.

Scholars systemized ethics into three categories: *virtue ethics, deontological ethics,* and *teleological ethics.* Ancient Greeks knew one could intuitively perceive virtuosity, and they believed it was also important to cultivate virtue, as ethics, through education and discipline. Of course, the early Greeks did not separate the spiritual nature from daily living. Therefore, when a Christian displayed the fruit of Christ's character, it testified that the Holy Spirit was active in that person's life. Deontological ethics professed that every person be honored and, when necessary, assisted, because humanity was created in the image of God. Moral action was a duty, instructed by reason and conscience. When one evaluated all the possible consequences of a decision before acting, it had a teleological orientation. (For example, before choosing a pharmaceutical product, its risks and benefits are weighed with the person's physical needs for the healthiest results.) In fact, moral architecture requires differing approaches because of the diverse personalities from whom and for whom the benefits are intended.

Henry Sidgwick considered a broad spectrum of morality across the history of ethics in pursuit of systemizing *right,* i.e., correct conduct for the instruction of others. He evaluated ethical antecedents in virtue, duty, practicality, free will, pleasure, political association, and intellect. He created a special nest for psychological issues because the intent and motive of a community's members shaped its moral disposition. Sidgwick also presumed God was present as a metaphysical construct.[7]

A more recent moral philosopher, Tom Beauchamp, evaluated the environmental aspects of psychological and political well-being. He concluded that a self-determining society seeking the ultimate good for all persons would derive the highest benefit for the community; however, individual interests might be sacrificed in the process.[8]

With his medical science students, Roger Crisp described ethical determination as choosing a lifestyle that adheres to consistent, general, and systematic principles. Since new discoveries are occurring daily in science, norms need to remain flexible and objective, but objectivity does not mean emptying oneself of compassion, especially when the products of science are tested on human beings. According to Hobbes, the lack of human sympathies caused dire consequences and created the need for moral structure, in the first place.[9] Hence, compassion is quintessential in making relationships meaningful and for motivating ethical responses.

Clearly, different types of people ask for distinctive ethical styles, ones that avoid arbitrary preferences. For example, women's values focus on relationships. Womanist principles could not transfer to the solitary lifestyle of a scientist whose inventions usually occur in a private laboratory. Indeed, all good values contribute to moral living, but they are affected by time, place, and circumstance.

So where does one begin to understand ethics? The options are dazzling. There is little doubt that modern reproductive medicine needs, at least, minimum boundaries on its practices, especially biogenetics, but there are a number of considerations one has to take on board before arriving at a formula. The early philosophies of ethics provided a basic understanding. In addition, human dignity, rights, and justice have become fundamental to Western moral concepts. This incredibly diverse world now understands that it needs to respect the differences of others as well as hold firm to ethics that shape humankind into the image of Christ for God's glory.

STEPPING STONES IN CIVILIZATION: VIRTUE ETHICS, NATURAL LAW, KANT, AND UTILITARIANISM

Description: Virtue ethics aspire to discover, describe, and teach human beings to model the highest likeness of God or the gods for the harmony of the community.[10] Teachings on Virtue from the Ancient Mediterranean World

As ancient Greek philosophers pondered the meaning of life, they lauded and sang of virtuous qualities in poetry, drama, and the ethics of the gods (ηθικα, in Greek). Greek gods were anthropomorphic deities. Hesiod played with their genealogy, while Homer dramatized the natural world as their dominion.[11] When Thales' Gnomic poetry (640-560 BCE) merged with Pythagorean verse (580-500 BCE), the classical world realized that poetry fed the soul with quietness of conscience. This made the whole body healthy. The ethic of the gods was known as ευθαμια. It intended the highest good (cf., Heraclitus, 530-470 BCE). The reward was happiness (cf., Democritus, 460-370 BCE).[12] Being human was understood in tangible, physical (*physikoi*, πηψσικοι) terms from whence gracefulness and order blossomed.[13] Sophist Protagoras of Abden (450-400 BCE) systemized knowledge about pleasure and pain. Socrates (47-399 BCE) educated his disciples about just and righteous acts using dialectics so as to harmonize differences and equip people with the knowledge to do what was good.[14] Antisthenes the Cynic reduced good to pleasure; he knew it was transient. Aristippus of Cyrene considered pleasure-seeking a vice that harmed the human spirit, along with prejudice and judgment.[15] Nihilism was antithetical. The Greek world desired to be fit as a matter of pleasing the gods who would in turn bless them with wisdom, reason, pleasure, and all that was good. The Greeks worshipped images of gods in statues and nature, presuming the spirit of the gods inhabited living bodies. Health had religious overtones.

A few philosophers had monotheistic ideas, which contributed sophistication and purposefulness to the mosaic. Euclides of Megara described one single, real Being who manifested excellence. Plato (427-347 BCE) perceived a Heaven of Perfection that surpassed human understanding. Side-by-side with Plato's spirit–matter dualism was Megara's metaphysic, wherein divine knowledge, wisdom, virtue, beauty, and wholeness were bestowed by divinity upon humanity. These gifts equipped one as an instrument in the divine plan, according to Protagoras. Indeed, Plato concluded that the physical universe was organized for an ultimate, divinely conceived, transcendent goal. Life yearned for its source and sought to know it through goodness and virtue.[16]

Discipline in both the physical and aesthetic areas plumbed the raw nature of humanity for its highest attributes. Human nature interested Aristotle (384-322 BCE) because each idea was novel, and moral consciousness burst into society through abstract thought, creativity, imagination, sensual experience, and emotion! The virtues provided a complementary genesis (Gk., γενεσισ). Wisdom (Gk., Φρονησις or σωΦια) was the greatest asset, and courage (Gk., ανδρεια) was the stuff of heroes. It meant strength that was open to reason. Temperance meant behaving in an orderly fashion. Justice and uprightness (Gk., δικαοσυνη) were social virtues, as was harmony.[17] The conscience tested and authenticated beneficence and virtue. Virtues attracted people to one another, and the highest result was love. According to Joseph Fletcher, being virtuous was prudent, because the attraction to love *is* the highest good.[18]

Greek philosophers, such as Plato and Aristotle, shaped society in virtuous living by discipline, incentives for happiness, and trusting the conscience (free will), but the Stoics (48-120 CE) wanted law, because conscience sometimes missed the mark. They believed Law had a cosmic nature with a universal integrity from a Higher Source. During stoicism, Roman law was reputed, and Jesus' teachings were only a budding new vine.

In the Southern Mediterranean, Egyptian philosophers also desired purity of the Soul. The mythology in North Africa foretold many miracles that were later described in the legendary story of Jesus. His wisdom fit well into the flourishing cult of *Gnosis* in Plotinus' time (205-270 CE). Wisdom and, therefore, God, were in *Gnosis,* even before creation, which meant it could overrule unwanted, natural human impulses (Gk., σωμα). Hence, the basest of all human behavior was destined to become virtuous, and it was hoped that, over the generations, humanity could be perfected and absorbed into the love of its Creator—subsumed into ecstasy![19]

Influential Teachings from Christianity

Jesus of Nazareth's birth, life, teachings, death, and Resurrection began a new calendar and gave birth to a new understanding about what *ethical living* was. As a Jew, Jesus' moral instruction was his emulation of the Jewish Law. Its Word, which he summarized, "You shall love the Lord your God with all your heart, and all your soul, and with all your strength, and with all your mind; and [love] your neighbor as yourself."[20] He was obedient for the sheer sake of love, and his adherence to the Word transformed him. Jesus fulfilled the Law, reconciled humanity with God, and revealed God's Promise! In part, Christ understood his role from things he read in Job, the Psalms, and Isaiah:

> . . . I delivered the poor who cried, and the orphan who had no helper. The blessing of the wretched came upon me and I caused the widow's heart to sing for joy. I put on righteousness and it clothed me; my justice was like a robe and turban. I was eyes to the blind and feet to the lame. I was a father to the needy and I championed the cause of the stranger.[21]

It sounds like modern social charity, but his association with marginal members of society was counterculture to first-century Jewish piety. Indeed, Jesus recognized that human physical needs had to be tended, healed, and brought to wholeness to prepare the way for the Lord.[22] Christ was a healer. His devotion to faith also meant that nothing physical could stand in the way of theological goals, because pleasing God outweighed earthly wealth, power, and domination. The Kingdom of Heaven was worth it! In fact, Matthew's Kingdom of God was for the poor, weak, sad, and humble who willingly forsook all other pursuits for the love of God.

> Blessed are the poor in spirit, for theirs is the Kingdom of Heaven. Blessed are those who mourn, for they will be comforted. Blessed are the meek, for they will inherit the earth. Blessed are those who hunger and thirst for righteousness, for they will be filled. Blessed are the merciful, for they will receive mercy. Blessed are the pure in heart, for they will see God. Blessed are the peacemakers, for they will be called the children of God. Blessed are those who are persecuted for righteousness'

sake, for theirs is the Kingdom of Heaven. Blessed are you when people revile you and persecute you and utter all kinds of evil against you falsely on my account. Rejoice and be glad, for your reward is great in heaven, for in the same way they persecuted the prophets who were before you.[23]

The blessing and consequences of encountering the Kingdom of God were recurring reminders that there was more to God's Promise than self-satisfaction. Humble forgiveness preempted retributive justice (eye-for-an-eye, Lat., *lex tallions*).[24] Pleasing God meant overcoming normal human behavior, cultural and religious, and becoming Christ-like. Jesus taught:

But I say to you that listen, love your enemies, do good to those who hate you, bless those who curse you, pray for those who abuse you. If anyone strikes you on the cheek, offer the other also; and from anyone who takes away your coat do not withhold even your shirt. Give to everyone who begs from you; and if anyone takes away your goods, do not ask for them again. Do to others, as you would have them do to you. Be merciful just as your Father is merciful. Do not judge and you will not be judged; do not condemn and you will not be condemned. Forgive and you will be forgiven; give and it will be given to you . . .[25]

Christ's strange economy became a proven reality when he was resurrected from the dead. Saul of Tarsus encountered Jesus' Resurrection and was transformed into Saint Paul the Apostle. Passion for God, sincerity of heart, and deep caring for others were characteristics that flowed from the heart. It was not a matter of simply checking-off the box next to each rule. Letters from the Apostles, especially Paul and John, carried a theme of friendship and a gentle loving kindness inspired by the Holy Spirit.[26]

Love is patient; love is kind; love is not envious or boastful or arrogant or rude. It does not insist on its own way; it is not irritable or resentful; it does not rejoice in wrongdoing, but rejoices in the truth. It bears all things, believes all things, hopes all things, endures all things. Love never ends.[27]

Christ's cross gave value to grief and emotions of all kinds, and it instilled both ontological and teleological hope in loving God and others as one loves himself/herself.[28]

Love is the centerpiece of the gospel message for many modern scholars. In view of a pluralistic society, Joseph Fletcher's *Situation Ethics* advocated disinterested love, being no respecter of persons. God's message mandated love for Christ's sake. Love was the motive, the means, and the end. Just as Plato and Aristotle maintained that any moral action required personal free will, Fletcher's duty to love was a matter of yielding one's own desires to the guidance of the Holy Spirit (bottom-up). Fletcher separated love from law due to the prescriptive nature of law and its resistance to free will. Only in freedom could the Holy Spirit abide with the human conscience as it weighed ethical choices.[29] Obedience to God's will prospered love.[30]

Stephen Pope considered healthy emotions and human biology in *The Evolution of Altruism and the Ordering of Love*. He had a strong sense of duty to the poor, homeless, and those without a voice of their own and, like Augustine, Aquinas, natural biologists, and evolutionary theorists, he knew that people needed intimacy, commitment, honor, responsibility, and care (human initiative). Pope saw Jesus' generous love shining through August Compte's ethic, which loved without reward. He also recognized natural prejudices, such as among family members who cared about their own first, before tending to the neighbors. After all, parents personally resemble their biological children and enjoy watching them. They provide for their food, shelter, clothing, socializing, supervision, care, and comfort. Children sometimes prefer one parent over the other. Family members want to be loved and remembered. Indeed, people base their actions on intentions, desires, and motives. There are also unconscious desires within biological counterparts, drive, instinctive proclivities, and inclinations.[31] Cynics, such as Richard Dawkins, argue that altruism of all kinds is motive-driven.[32] The truth is that all relationships are interdependent, and simple acts of kindness are woven into daily living.

Christian charity does not depend on rationalized behavior because it thrives on intelligence, freedom, and creativity while exemplifying humanity and God.[33] God loved and trusted humanity enough to allow free choice, fed by the Holy Spirit. Pope earthed religious motivations with biology, emotions, and sociology. Fletcher and Pope conceived of human beings as initiators of a love that was completed by Christ.

For Stanley Hauerwas and Henry Sidgwick, Christ *instigated* altruism and enabled love (top-down). Christ made moral behavior attractive, and the Holy Spirit revealed the truth to the person. *The Peaceable Kingdom* told of God's gifts and transforming character coming to individuals from on-High, as well as in human relationships. Hauerwas stayed close to the incarnational theology of the first century that brought divine activity into nature so one could become God's loving activity in the world through Holy Spirit.[34] Similar to Aquinas, Hauerwas had a hylomorphic, holistic idea of the divine–human metaphysic.

Sidgwick's history credited the Holy Spirit with inspiring faith and obedience through the Sacraments.[35] The Christian was cultivated through benevolent conformity, purity, humility, and counsels of perfection (for those in the devotional life). Many of his ideas were cut from the same cloth as the classical Augustinian, neo-Platonian views. God was distinctly Other from His creation, remaining sovereign over all.

The differences between Fletcher, Pope, Hauerwas, and Sidgwick have to do with divine–human homeostasis. Monotheistic views of Plato's dualism meet Aristotelian natural ethics or the School of Alexandria meets the Antiochene School. It happens repeatedly. There were debates at the early Ecumenical Councils, and medieval philosophers kept a respectable divide while exploring God's activity in human bodies. Today, we see God trusting humanity to perform God's activity on earth. Some believe altruistic behavior is bottom-up, and others think love is top-down. The debate is one of theology—*how* God worked out his redemptive plan. In singularity of purpose, scholars and ministers hope to effectively articulate values that lead to a virtuous, transformative community.[36] The undisputed Christian values are faith, hope, and love, which manifest wisdom, harmony, righteousness, justice, and temperance—a regal bequest, known first by the ancients and still honored by many in this millennium.[37]

Christian Values Progress to Modern Times

Before moral theology and philosophy were systemized, the general rule was simple—life was desirable and death was to be avoided.

In the early years, people associated death with divine judgment as seen in weather, water, fires, and wild animals. There was a universal understanding that there was Power greater that humankind.

By the fourth century, the myriad of polytheistic cultures in the Roman Empire gave way to Emperor Constantine after he saw a luminary vision of the Christian symbol (Xρ) in the night's sky and waged a victorious war in the name of Christ. This created an organic relationship between the Church and society.

Christianity was proclaimed the imperial religion in order to sustain peace, unity, and ethical harmony. Doing what was right was integral to the Christian faith—it was a duty owed to God and to the emperor. Outward ethical behavior was evidence of Christian character; hence, people strove to be obedient, patient, benevolent, pure, and humble.[38] As the faith became systemized, moral law and temporal sanctions became Church Doctrine. The Christian world was also a learned one. Clergy and philosophers contemplated and debated the power of divinity within human reason and nature.

Natural Law

Definition: Natural law is a duty-based ethic. It presumes universality, reason, innate moral duties, common obedience to authority, and ethical relativity, but it does not make all things permissible.[39]

Aristotelian philosophy was popular during Thomas Aquinas' university years, and he found it refreshingly pragmatic compared to the neo-Platonian attitudes, which the Church had inherited from Augustine. He recognized a connection between inward transformation, in the theological sense, and the primacy of vii ue in Greek philosophy. Christianity was part of the natural world since God was the Creator of nature and the Universe. Aquinas wrote about human consciousness and intellect in a way that made God manifest to the Soul.[40] He understood two expressions of morality. One came from an educated intellect; the other was God's inspiration of ethical principles.[41] Jesus was hylomorphic, which meant the divine and human were integrated—on some level. Anthropologically, the physical body used the senses and raw intuitive reactions, like birds or animals. Yet, unlike any other creature, humanity possessed conscious reason.[42]

Medieval scholars preferred nature-oriented interpretations to Neo-Platonic dualism. Christians, Jews, and Muslims desired a better understanding of God's communication with people. Averroes, an Islamic Scholar, said that God was one all-authoritative Agent Intellect (AI), but Aquinas could not fathom a single overarching Intellect for all people. Rather, God entered each human mind to reveal the things of God in the natural world; consequently, men and women interpreted ideas for themselves. Aquinas decided Spirit guided decisions were "fixed by intention, aimed at by the will, while under the influence of practical reason."[43] Thomas also recognized that human beings were flawed and needed law to shape habits and direct good behaviors.[44]

In his *Commentary on Ethics,* Aquinas made it clear that a person who patterned her/his life after ethical teachings would develop moral skills. Some people did evil because they were confused and thought it was good. Education taught discernment of just and virtuous principles, while recognizing personal limitations. Moral science encouraged reason and discouraged emotional reactions.[45] The conscience was the key mediator between human nature and Eternal law.[46] Those who were rational and conscientious knew the difference between natural law and error (e.g., Aristotle, H. Grotius, and Richard Hooker). Having opened the door to metaphysics, philosophers pondered God's influence on the mind as well as biophysics.

Kantian Metaphysic Moral

Definition: Kantian moral theory proposed a deontological premise, a duty, styled as a categorical imperative. One "ought" to act regardless of the intended results and to do it as if it applied to all situations and persons, universally. Ethical actions, desires, and instincts had to be freely chosen and based on experience.[47]

Kant's metaphysic moral was a response to the scientific empiricism of the eighteenth-century, which questioned all accepted values, and Kant also took a strike against intuitionism, made popular by the Enlightenment. In typical German fashion, he held to an immutable standard of right.[48] *Deon* meant binding duty (in Greek). Syllogisms frequently expressed universality "*if* this, *then* act." The duty (the *oughtness*) was imperative and was not contingent upon consequences. It was nonteleological.[49]

Kant's philosophy was fed by logic, physics, and experimentation. Logic provided the nonempirical *a priori* evaluation. Physics and experimentation were the empirical tests. He weighed material evidence with *a priori* data, concluding that in order for a choice to be truly ethical, it had to be experience-based and volitional. Hence, one ought to do what was right, but it was both practical and moral that it be done willingly.

Ought was the categorical imperative in which a person had a duty to be objective; otherwise, the principle would be weakened by self-interest or personal gain.[50] Conforming to a relevant precept was acting rightly. One's debt to others was a "perfect, unchanging duty" that sought a universal harmony of purpose. The difference between a perfect and an imperfect duty depended on "how" and "by whom" the act was to be implemented. Volition was at the heart of every moral action.

Personhood was regarded so highly that each person was the *end*. Humanity was not to be used as a *means* on the road to someone else's goal. The formula of autonomy was necessary for the "kingdom of ends," which was only attainable when *all* people exercised the same values pursuant to the same *ends*.[51] Kant presupposed that moral law was recognizable—even before it became of interest to us. It was a substrate of our conscious awareness and proceeded from our own intelligent will. The fact that the world was intelligible helped humanity recognize and esteem one another.

Utilitarianism

Definition: Utilitarianism proposes consequentialist ethics. Moral actions need to have a desirable outcome for the community. There are no universal presumptions—it is consistently relative.[52]

Utilitarianism prioritized happiness above duty (Kant's trademark). It was a British recipe featuring: (1) Mr. Paley's "common sense," (2) a philosophy based on empiricism by Jeremy Bentham, and (3) John Stewart Mill added a sophisticated version with sanctions for wrongdoers and a crescendo whereby one is happy to sacrifice for someone else's benefit.

Paley preferred a moral code that brought the greatest pleasure to the greatest number of people, without dismissing private happiness because, like Abraham Tucker, he believed that God willed happiness equitably. There was neither free will nor deserts.

Jeremy Bentham, influenced by Hobbessian materialism, used the community's collective experience to discern good and pain. Hence, consequences were empirically testable. Evaluating good and bad behaviors of the whole population revealed the greatest happiness for the greatest number. The calculation included alimentation, sex, senses, wealth, power, curiosity, sympathy, malevolence, and social and individual goodwill, with corresponding unpleasantness from manual labor as well as organic disorders (i.e., illness, etc.). These calculations were intended as the basis for law and civil codes, but Bentham suspected that government leaders might have personal motives. Therefore, he encouraged public participation.

John S. Mill calculated the overall aggregate happiness without neglecting the felicity of individuals. He was midpoint between altruism and Bentham's egoism. His standards were derived from case experience, the potential consequences to the community, and its unity.[53] Moral sanctions instructed and encouraged a higher personal norm, but, in time, a morally mature individual would gladly suffer for someone else because human nature delighted in virtue, even self-sacrificial love. Utilitarian motives dissolved in the face of moral perfection since it was the penultimate value. The conscience provided a reliable guide for ethical decisions, usually due to the understandability of competing challenges, such as stealing to eat in order to survive.[54]

Utilitarians were split as to whether one simply acted as needed or went strictly by the book. Act Utilitarians desired the most expedient choice. Rule Utilitarians thought one ought to always stay within the bounds of the law or, at least, change the law before proceeding. Of course, one had to act in some situations or they could be criminally negligent. The rule was to modify the program before neglect or inappropriate behavior brought harm to an individual.[55] Both Act Utilitarians and Rule Utilitarians believed the particulars should be put into writing.

Due to the rise in science and its ever-changing scope, the Benthamite system was favored because of its empiricist and teleological aims. It suited the objective, highly material, and intellectual climate.

Biological concepts, such as quality of life, replaced references to good and bad behavior, pleasure and pain, as well as moral sentimentality. Ethics was being earthed, and the precepts of scientific method bled into other fields. When science began to draw analogies without differentiating between each species, the boundaries between humans and other animals were blurred. The order of nature was skewed. Churchmen either denied or ignored the impact that science was having on faith-based morality. Although many supported the Benthamite approach, the idea of the greatest good for the greatest number did not work for minorities and the poor, who were easily swallowed up by majority rule. It flatly contradicted an equitable and truly moral society.

Sidgwick added common sense to Utilitarianism as well as Marineau's psychology. He referenced Butler's principles, which affirmed individual needs and the duty to take care of one's self. Universals existed by virtue of moral intuition and the natural desire for happiness. Common-sense moral philosophy curved Utilitarianism back toward truth and good, with a personal touch. His new theory embraced prudence (rational egoism), justice and equity, and good behavior directed by reason (a logical benevolence).[56] Ideas of conscience, the human personality, and moral authority were accentuated by Marineau's psychology.[57] In acquiescing to the dignity of humankind and finding the conscience a suitable mediator, human reason was deemed capable of formulating ethical values.[58]

MODERN ETHICS: PRINCIPLE-BASED ETHICS, WOMANIST ETHICS, AND MESOETHICS

Introduction

People from several cultures contributed valuable insights to this discussion, including those from classical Greece, Judaism, Christianity, Germany, the Enlightenment, and England. The information traveled across centuries and, indeed, traversed the globe, but the original values arose primarily from theologians, scholars, and philosophers living in homogenous societies. Foreign wars and international migration led to cultural microcosms; therefore, behavioral norms were localized. Segregation remained with an "us–them" mentality.[59]

Ethical principles would have to be revamped to deal with inequality and the moral uncertainty of today's world.[60] To arrive at democratic civil codes of conduct, groups had to negotiate, but symbols and language did not always mean the same thing. Still, respect was a universally accepted principle, and "honoring thy neighbor" became politically correct (PC) in terms of acknowledging and tolerating many differences.

Principle-based ethics formed the moral toolbox for the era of modern reproductive technology. Innovative therapies created hope for human health issues, and it confronted accepted traditions in the process, which accentuated the need for ethical definition. In biomedicine, professionals followed four basic principles: respect for persons (also known as autonomy), beneficence, nonmalfeasance, and justice. Since *justice* and *rights* continue to be in tension, it is worthwhile to discuss them from a Mesoethics perspective. Patients and doctors need both rights and justice. Rights must be unmasked to protect pregnant women and the weaker members of society, such as children and the infirm (in various stages of illness). Justice is needed to ensure egalitarian distribution of services.

Reproductive technology applies to women's bodies, so *Womanist Ethics* gives voice to what is a uniquely female understanding of values, especially since ethical scholarship has been predominantly male. Mothers gave birth to everyone in the world, yet mothers-to-be and fetuses are now subjects of research, experimentation, and untested therapies. In material terms, they are little more than embodied test tubes, which is absurd in a society where women are educated leaders, teachers, hold a large percentage of the health care positions, provide natural empathy, and guide the rights of passage for young and old alike.

Principle-based ethics, Mesoethics, and Womanist Ethics contribute an organized collage of standards, without losing sight of the traditional foundations. Humanity needs to participate in its own health care and deal directly with professionals. Understanding the vast array of moral precepts provides insight into effective ways of knowing and deciding.

Principle-Based Ethics

Definition: Principle-based ethics have four fundamental principles often considered universal ethics. Respect for human life (dignity) is the foundation. This includes: (1) respect for persons, including autonomy for capable persons and protection of persons incapable of autonomy; (2) beneficence, maximizing good; (3) nonmalfeasance, minimizing harm; and Justice (below, in its own section).[61]

In attempting to delve deeper into the treasures of what it actually means to be human and how to appreciate and respect humanity, Christians promoted a hylomorphic divine–human hypostasis wherein people shared in the properties of God—to direct conscience and sympathies, but the academy also studied the secular components of moral philosophy, such as human personality, physiology, intelligence, psychology, and memory, as well as conversational and symbolic aptitudes. The paradigm shifted as curiosity grew in the sciences.

Respect for Persons

For centuries, it was unequivocally understood that God bequeathed piety upon the faithful. Secular piety became fashionable when Deist's exercised their free will in an age of science and rampant individualism. It emancipated rights language.[62] Natural rights and freedom of conscience challenged natural law. Early Christian liberals presumed that humanity was made in the image of God and preferred rights language.[63] Although *imago Dei* was not wholly empirical, it was the *raison d'etre* and necessitated dignity, mutual respect, and autonomy.[64] J. Fletcher described certain features that distinguished human beings from other species *sine qua non* (without equal): self-awareness, human relationships, affection, spontaneous happiness, abstract thought, duty and responsibility, the balance between reason and feeling, a sense of time, curiosity, self-identity, self-control, and the ability to change.[65] William May upheld humanity as a unique biological species, full stop.[66] Indeed, human beings have an elegant consciousness that instantiates respect and awe.[67]

Conscience and reason presume respect and autonomy (self-determination). In fact, according to C.A. Pierce, conscience itself was a reflexive verb—it acted upon itself. Conscience was innate, perceivably from Christology. Philo and Polybius feared the conscience (*sunedis,* συνεδις) as an internal judge to be dreaded, convicting every wrong-doer. A guilty conscience was considered a disease. Orestes's terrible crimes made his conscience (Gk., συνειδεησις, *suneideasis*) an ulcer of the flesh (Euripides). (The reason for two different Greek words is unknown.)

By the first century, people were ready for Faith in Christ to re-deem their guilt. Paul admonished Christians to be blameless and not to burden the conscience of others by calling down blame upon them (Gk., αμαρτανω). Aquinas taught that conscience inclined toward the good and away from evil. In natural law, conscience and reason teased out choices, mediated duty *(deon)* according to God's will *(telos)*, and opted to accept or reject ideas *(liberum arbitrum, electio)*.[68]

Gabriel Biel, Martin Luther's mentor, considered conscience mu-table and subjective. It delivered practical and self-evident decisions. Luther did not believe that the conscience inclined toward good be-cause humanity was corrupted by sin, but the erring conscience could repent and change when instructed by Scripture. In order for a person to be morally responsible, the person had to make his/her own de-cisions. This mandated freedom of conscience.[69] J. B. Lightfoot crowned conscience as the most important word in ethical nomencla-ture. The average person presumed it was common sense, and some human rights advocates considered liberty of conscience as the cor-nerstone of all freedoms.[70] God entrusted humankind to make deci-sions, and that was worthy of respect.

Moral Autonomy

The technicalities underlying moral autonomy have generated much discussion. R. S. Downie and Elizabeth Telfer considered feelings, intentions, and motives as the driving elements in decision making. Emotion is parleyed by noncognitive biochemistry and environmen-tal forces, yet true responsibility has to be free of external controls.[71] Gerald Dworkin radically stood by the importance of having values originate with the person (i.e., not susceptible to the persuasion of an-other) because of the binding effects as well as the burdens that unre-servedly rest upon that person.[72] W. D. Ross thought total autonomy was impossible because circumstances interfere, as do certain priori-ties. Examples are safety over happiness, nondiscrimination, etc. Did

a previous promise exist that created a responsibility? Did careless-
ness necessitate reparations? Does self-preservation take priority
over improving the life of another?[73] When charged with the care of
an incapacitated person, one has to try to imagine what that person
would wish as well as the insults to their dignity.[74] Rarely is one able
to fully understand everything in another person's life, especially
someone incapacitated. These issues indicate the importance of respecting autonomy as well as recognizing its limitations.

Beneficence

Beneficence vis-à-vis autonomy are conflicting and competing
values. Edmund Pellegrino and the late David Thomasma consider
beneficence the central moral principle of medical ethics. On the
other hand, Robert Veatch does not agree that physicians should presume to decide what is best for the individual. He stands staunchly in
favor of giving the patient the last word. The real conflict is not between beneficence and autonomy, but resides between autonomy and
paternalism. Paternalism is when the doctor imposes his prerogative
above the patient or her family's choices.

Some have proposed structured doctor–patient relationships. James
Childress defined objective, neutral perimeters using rules, guide
lines, procedures, and strictures. MacIntyre preferred a bargaining
process solidified with a doctor–patient contract. Thomasma and
Pelligrino disputed reducing ethics to contracts. Veatch lauded human values over holding to a set of technical rights and duties.[75] Patient–doctor integrity has, historically, placed the personal above
mandates and mechanics.

Some physicians doubted whether a women patient could make
competent medical choices. Arguably, imbalances in biochemistry,
anxiety, drug therapy, or general discomfort affect competent decisions
(in addition to socioeconomic factors). The physician knows body
chemistry and recognizes emotional anxiety affecting capacity, but
the doctor is also prone to long hours and operates at low levels of
energy. In fact, no one can make a fully informed decision. There is
more than physics to consider, such as economic, family, social, religious, and spiritual values. The basic rule has been for fit patients to
choose when the diagnosis and options are clear and well documented,

but not when little is known about a disease, its prognosis, and it has a marginal or dubious therapy.[76]

Physicians risk lawsuits from emotional parties, so it is wise to document case details. Paranoia has also driven doctors to eliminate potential lawsuits by advising treatments or abortions that remove "possible" birth defects, according to Israel Nisand. Institutional coldness and killing have not been openly discussed since the Nuremberg Doctor's Trials. Practically speaking, patient autonomy reduces a physician's legal liability.

Morality will be discovered not by recourse to formal laws, moral rules, or moral principles, but rather in the context of the physician–patient relationship itself.[77] Both doctor and patient are moral agents, and both are obligated to make informed decisions. The physician has more extensive education and experience, which yields a higher accountability, but the professional code requires the physician to respect the patient's wishes and commends moral integrity and compassion. Bernard Mayo insists that the doctor have a strong moral character, good discernment, and a mature value system. In Beauchamp's eyes, good character stems from an intuitive sense of right for the welfare of others—apart from thoughts about God. Other ethicists identify beneficence with Christ's character.[78] The beneficence-in-trust model reflects stability because it presumes good character, a mutually agreeable health plan, and tentative strategies for problems that may arise.

Nonmalfeasance

Based on Hippocrates' mandate "Do no harm" *(prima non-nocere),* nonmalfeasance directs the doctor to practice medicine so it benefits the patient.[79] Often, a choice has to be made from the lesser of two harmful alternatives—also known as the benefit-detriment or double-effect method. Questions include:

1. Will harm be incurred by the treatment (death to the fetus, danger to nonconsenting individual, imposed sterility, dysgenic male, etc.)?
2. Is harm a by-product of treatment?
3. Are the procedures considered extraordinary means?

Richard McCormick evaluates "extraordinary means of therapy" in light of the person's ability to engage in meaningful relationships with others and with God. When the lifesaving or sustaining measure usurps the patient's personality and the technology becomes the ultimate value, then the person's life has been distorted beyond its own context.[80] Double-effect is an absolute principle. It requires a minimum standard of care, and the doctor is asked to examine his/her own motives.[81] The lives of women and their infants touch many, and respecting their dignity is legally protected by the Sixth Amendment, U.S. Bill of Rights.[82]

Mesoethics of Rights and Justice

Definition: Mesoethics defines and gives context to justice and rights by studying the intent of its formulators, ensuing development and progress. It is practical for guiding administrative decisions in health care policy and law.[83] The foundations of Rights and Justice demonstrate the cosmic significance of moral selfhood.[84]

This analysis gives special attention to freedom of conscience, personal autonomy, and equality. There is an age-old tension between individual rights and social well-being. Freedom of conscience guarantees both individual liberty and protects public morality.[85]

The community good can compromise individual interests. Biomedical issues concern babies, women, children, those infirmed by racial or geographically related illness (sickle cell, Tay-sachs disease, etc.), the weak and unhealthy, the poor, and the elderly. Justice requires that these minorities be defended and protected against all forms of marginalization. The public conscience legislates human rights, and law enforces these dynamic ideals. They are all works-in-progress.

The Mesoethics of Human Rights

Definition: Right has been defined as the highest possible good. Absolute rights affirm the inviolability of life and presume liberty. For Libertarians and moral pluralists, the right precedes rules, keeping minimal government interference. Rawlsian theorists place rights before general or material goods. Ruth Benedict defines good as a habit one learns.[86]

Human rights developed through religious, historical, social, scientific, health, and security sources. Jean-Marc Chouraqui traced human dignity to the Jewish *Torah,* in which humanity was created in *Eloheim's* image and strove to emulate God's righteousness.[87] As the only species that was aware of God and self-conscious, human beings were ontologically equal.[88] Similarly, the conscience inspired and discerned right behavior without rigorous constraints.[89] *Torah* acted as a written conscience and described the rights that governed a divine covenantal bond.[90]

In *Introduction to Romans,* Robert Morgan exposed the intensity of a covenantal relationship. Paul, a Jew, experienced God directly when divine righteousness was poured *into* his human heart. In Paul's letters to Christian communities, he used *pistis Christou* (Gk., πιστις Χριστου), which implied faith was both descending and ascending. Descending from God, righteousness was deposited *into* the believer, so her right[eous] decisions were divinely mediated. She had the faith *of* God. The ascending position considered her to trust in God's word. She had faith *in* God. When Paul penned his letters, it seems that he intended faith "in *and* of" Christ. The Evangelists also put *pistis Christou* on the lips of Jesus. In Christianity, freedom of conscience was inextricably tied to the inviolability of the mind of Christ, which was worthy of protection.[91]

Derek Davis, James E. Wood, John Witte, Johann D. van der Vyver, and a host of other theologians, ethicists, and political scholars dedicated their lives to the centrality of conscience to religion, human rights, and the hope for universal harmony. Religion has been persecuted for "marching to its own drummer" and has, at times, been frothily intolerant. Well-learned lessons made liberty of conscience essential, and it is the foundation of all other human rights.[92]

Jean-Pierre Imbert, international expert on law and tolerance, remembered John Locke's sixteenth-century *Letters of Intolerance* and how scholars such as Jean-Jacque Rousseau and Charles de Montesquieu fought for freedom—limiting both government and church strictures. These were keynotes to eighteenth-century liberalism, with the American, French, and English Revolutions spelling out the bloody drama to freedom. The American and French Declarations transfused the stalwart struggle for individual and independent liberties into the *de facto* implementation of human rights.[93] These foreign wars accentuated the plights of war victims. Human rights activists crossed the frontiers to care for victims of violence and torture. Jean-Henry Dunant, a Swiss war journalist, published *Un souvenir de Solférino,* describing the disregard for life, making health and safety issues a governmental priority. The International Red Cross established precedents confirmed by the 1863-1864 Geneva conventions, the Hague (1906), the 1949 Geneva convention, and the 1969 Vienna convention (Article 60, paragraph 5).[94] Several human rights tributaries grew from pursuing freedom of conscience, with cooperation between governments, professional nongovernmental organizations (NGOs), and lobbying churches, which encouraged the moral dimensions of global civilization. Rights language formed a cosmic personality to alleviate suffering, be it antigenocidal campaigns, the rights of parents to direct the religious education of their children, or prohibitions to discrimination.[95] Respecting and protecting personal freedom was the first responsibility of the government.[96]

Respect for human dignity reflected the preciousness of human life and health, while honoring the primitive, Christological birthright. Overt religious tones had to be softened to cultivate a worldwide acceptance for protecting and providing for the weak as well as giving minorities a voice.[97] Creating written rights documents simply acknowledged that reasonableness and unreasonableness coexist. It was *déjà vu* of Spinoza's correction to natural law. The human rights campaign cut through the coldness of science and manifested the need for physicians to be sensitive to the patient's desires. To gain multinational acceptance, human rights legislation sought broad, loosely defined, nonaggressive, rational resolutions. These had facts and statistics to avoid competing claims and divisions of purpose.[98]

Authenticating human rights proved *just* for both the private and public sectors, which also had competing values—one judging by consequences, and the other valuing personal relationships, friendship, love, integrity, and fairness. In the eyes of Ronald Dworkin and T.M. Scanlon, neither civic welfare nor autonomy were to be sacrificed.[99] Guaranteeing rights was a step toward freedom *from* want and fear, as much as it was to guarantee welfare for the sustenance of life, providing access to food, medicine, shelter, and employment.[100] Rights to goods and services as well as proprietary development affirmed human dignity.

When people believed they were entitled to certain goods and services as rights, this inadvertently meant some professionals had to sacrifice personal income to public welfare. R. Sade and Robert Nozick staunchly disagreed, saying, F. D. Roosevelt perverted the "freedom to pursue something" to the "right" itself. The purpose of having limited government was to allow individuals private goals according to their ability, while protecting the public from harm. Libertarians believed the excessive conversion of private resources (i.e., taxation) for public distribution violated personal rights. This included purchasing hospital facilities, research funds, and educating medical personnel. Nozick and Sade argued in favor of a market-driven health care system, presuming people would conserve consumption if they had to pay for it personally. In addition, it protected physician's rights, intellectual property, and professional diagnostics.[101] The fact that society provided public money and universities to educate physicians may have been overlooked because of their privileged backgrounds and private schooling.

Mesoethics of Justice

Definition: Justice is fairness, credibility, self-government, and a universal truth.[102] Justice can only come from measuring like cases by like cases. A just society democratically decides the equitable distribution of benefits and remedies, including access to reproductive health care services. Justice, as mercy, forgives without retribution.[103]

Aristotle believed justice contained all the virtues. Over millenniums, civilizations have sought rules that are harmonious, consistent, and universal.[104] His *Nichomachean Ethics* advocated justice in law—with equity in trial, distribution, exchange, and correction, preferably in place of retribution. Ancient tribes entered into mutual covenants with their chieftains (an early form of constitution). The Roman Empire merged tribes, cultures, and religions—blurring prejudices.[105] But for brief periods, the expansive Persian and Roman Empires satisfied the differing cultures of Jews, Greeks, Arabs, and Egyptians by allowing a certain amount of autonomy in religion and self-rule—until Constantine made Christianity the dominant imperial religion.

Christian principles filtered through time in the Western English Chancery, which established Courts of Equity. The three main principles were: (1) the poor must be protected from the powerful; (2) agreements based on trust were enforceable; and (3) disputes were settled based on the merits of the case, not general laws. Judgments were enforced.[106] *Ad hoc* favoritism challenged true justice, so legal institutions were established to articulate and negotiate fair decisions. The philosophical movements of the seventeenth and eighteenth centuries emphasized individual rights, such as freedom of conscience, freedom of speech, freedom to own property, freedom of political participation, and freedom from arbitrary arrest and judgment. These are today's constitutional liberties and protections.

For the sake of democracy, Libertarians fought against radical autonomy. Competition for power and possessions frustrated the balance of limited resources.[107] John Rawls proposed society view the world in an original state of nature. His way presumed equality and played ignorant to social hierarchy. The individual's right to his/her fair share would not be sacrificed for the general good. Rawls's right preceded good.[108]

Robert Nozick and Michael Walzer could not fathom Rawls's self-imposed blindness because most resources were personally owned—whether material, knowledge, intellect, or a physician's skills. There are "haves" and "have nots."[109] Equitable distribution was only just if it were voluntary and not compulsory. Otherwise, free will was quashed, and, along with it, so was one's dignity.[110] Sade, Walzer, and Nozick's anarchistic laissez-faire social contract lacked public participation (no legislation).[111]

Gerald Dworkin described the need for social accountability to victims of accidents, catastrophes, sudden handicaps, and birth defects.[112] The moral response was to have a mechanism in place, such as public insurance, and not wait for a charity drive. Assessing how much a person contributed to his/her own misfortune identified persons who took advantage of the system and fraudulent claims (cf., contributory negligence).[113]

There was a Trilemma facing egalitarians, which Williams described as sovereignty, security, and sufficiency. *Sovereignty* affirmed the right of people to control the use of their property, providing they did not jeopardize the fair shares of others. *Security* provided just recourse in cases of unfair distribution. *Sufficiency* set a minimum standard of living for disadvantaged individuals.[114] Circumstances beyond a person's control can result in arbitrary suffering and missed opportunities, such as a child from an impoverished family being deprived of an adequate education to get a good job or becoming the victim of a bad medical decision.[115] Individuals have the right to choose, but circumstances, inadequate information, and mental capacity inhibit success. Poor professional advice worked to the peril of many as well as other causal laws in the universe. Religious or symbolic reasons were valid rationale. One had a right to factor these into his/her choice or rejection.[116]

Justice in medical agreements needs to consider individual liberties, freedom of conscience, autonomy, equity, right relationships, and motivation. Medical authority can be descending, ascending, or shared. Patients may fall under the jurisdiction of contracts handed down (descending) from a hospital or physician's management corporation; the doctor's charges may be dictated by the patient's insurance company (ascending); or, when possible, Veatch advises the physician and patient discuss and spell out potential decisions (shared consent). Bill May preferred the covenant form, because it was mutual and also recognized the doctor's superior position. Weighed in the balance, Veatch was too reductionist and May's code echoed egoism, but had no teeth. In Dan Clouser's opinion, recognizing the doctor's extensive education and experience was the most straightforward because the physician needed to do whatever was necessary, without deception, to save life, alleviate pain, and comfort distress.[117] A professional may have to weigh a patient's needs to determine the best use of limited economic and technical resources. Since medicine was institutionalized, the Trilemma affects the corporate realm, fiduciary relationships, and extemporaneous circumstances.

William Clinton's Commission for Biomedical Ethics used statistics to estimate equitable health care and to create a mechanism for organizing shared costs for the less fortunate—while determining a manageable budget and resources for social services.[118] The U.S. Presidential Commission depended on taxes to ensure fair health practices, not unlike Britain's national health insurance. The doctor's time and income were regulated, but government paid for legal counsel in malpractice cases, so costly malpractice insurance no longer burdened the doctor's budget. Patients incurred lower medical expenses, but carried higher endemic institutional risks, because physicians had less time to devote to patient care, review the prognoses, and evaluate pharmaceutical effectiveness. True justice in health care is also at a quandary because services and technology are still at the mercy of a market-driven economy. Health, in its business suit, has to watch its bottom line as well as the interests of its professionals. There are stockholders to satisfy, a high demand for pharmaceutical products, individuals motivated by wealth or status, prestigious university research grants, and political lobbies, often for orphan diseases. One wonders if the availability of health care resources can be just or even adequate.

In Kant's theory, "justice must never be accommodated to a political system, but always the political system to justice."[119] Public responsibility had a duty to social welfare and personal free will while maintaining a stable free-market economy. Justice suffers when governing authorities support prestigious research over common health care. Health services are downgraded. Government health services have to respond to mentally, physically, socially, and economically disabled human beings.

Moral principles, according to H.L.A. Hart, are rooted in positive morality, with internal checks and balances on the practices of the social institutions.[120] Society develops a sophisticated moral conscience by defining its norms, responsibilities, and establishing guidelines based on a complete and well-balanced collection of cases.

Womanist Ethics

Definition: Integrity, care, and fidelity are essential to ethical behavior. Persons are ontologically equal, relational beings who are entitled to liberty, justice, and peace.

Introduction

Thus far, the promenade of ethical valuations has visited: classical Greek virtues, Christian Ethics based on love, natural law's rational approach to God's moral will, Kant's moral metaphysic, Utilitarian ethics for the public good, principle-based ethics, and the Mesoethics of Rights and Justice. These moral and ethical constructs had unresolved tensions between Spirit and matter, religion and philosophy,

God's law and human reason, duty and free will, social goods and individual rights, paternalism and free choice, distributive justice and radical *laissez faire* policies, to name only a few. Across the generations, *men* wrote ethics and moral philosophy. They presumed the myth that men had a spiritual status greater than women. Often, authors believed women were not capable of self-determination and needed to be protected from supposed gender-related inabilities. Women scholars have since corrected some of the gender-biased conclusions.

Values differ considerably from a woman's point of view. A woman's natural inclination is to be conscientious about the welfare of her family members, neighbors, and her community.[121] She is a relational, social person, who freely exercises compassion. Studies about women support the finding that a woman's ethical value system is coherent, internally consistent, cohesive, and universal. What she does, she does with a passion. Womanist ethics are sufficiently grounded to stand next to the classical, traditional, and principle-based models, since it is sensible, realistic, sensitive, holistic, and, like Christianity, seeks to teach morality and transform others. Beyond her biological responses, a woman's natural character is gentle, creative, kind, compassionate, loving, as well as thorough, conscientious, mindful of other's feelings, and vigilant—like Christ.

The portrait of the Womanist Ethic is examined in light of: (1) values, goods, and affection; (2) psychology for holism; (3) duties and responsibilities; (4) reason, conscience, and rationale; (5) free will (choosing options); (6) politics; (7) metaphysics and universality.[122] Each group of qualities was associated with one of the previously discussed ethical theories. A woman's natural ethic tends to showcase all of them in one unique and sensitive style.

Values, Goods, and Affection

Integrity, truth telling, and fidelity are the core values for healthy, ethical personalities, because these create trusting relationships and build bridges for a more transparent society. Women desire an environment in which it is safe to express feelings and genuinely care for others—caring is the watermark that a woman uses to measure her own importance. A woman strives to please others by setting a virtuous example while respecting people for their unique qualities, being consciously aware of the whole person—physically (bodily), psychologically (mentally), and spiritually (Soul). Value is not simply an ability to treat someone. Since people are interdependent, showing fidelity and honor for one another sets the stage for a harmonious community. Unity-in-diversity harbors a resounding "yes" in this pluralistic world, but culture continues to educate people into specific gender roles.

Interestingly, natural drives and affections intimately connect human lives, regardless of gender.[123] A husband cleaves to his wife, in body and emotion, to create a baby. The womb is a sanctuary for mother–baby nurture and reciprocity of feelings, and, although they live in the same body, the mother and baby are distinct individuals. After birth, the two continue in a close relationship that extends to grandparents, relatives, neighbors, and social groups—each relationship having its own starting point and purpose.[124] In Mary Midgley's observations, children imitated behavior, language, facial expressions, and believed what others said to them. The opinions of others often became his/her self-image as "clumsy and dumb" or "graceful and beautiful."[125] Since people are truly affected by the impressions of others, then the best practices are to be respectful, loyal, to boost confidence, and to show affection.

Those who have been sculpted to live in charity, humility, and self-sacrificial love, according to Mary Daly, present behavior models conducive to a healthy life, a well-balanced family, and a successful community life.[126] Being considerate of others is a fruitful means to a desirable end. People should build up others, according to Eleanor Haney, not create guilt or blame (i.e., counter retribution).[127] In a woman's worldview, interdependent relationships are cyclical and contribute to one's own character and to the development of others. Awareness of the dynamics in a relationship signals the right response for each occasion and helps avoid harming others.[128]

Psychology for Holism

Maintaining a holistic worldview means appreciating both intelligence *and* emotive responses. Taking pleasure in the accomplishments of others displaces self-centeredness with compassion.[129] This is not self-exclusive, but self-responsible. Caring about someone else generates a self-perpetuated duty in which one finds pleasure and satisfaction. It opens the door to self-awareness and integrity as well as fidelity, mutual respect, and responsible autonomy.[130]

Self-knowledge develops through interconnectedness, experimenting with ideas and values, and making reasoned assessments.[131] Intelligence, sensitivity, and experience equip women's moral discernment—together these empower doing God's activity in the world.[132] The power of God is in many things—lightning in the sky, the spark of life in a newborn, and inclining one's best efforts to care for others.[133]

Duty and Responsibility

Providing nurture, care, and protection is a duty, especially since these enable others to develop as independent, autonomous individuals.[134] Carol Gilligan found that autonomy was differentiated during childhood, based on gender. Mother–daughter identity echoed in-continuum, the perpetuity of mothering from grandmother to daughter to granddaughter. On the other hand, boys were directed into relationships with other boys, away from mother's feminine traits. Having been separated from natural emotion, most men do not respond until midlife with the level of intimacy, relationship, and care that women possess naturally.[135] Men identify maturity with independence and tend to view women as immature because they have continuing relationships and express emotions when, in fact, the womanist ethic expresses moral maturity.

Reason, Conscience, and Rationale

With the rise of Western intellectualism and scientific method, men's scientific discussions were known for their reasonable, sterile tones, and mechanistic attitudes. The public image of a successful individual consisted of dispassionate, neutral confidence, which appeared devoid of care.

The medicalization of reproduction routed maternity and procreation into a culture of cool sterility, which is contrary to a woman's nature and offends her ethical standards by disregarding feelings.[136] Some physicians treat patients as if they had a plumber–plumbing relationship, like fixing machines or computers. This is counter to reason because the skills for doctoring come from sentience—creating the feelings in the hand to grasp the surgical instrument and the feelings to conscientiously guide it.[137] Medical and scientific cultures, not the women, need oversight—to protect justice, human rights, and liberty of conscience. Medical professionals, protocols, and legal documents should acknowledge women's bodily integrity. Self-determination is not something someone else has the right to bestow as a good among other goods. A woman's personal choice is a matter of conscience and an inviolable right.

Free Will (Choosing Options)

The Womanist Ethic uniquely places sensitivity, experience, and relationships side-by-side with intelligence and reason, insisting on volitional, autonomous self-determination. All human beings develop discernment gradually through trial, error, reward, and life's experiences. All decisions, freely made, authenticate morality. The ethics of the reproductive process depend on mutual consent as the individuals move through courtship, conjugal love, conception, gestation, birth, and nurture. The relationship of a man and a woman as well as mother and baby experience love, pain, joy, fear, and happiness.

Sometimes women are asked to be surrogate mothers for infertile family members or for money. A duty to volunteer reproductive services/organs may be presented under the guise of altruistic love—manipulating a woman's desire to help in a caring, responsible way. Surrogate parenthood challenges bodily integrity, authenticity in character, self-care, and fidelity to God's vision for the persons involved.

Janice Raymond strongly dissuaded women from submitting to the role of a breeding machine.[138] Paid reproductive services allow others to presume they can direct maternity behavior. Difficulties are encountered when nature and nurture do not want to give the infant away—or take the role of the baby's "auntie." The Old Testament established monogamy after Jacob had twelve children with four different women because too many parents confuse and harden relationships. In order to behave in a caring way, to truly *be* as caring *is,* there can be no coercion, intimidation, or compulsion.

Adoption is still a loving option for infertile parents who desire families. It gives place to children who have no parents. In revealing God's being, Jesus freely responded to each relationship with love and the appropriate type of care for children and women.

Politics

The ethics of the community are displayed in the law system of a well-hewed political body that is squared in liberty and integrity. Constitutional law and politics are the cradle for the protection of human rights, dignity, and conscience.

What happened in the case of constitutionality and biotechnology? Science became so advanced and complex that legislatures hired scientific experts to analyze situations and make recommendations. The problems with this were many. As professionals, scientists viewed biology for its mechanical function and manipulative potential. Medical scientists applied an objective, clinical approach to reproductive biology and womanhood. In some cases, women were treated as merely a reproductive resource, a conduit through which life passes.[139] That amounted to the instrumentalization of tender, sensible human beings and had strong commercial overtones.[140] Lawrence Kohlberg and Richard Kramer described women as "powerless and less responsible" because woman advocated nonviolence and avoided harm.[141] This presupposed some type of masculine decision-making superiority, but it placed aggressive behavior on a podium while defying reason and many other moral and legal principles. Such coldness made one reconsider whether the bar should not be raised on nonmalfeasance and changed back to "do no harm."[142]

Respecting human dignity resounds with a proclivity toward the natural sensitivity associated with the birth process. Gestational cycles from conception to the delivery of a baby nurture a deep appreciation for life. Physician–patient relationships are long-term relationships, especially when genetics are concerned, so the patient needs to trust her caregiver to organize, supply, and present all the relevant information in a fashion that is understandable and conducive to making a fully informed, volitional, and conscientious decision.[143] Scientists have no obligation to the voting public and are interested in academic freedom and personal success, whereas the political representatives were elected to preserve and protect freedom of conscience. In the U.S., "assault and battery" remains the only legal protection in cases of assisted reproduction. The delicacy of maternity has been left wide open to research.

Metaphysics and Universality

The description of humanity created in the image of God, *imago Dei,* highlights the suspense, depth, and complexity of human life and, as a result, "materialist-only" views lack sufficient dimension to make a well-rounded contribution. Christians understand God in a multidimensional formula—One God expressed in Three Persons. The Trinity is equal, nonhierarchical, and coexists in community. God is a plurality of expression. God, the Creator, shows God's perfect character in Jesus, the human being. The historical Jesus had a divine–human hypostasis—two natures.[144]

Many women theologians emphasize the earthly spatial, natural life of Jesus because it connects his social, historical, and cultural existence to the God's redeeming activity in the world.[145] Christian texts illustrate Jesus' redemptive work coming through his own body and blood. This offers an invitation for natural beings to partake of God's Eternal nature, so the Holy Spirit can transform the believer.[146] It was the sacramental shaping and integration of mind, body, and spirit for the purposes of Christ.[147] Being faithful to the Christian Promise affirms the believer, honors fidelity, and empowers the social order of the community.[148]

CONCLUDING REMARKS

The intrigues of human life have woven much into the ethical landscape, with each successive generation contributing to its dilemmas and solutions. Ethical scholarship is greatly indebted to the analytical work of Henry Sidgwick in developing a very thorough history of ethics. His writing examined the ancient and modern philosophical ideas behind the virtue ethics of his era while wrestling with Kant. Sidgwick, as a Utilitarian, was faithful to his culture's sense of practical responsibility, as well as to Christian values.

This chapter also has presented and integrated the formative ethical theories of several noted scholars, including medical ethicists such as Tom Beauchamp and Robert Veatch, to bring the perspectives into the twenty-first century. It bridged the ethical analysis of the specific disciplines with which molecular medicine and its patients were concerned.

Indeed, the issues introduced by modern reproductive technology and genetic medicine needed a pragmatic and physicalist perspective, but a person is more than *just* a body, which is the reason behind any and every ethical inquiry. Human beings bring new life into the world, and they suffer and laugh with one another until death. Each life has convictions and values, and acts as a symbol and teacher of moral intent for other people. It was not only reserved for heroes and saints. The present chapter shows that Christian ethics involve a high barometer of love, Womanist ethics promote care and nurture, and that virtue and principle-based ethics prudently expect right[eous] behavior.

The discussion is both subjective and objective—it cannot be devoted exclusively to one or the other. In many cases, it addresses women and children who could be our mother, brother/sister, or neighbors. They are people with a history, a past, present, and future. The entire family structure is involved in reproductive medicine, and with family comes the community in which it dwells. In fact, certain genetic aberrations affect whole races of people (i.e., Tay Sachs and sickle cell anemia), and that means *all* the neighbors. Decisions must be fair because every life is valuable.

Fortunately, civilization has formally recognized human dignity and respects autonomy. Despite religious precedents in common with human rights and justice, the relevant issues hold a double-edged sword. Research into Mesoethics delved into etymology that demonstrated an overall social responsibility for health care. Ethics can only be systemized to a certain extent since the issues are so complicated; there is rarely a quick answer. True equanimity will most likely be achieved when the parties courteously listen and take the time to assess the issues from a variety of ethical perspectives while valuing each life. This scholarship was purposed to provide a wide range of information.

The next chapter examines how ethics is played out in law and politics. A religious person is affected by canon law. Her address determines whether she is under civil law or common law. Some jurisdictions serve human rights, and others uphold constitutional provisions. Legal history explains to the Christian that Christian principles are embedded in the systems themselves; therefore, although the language is secular, the intent is fruitful.

Chapter 3

What Politics?
Which Legal System?

INTRODUCING THE SYSTEMS OF LAW

Innovative reproductive technology has sparked hope, intrigue, drama, and controversy. The previous chapters discussed Christology, theology, and the ethical theories most influential in guiding personal decisions about difficult pregnancies in this age of biotechnology. The personal decisions made by expectant parents also affect fellow members of their communities because medical assistance is expensive, and circumstances may require special services and education. Legal entitlements and obligations change according to the legal jurisdiction.

Religious law, codified law, common law, human rights law, and international law are the major legal systems that have something to say about health regulations. Each legal system has evolved over time and in its own geographical context. Precedents from common law do not necessarily cross into civil law or other systems. To have legal rights in any law system requires citizenship or legal personality. Going to another country for therapy probably does not protect the patient or the doctor in cases of medical injury or mistakes.

In this chapter, the development of law into systems shows a maturation process. Community rules began with mythology and intersected several cultures. The principles supporting liberty of conscience and human rights existed before the terminology. From a Christian perspective, the conscience tested faith and right[eous] action. Hence, the protection of rights, such as the right to worship and to practice one's faith, was essential for Ultimate issues. Of course, Christian ideals found their way into statutory law.

Counseling Pregnancy, Politics, and Biomedicine
© 2007 by The Haworth Press, Inc. All rights reserved.
doi:10.1300/5697_04

Every legal value system has elements of myth, religion, and ideology. Tribal chiefs, sages, kings, bishops, and community leaders who were also believers wrote the laws that evolved over time. As knowledge increases, so does the potential to do good and to do harm; therefore, values are continually being defined, updated, and incorporated into law. Knowing whole communities deliberated legal and moral dilemmas over decades, is consoling when one is faced with making tough decisions.

Many European countries operate under civil law, which describes the right or restriction *in advance*. The American and English common and customary law systems define norms *after the fact*. Court decisions are handed down, *stare decisis*. Nonetheless, civil codes and statutes can and do function in tandem within common law societies (i.e., traffic laws, etc.), so cooperation exists. The divide widens, however, when scientific issues are involved because science and law are strage bedfellows, much the same as are science and religion. Science thrives on research, whereas law is carefully defined and limited.

Reproductive technology introduced a whole new era of law review—by its content and the level of the expertise involved. Politicians had no option except to retain scientists who were trained to interpret medical technology. The representatives were ill equipped for such a daunting task, but voters empowered the legislators to make moral determinations, not scientists. Scientists are under no obligation to represent voters, and need freedom from laws in order to be creative. Leniency in self-regulation is the order of the day.

One example of impropriety arose when constituents requested cloning bans from their senator due to the sheep cloning (named "Dolly" for Dolly Parton since the cell was taken from a sheep's mammary gland). A well-intentioned California legislator invited a scientist to describe the biochemical and scientific method used in cloning, so that his proposal to ban human cloning could be scientifically accurate. The scientist's description was outmoded and deceptive. The average legislator simply cannot interpret highly sophisticated medical treatments. In short, he is easily duped.

Medical and scientific professionals have different ways than politicians for drawing the right conclusions. Political and juridical agents think in terms of law, psychology, or the philosophy of law. Physician–scientists use a physics-based, scientific, and moral rationale, based on palpable values. Descartes insisted that philosophy and tangible truths were exclusive of one another.

To complicate matters, rights, privacy, protection of intellectual property, and confidentiality prevent intrusion into scientific matters. If a scientist's copyright, patent, or intellectual property is threatened, he or she simply goes underground or even moves to another country. Hence, biotechnology and its discoverers are internationally mobile.

Fortunately, the 1948 UN Declaration of Human Rights set forth international goals in maintaining human respect, which now includes a person's gene set. The fact that there are international governing bodies working specifically on reproductive ethics sends the message to ruthless, individualistic enterprises, warning that unscrupulous practices will yield unpleasant consequences. Hence, the ethics of what one does to the human body is recognized by legislators.

Life and breath have been recognized as a sacred mystery since the dawn of time, and law has always been considered a *living* system. One very significant contribution made by religion was its insistence that every person had great potential because he or she was created in the image of God, *imago Dei*. In the early years, human rights advocates wrote several legal instruments, which presumed that humanity had an innate dignity, not to the detriment of other species, but to be stewards over them.[1] When it came to bioethics, policymaker–scientists preferred physical descriptions as a matter of utility, but this can marginalize people with severe heritable diseases as well as their parents and siblings.[2]

The section on religious law considers the relationship between human rights and Christian faith, partially due to the conscience factor. Faith in Christ, *pistis Christou* (Gk., πιστις Χπιστου), has a corrective or righting (Gk., δικ–) task. Being able to exercise faith (Gk., πιστις) is essential to having a clear conscience and living a full life. Therefore, people are entitled to certain *a priori* human rights. Turning back the pages of history, the reader will find Christianity played a major role in developing legal principles.

RELIGIOUS LAW: A "LIVING" STANDARD

Definition: Religious law systems consist of interpretations of sacred texts by special interpreting authorities and opinions about the transmission of faith.[3]

One way to review ancient religious law is to temper history with the wisdom factor. Nature and myth merged to establish the preeminence of the sage–leader, first as the family's grandfather and, as families grew, the leader was the one chosen as the tribal wise man or sage. The chief was vested with mystical authority. As civilizations grew, so did the corporate religious personality and his authority. The Elder's favor with the gods provided the defensible power of the group. Since warfare constantly brought conquered people into the tribe, codes of behavior had to be established.[4] For example, Codex Hammurabi codified the behavior for several Middle Eastern tribes.

Abraham, patriarch of three world religions, and his family dwelt in the Middle East and knew the customs and social expectations well.[5] Abraham lived a good life, and people followed his lifestyle because it was righteous (Gk. δικ−). Abraham's grandson fathered 12 tribes that grew into millions, all of whom were taught to emulate Abraham's lifestyle.

A few hundred years later, God sent Moses to these people, now called Hebrews or Jews, with the Ten Commandments. They were to follow those laws because God Himself saved them from Egyptian slavery, through the hand of Moses.[6] Moses was a sage with a genuine personification of the divine. He was ethnocentric rather than egocentric, and he taught others about God's unusual economy, using law, life, ritual, and celebration. The laws were showcased by stories about how people lived in response to God's Commands and provided narrative examples *(Torah)*—these were "living oracles."[7] The two tables of the law described attitudes and behavior. The first table recalled that God delivered the Israelites from slavery; therefore, God was the only true God and there were to be NO other gods or images—devotion was solely to God.[8] The second table protected human health and behavior. It asked the people to rest on the seventh day, in honor of God, and to honor parents and neighbors by not killing, stealing, defaming, or being envious—obedience was conducive to a harmonious society.[9] The Hebrew elders acted as courts for arbitrating disagreements.[10] The Law was Holy to God and was kept with great reverence despite foreign influences.

In addition to having sages, as lawgivers, religious law consisted of promises by and between God and His people. Yahweh promised Abraham a son of his own flesh, land, and a peaceful community. To

Moses' people, God promised a Law aimed toward communal solidarity as the Jews journeyed toward the Promised Land, filled with
milk and honey. Over time, Jewish authorities meticulously detailed
the meaning of the Ten Commandments and *Torah,* which led to 619
rules.

Jesus, a Jew born in the first-century to the tribe of Judah, simplified *Torah.* He formed a community and taught by example, much the
same as Abraham and Moses had done. Jesus' disciples emulated his
moral and holy lifestyle as best they could, as a matter of heart, which
differed from simply following rules. For example, Christ taught complete forgiveness of offenses, to pity the offender rather than judge
him. He showed compassion, rather than judgment toward the af-
flicted, ill, lame, and blind and cared for the lower members of the
social ladder (comforting the poor, widows, and the fatherless). He
encouraged those who had lost confidence in their own abilities
(rather than criticizing a weak spirit), and advised several other methods for improving living together—all intended to fulfill religious
law.[11] Indeed, Jesus simplified the ten [or 619] commands into two
commands: "love the Lord your God with all your heart, and with all
your soul, and with all your strength, and with all your mind" and
"love your neighbor as yourself."[12] His teachings promoted charity
and egalitarian treatment and were quite revolutionary for his day.
Dramatic social change was taking place as he condoned and, indeed,
encouraged clemency from Jewish religious rules and raised the dignity of the underclasses, such as women, children, and those who had
fallen into ill fortune (health wise or economically). Jesus' teachings
were well received. His students became apostles and ministers who
showed others how to follow the way of Christ via this exemplary,
narrative-style religious law.[13] The records of Jesus' teachings were
written by his Apostles and consolidated into the New Testament.[14]
Christianity spread easily, since the Roman Empire had well-developed trade routes and was tolerant of different religions because Roman citizens came from several lands and had many traditions.
Religious neutrality nurtured loyalty.

St. Paul, a Roman citizen, used the citizenship theme for the
church—albeit in a heavenly dominion held in place by an earthly anchor. Citizenship with Christ did not compete with Caesar's hierar-

chical world—and Paul taught nondiscrimination.[15] In fact, the Roman
world and Paul's religious aims were quite distinct from one another.

Robert Morgan discussed Paul's "rights" language in light of Roman customs in *Romans: New Testament Guide*. Paul used the Greek
dik- words morally and forensically (c.f., law courts).[16] Paul developed rights as entitlements—easily corresponding with the customary law approach to dignity and rights. Morgan examines Paul:

> Both aspects [religious and forensic] imply right relationships . . .
> "in it (the gospel) *righteousness* of God is being revealed from
> *faith* to *faith* [from God to humanity, from Jews to Christians,
> from community to community, etc.], as it is written the *righ-
> teous* one shall live from faith." What exactly Paul's phrase
> "righteousness of God" means has been debated since Augustine
> made it central for the Middle Ages, leading to its impact on the
> young Augustinian monk Martin Luther. They all used the word
> *iustitia,* justice, still preferred in some English translations,
> which suggests the stern philosophical meaning of giving ev-
> eryone their just deserts rather than the [correct] passionate reli-
> gious connotations it often has in the Greek Psalter and Isaiah.
> Luther found his understanding of Christianity revolutionized
> by taking the ambiguous "[faith] of [Christ]" as righteousness
> *from* God (c.f. Phil. 3:9), that is, a *gift from* God rather than a
> *quality of* God (his character). He had been taught that God was
> just and would therefore punish sinners, but he noticed that
> Paul's context implies a positive sense referring to salvation,
> and so interpreted the phrase in connection with faith, as the sal-
> vation God gives.
>
> But why does Paul use this judicial metaphor suggesting vindi-
> cation in a law court?
>
> We can see from his quotations that the origins of Paul's "right"
> language are biblical . . . What exactly this [righteousness and
> salvation] means for them is not explained, but like most of
> scripture it refers to human life *in this world* [emphasis added]
> and Second Isaiah is widely admitted to contain a key to Paul's
> use of the verb "to put right, vindicate or justify" [the main
> source is not considered to be the Psalter].[17]

Paul was trained in Jewish law and, originally, believed obedience to *Torah* justified the believer, but Paul struggled with that interpretation after his Damascus experience.[18] Paul, like Jesus, believed God did not intend a rule-intense culture.[19] Morgan reconciles *nomos* (Gk.,νομως) law with rights language and points to its necessity for morality and Ultimate issues—one must be able to live according to his faith *in* Christian principles (i.e., the same principles as Abraham, Moses, and Jesus). A believer's heartfelt love for God, *chesed,* drives his or her moral behavior—not unerring duty. In a Hellenistic culture, Paul easily exchanged the Greek *pistis* (faith) in place of the Hebrew *chesed* (God's steadfast love), thus, importing *chesed*-love into the meaning of faith. This is a far greater dimension than any modern English translation can convey about faith.[20] Paul linked *pistis*-faith with a volitional understanding of improving character, δικαιος—for the purpose of being made righteous by God. This way, obedience stems from desire, rather than from duty. It is a two-way flow; God's own faith (faith *of* Christ) was made manifest first in Jesus Christ and then through the Holy Spirit, *in* humanity (as *imago Dei*). Thereby, *pistis*-faith, together with the righting verb (Gk., δικ–) created an ethical response *because* it was volitional. When faith drives morality, one is entitled to it.

Logically—Jesus freely chose to respond to God by following Torah—*of* and *in chesed*-love (deep commitment). His faith was personal as well as a quality *of* God—it was the *imago Dei* that also was himself.[21] Jesus' own faith simultaneously revealed God *in* Jesus as (1) the goal of the faith and (2) the fulfillment of the law (Gk., πιστις Χριστου, the faith *of* and *in* Christ).[22] *Torah* provided the framework to embody Christ, but fulfillment was motivated by love and faith, not rules.[23] The crescendo of Jesus' ethic and glory was when the full incarnation of Christ ushered him through death to resurrection—fully subsumed in God's life. Jesus Christ made the Truth clear when he ennobled *imago Dei*.[24] Becoming fully human (as embodied *imago Dei*) was dependent upon having the right to practice faith.[25]

Morgan shows how the *right*ing (Gk., δικ-) language and the *good* (Gk., ευ-) words reckon righteousness as a property of *logos* (Gk., ελογισθη).[26] A person chooses, by faith, to live ethically and is made sufficiently righteous to be justified for God's ultimate Promise—ascending with Christ into the Kingdom of Heaven and conformed as *logos*. When choice and development of faith keenly tie ethics to Ul-timacy, it qualifies as an entitlement right.[27] In the wider sense, free-dom of conscience or faith becomes an essential component for a moral community.[28]

Freedom is the principle that honors personal responsibility, espe-cially that of a pregnant woman whose pregnancy has serious ques-tions about life and death. God brought the Jews out of Egyptian slavery into a free and lawful community. It was an archetypical sym-bol of the redemption available to *all* humankind. Every human be-ing, regardless of one's culture, gender, or social status, was entitled to live his life fully and completely and to change course at any point along the way (as many scriptural exemplars had proven). Several theologians and political philosophers agree with James Wood, Jr., that freedom of conscience was the seminal right of all human rights.

Conscience was essential to character formation, and Paul differ-entiated between law as a living faith (i.e., Jesus' character) and law as a system of religious ritual.[29] The law in its exemplary and narra-tive form inferred that doing what was right was in conformity to principles. Acting on principle was volitional, a matter of free will, and was conscience driven. Dignity was inherent to the concept, be-cause it demonstrated that God trusted the faithful to make decisions as much as the faithful trusted God to fulfill His Promise. Living the *nomos* (Gk., νομως) law, in principle, endowed one with the respon-sibility to act in legal agency (i.e., to do exactly as the Exemplar would do).[30] Modern constitutional concerns for freedom of con-science are embedded in these early religious precepts.

Religious rituals, when not used as pedagogical tools or devotional acts, can become mechanical and prescriptive (with minimal value to faith and *praxis*). When the faith community followed *Torah,* pre-scriptively, including the Pharisees, Sadducees, and Scribes, people did not think for themselves. This meant rule-bound law was *not* ef-fective in discerning right action or promoting faith, but merely con-formity to statute.

In the Protestant reformation, Luther's "justification-by-faith" doc-trine came out of his frustration—when he realized that it was humanly impossible to follow the myriad of rules that had been formulated by the church's interpretation of scripture (c.f., the Pharisee's legalism). Luther was swift to point out that Paul himself denounced the observance of circumcision and food laws for the Gentiles (i.e., *Torah*) and chose to focus on Abraham's righteousness "based on faith" (trust, as his response to God). Faith superseded ritual.[31] (Morgan noted the double entendre wherein Abraham, the receiver of the circumcision, was justified by faith, not ritual.) Luther cited Romans 4 and 5, which referred to Abraham's aging body because it provided the explicit evidence that Abraham was unable to generate progeny—apart from believing God promised him children of his own flesh. Luther refuted any suggestion that a right relationship with God could, somehow, be earned by religious legalism (he condemned James' epistle because he thought it gave this false impression). Nonetheless, Jesus taught followers to be doers of his teachings—those written in the Bible.

Abraham and Sarah, though they were old and she was infertile, propagated a biological son in a physiological sense (not symbolically). Paul's God was still a God in covenant with his chosen, rendering a concrete mutuality between God, i.e., YHWH, and His community.

Luther and Paul could both agree that Abraham's righteousness was based on his trust in God, not written codes, and here is where it seems Paul was making his distinction. A more probable examination of the text would show that the Pauline corpus and, especially Matthew's gospel, constantly referred back to the old patriarchal narratives in the law (which was authoritative for them) as evidence that Christ's life was fulfilling *Torah*'s prophetic path.[32] Christianity retained the Jewishness of Christ, as *Torah*, without its legalism, since it was through radical liberation that Jesus' activities brought about human freedom from the slavery of overzealous religious interpreters and guilt under the law.

In summary, the religious law that Paul wrote about embodied rights, principles, entitlements, egalitarianism, the freedom to respond (consent), free will, and freedom of conscience. Justice was also deeply embedded in the faith, which Paul referred to as mercy.[33] David Réne summarized the original law, *Torah*, as one to be remembered for conciliation and peace.[34] Jesus himself said that he came "not to destroy the law but to fulfill it," and he taught justice, mercy, and faith, as the ways of peace—and the new law.[35] Paul's religious law was a living law because faith transcended time—it communicated God's Promise to humankind across the ages.[36]

There were many divisions and power shifts before the Roman Empire embraced Christianity as its official religion (i.e., 313 CE), but in so doing, it had a healthy role in bridging Judeo–Christian morality into our current legal systems *via* the Justinian imperial reform. The synthesis of cultures naturally congealed religious norms into legal principles.[37] Constantine used the faith to unite his empire for the sake of peace and also because proclaiming the Kingdom of God on earth fit neatly into the Emperor's personal vision as an icon of God on earth.[38] The Emperor was consecrated into office as "bishop to the unbaptized" (similar to a prelate, τῶν εκτος). He embodied religion and law so when conflicts occurred, he convened a council to make decisions with him on religious issues. Hence, orthodox (right) conduct was organized, creedalized, and canonized into a legal structure.[39] From Constantine onward, Roman law consisted of a mixture of principles, rules, and concepts—gathered from a righteous lifestyle based on transcendent principles and suffused into imperial dominion. Geoffrey Sawer rightly observed that Roman law had developed a legal system comprised of autonomous, complex, human relationships experienced through the centuries.[40] Law seemed to be revealing itself as a transfinite conscience of humanity.

CODIFIED LAW ENUMERATES RIGHTS AND RESPONSIBILITIES

Definition: Codified law, derived from the historical–socio-religious–cultural values of the Roman empire, formed a code of rights and duties legislated by the highest authority, whereby all legal entitlements must be inferred by an expressed right or duty, or it does not constitute a legal right.[41]

The Justinian Code (534) made Roman law coterminous with Christian morality. Toward the end of the empire, these laws were officially expressed in the *Corpus Juris Civilis,* supplemented by the *Digest* or *Pandects* and exemplified the legal interpretation of the Byzantine church–state alliance (caesaropapism). The laws remained relatively few and dealt with the administration of justice; they were not mere rules.

Civil authorities still had to conform to divine law and custom. The law was above humanity, and, therefore, judges did not have creative power. Law was still seen as an oracle and a vehicle for justice. Réne considered the difference between the professional administration of law and Canon law as the business of the church.[42] Gratin synthesized Canon law in *Concordance of Discordant Canons* (1140 AD, *Decretum*). Réne saw the *Concordance* as an extension of law into church instruction and sacraments. Customary law and ordinances conformed to divine law or were emptied of authority.

As the empire grew, the Church and politics polarized into two bodies—forming the eastern and western segments of the empire—and the Church. The East continued with Justinian Code, but Charlemagne, who was consecrated in Carolingen Europe, designed his own meticulous legal system wherein, secular and sacred authority continued to coexist in a state of tension.[43] Law was inseparable from culture. The rules had to fluctuate to meet the changing character of law. Geoffrey Sawer noted that there was an increase in attention to fairness and equality.[44] Naturally, expanding cultural and geographical influences promoted equity and also brought it under scrutiny. Women were conducting business, despite their dubious social recognition (apart from marriage).

Sawer explained how such changes created legal personality and gave each person the right to appear in court. Where legal personality had once belonged to the father, it later extended to other family members (aka, *paterfamilias,* i.e., the first born, his wife, c.f., Gal. 3:28). Society was educated in egalitarian responsibilities by lay advisors, tutors, and curators who assessed age, mental condition, and one's ability to preserve the family estate. *Juris* consultants gave advice by general, abstract guidelines.[45] Broadening legal capacity reflected a greater awareness of the importance of nondiscrimination, elevating standards for human dignity one more notch.

In the eleventh and twelfth centuries, schools formed around legal scholarship, such as at Bologna. These blended culture, social morality, judicial insights, and Christian social ethics into a Greek philosophical context. About the same period, Thomas Aquinas studied Aristotelian concepts about nature, refocusing attention away from the Augustinian heavenliness back to an earthly reality. His introduction of Greek precepts explained religio-moral and legal standards in terms of natural law (i.e., *Summa Theologica*). Aquinas' writings contained a metaphysic that was highly anthropological, and decisions were based on reason. It was an understanding amicable and equitable to most cultures. The community, which embodied the law, was beginning to awaken to the idea that those in authority were also "subject to" public law.[46]

As the Middle Ages progressed, the humanists made a scientific study of the Justinian texts. Higher Law was segregated into a separate field because there was no way to verify theological hypotheses, but law itself consisted of many unmarked religious principles.[47] Humanists believed God gave human beings free will to act and change their own destiny using discernment, reason, and conscience, so men and women had the right to exercise their own judgment. Church leadership was offended. Nonetheless, imagination was given free reign in art, music, science, and law.

The new vision for society that came with the Holy Roman Empire was the scientification of codified law, politics, natural law, and better communications. University scholars wanted to professionalize law. The collection of written rules: (1) made law more intelligible to ordinary citizens, (2) protected against a professional domination by lawyers, (3) extended to many generations, and (4) categorized law by subjects. Classifications included private law, commercial law, criminal law, labor law, etc. These were then cross-indexed into theories, principles, and interpretations. Theories predicted the consequences from various actions. Principles governed ethical response. Public and private law were separated from one another, *Summa diviso,* so that private enterprise could maintain a fluid entrepreneurial nature.[48] Fourteenth-century post-glossators created a system to reference particular cases.

Natural law reorganized religion, identifying common features between God, humanity, and society, while creating symmetry and harmony—it made God's activity in the world more understandable. Greek virtue was mingled with Roman ideals, like simplicity and consistency. Harold Berman concluded that much of medieval canon law actually passed into state law.[49] As a result, the principles of the Western Catholic faith remained influential in civic practices.

The participation from ordinary citizens was minimal, but as communications and literacy improved, the public, however meager their skills, began participating in the political and legal decisions affecting their own lives. Tension between social classes, literacy rates, as well as persecutions of religious nonconformists brought about harsh realities that led toward a more republican government—after many lives had been sacrificed in the process. Unfortunately, church rule had not guaranteed virtuous government or a happy citizenry, and, as Bruce Thompson wrote, "the universal empire collided with the demoralization of the church, nationalism, humanism, the Renaissance, and the Reformation."[50]

COMMON LAW: THE LAW WHERE PEOPLE LIVE FROM DAY TO DAY

Definition: Common law or customary law develops when preferences and particular values (i.e., religious, economic, altruism, etc.) evolve over time. A democracy legislates acceptable and prohibited behavior. Breaches of law are brought to court and arbitrated. The decisions form profiles for normative case law.[51]

Codified law fared well in Italy, France, Spain, the Low Countries, Germany, and Scotland, but the rest of Western Europe and England headed down a different road. It was an odd mixture of customs and Roman law, which led to the common law system. Culture made a significant difference in behavior; therefore, during the twelfth and thirteenth centuries, "customs" were unwritten. Preserving customary laws was a matter of justice and identity. French legal scholars went so far as to say that, if customary laws were written, the custom could lose its unique identity.[52] There are several examples of customary law. In the thirteenth century, the German School mixed Romanized canon law with *sachenspiegel* (German customs). The English judiciary used their basic Roman law in cases of equity and ecclesiastical jurisprudence, but, in navigation, nautical, and admiralty cases, the decisions were made case by case.

Judges sometimes changed the custom by their interpretation of it.[53] The English Chancery (influenced by the Roman Catholic Church) did not focus on the allegation, but on the person's conscience—duty was the common law standard. The underclasses were, primarily, protected by equity courts influenced by England's affiliation with the church.[54]

Judges and lawyers tended to interact in English courts, whereas the other European courts functioned in an administrative (autocratic) manner—organizing cases into a portfolio. English politics and society preferred the customary method, which was uncoded and unwritten. Lord Chief Justice Mansfield (1705-1793), who was educated in Scottish Roman law, blurred German–Roman law and common law.[55] Blackstone's *Commentaries* (1765-1769) accentuated the principles behind his legal reasoning. It was not until individual lawyers in England took the initiative that a yearbook of cases was created (circa 1800). Being historically based, case law avoided discrimination and circumvented abstract logic. Lord Chancellor Halsbury succinctly stated: "A case is only an authority for what it actually decides. I entirely deny that it can be quoted for a proposition that may follow logistically from it."[56] Casebooks extracted principles that were common to several cases. But it was the popular will, through Parliament, that determined general principles.[57] There was widespread use of jury trials to prevent too much government control. The English wished to avoid issues on its indifference to class struggle, which they observed on the continent—they also wanted to protect England from foreign influences.[58]

In the seventeenth century, Sir Edward Coke influenced English law, as did the Anglican *Book of Common Prayer* and Calvin's *Institutes*. John Locke and Isaac Newton promoted human interests. Systemized studies of criminal and civil law, by Matthew Hale, incorporated piety, order, discipline, and moral responsibility into the law.[59] Law remained grounded in rational decisions, but the philosophy of the age was also the recipe for civil rights.

Continental philosophers supported the decision-making capacities of the people, since they had the power of reason and the promises of science. Montesquieu contributed *The Spirit of Laws* (1748), Diderot wrote *Encyclopedia,* and Jean-Jacques Rousseau delineated civil responsibility in *Social Contract* and *Confessions.*[60] Such philosophies refuted religious claims of moral paternalism and challenged aristocratic traditions, such as primogeniture. In order for the public to exercise their natural abilities, there had to be a forceful confrontation with the aristocracy.[61]

Revolt erupted against the churches and the monarchies. Three major revolutions were rooted in antiecclesiastical and antiaristocratic sentiments—England's Glorious Revolution of 1688, the American Revolution of 1776, and the French Revolution of 1789. The people wanted to be treated with respect and fought for civil rights. Berman referred to this as an "ancient common law constitution." John Locke's *Treatises of Government* advocated mutual restrictions for the ruler as well as the citizenry. Protection of individual property, contract rights, jury trials, and defenses against cruel and unusual punishment were the first fruits of constitutional rights. Government was aware that the public was watching.[62]

Natural law presumed natural justice, and the written constitution supported this. English jurists Coke and Blackstone buttressed common law with the saying "reasonable conduct for reasonable man." Eighteenth-century natural law, based on reason, merged into natural rights. When reasonableness informed natural rights, the people deduced that revolution was rational, even religiously justified.[63] The Americans enumerated these natural rights in the *Bill of Rights,* and the French echoed the transaction in the *Rights of Man.*

MODES OF LEGAL INTERPRETATION AND CONVERGING SYSTEMS

American judicial practices grew up differently from their European ancestry. The courts looked for judicial precedents, *stare decisis,* but professionals continued to draw general principles from codified law, as professional literature. American judges had more authority and power than European jurists did. Legal autonomy was fashioned by each provincial government—with an eye on local justice.[64]

Discovering the new continent, revolutionary takeovers, and new governments contributed to different legal approaches. Many believed the changes ate away at public morality. As Alaisdair MacIntyre reflected on today's morality, he was disquieted by the damaged state in which sociopolitical and economic structures found themselves.[65] Yet, this restructuring engendered striking and very positive personal freedoms. When people were trusted, they acted responsibly and made choices driven by good conscience, rather than by threats and intimidation. For example, the separation of governmental powers (executive, judicial, and legislative) and public participation increased the opportunity for fair legal decisions. Egalitarianism formed a collective economy and confronted hierarchical society, and dissenters challenged insincerity in the traditional church. Americans and others worldwide wanted to make personal choices.

Legal and political philosophers believed governmental neutrality to religion protected personal freedom and faith. Writings of Jean-Jacques Rousseau and his colleagues placed morality squarely in the heart of the person.[66] Being objective was becoming the tenor of the courtroom, as well. Jurists thought legal decisions should be limited to the facts and moral determination left to individual conscience.[67]

Nonetheless, the law had evolved from principles, values, and policies that had religious origins.[68] Scholars were divided as to whether moral neutrality was even possible in the judicial setting (or anywhere else).[69] Legal philosophers watched as positivism divided into "substantive rules" and "analytical concepts"—pragmatic to the core. Legal evidence grew in popularity, and legal scholars, such as Savigny and the German historical school of law, continued to consult Roman law, treatises, and ancient texts. Empiricism incorporated history into the organic community the way early Rome focused on the *ius commune*. The idea was to integrate communal values, law, and national consciousness—to protect the law from a frigid positivism. Berman credited German Historical Positivism with the prevention of capital punishment and genetic engineering, following the atrocities of World War II. In fact, empirical and positivist attitudes were just inches away from desensitizing human values. As the legal system matured, its framework became more technical than symbolic.[70] Acting upon the literal words of the law meant more than the situation it tested.

John Austin's school (1790-1859) rested on "necessity" as the measure for legal rational hence, the term "imperative." Procedural and substantive law standards were utilitarian, judging according to available remedies. Oliver Wendell Holmes made law out as the bad man who cares only about material consequences, not as a good guy who desired to explain the decision rationally and in good conscience.[71] Valid law, for H.L.A. Hart, expressed acceptable social norms. He believed that even with its mechanical tendencies, the law had not forsworn its living character. There will always be factors beyond human control, capable of interfering with the projected outcome and influencing the legal structure.

Berman saw the overall picture thusly: positivists relegated authority to the lawmaker, historicists based it on national character, and naturalists stood by reason and conscience. In an attempt to be just, morally neutral, and autonomous, jurists tried empirical, positive, and imperative interpretations. Sawer was looking for the methodology that helped the public internalize the law—that is to live rightly and naturally.[72] Civil codes, judicial persuasion, and legal systems were converging. Legal precedents and statutory specialization helped codify several solutions.

In these times, the legislature and judiciary are being asked to function in an evidence-based society—one that is about high technology and human health. The major exception to legal rules remains in the area of innovation. Scientists and other artists do not trust restrictive reasoning—they operate best when structure is minimal.[73] The experimental nature of medicine and the framework of law are worlds apart. Public health is both legal and medical—who bows to whom?

RECONSTRUCTING LAW TO FIT BIOMEDICINE

Roger Dworkin declared existing laws pregenetic and advocated reshaping law so as to include biomedical technology—construing genetics narrowly and cautiously. Law normally addresses and resolves public policy disputes, but people in many fields have opinions about the right approach to modern reproductive technology. Dworkin's observations constitute an organized assessment of some of the intersecting areas from law, politics, ethics, science, and medicine in Exhibit 3.1.[74]

Clearly, legal writers need to be familiar with differing subject matter and methodologies if they are going to communicate just and effective standards in reproductive technologies. There are different schools of law and different ways of practicing medicine.

- Take law for example; students of law in Europe receive an education in civil, prescriptive law. English and American professionals are educated with experiential, common law case studies.
- Biomedicine needs formal instruction, practical clinical studies, and philosophical hypotheses in order to be effective, especially since genetic science is still very young and has already developed alternate philosophies of practice.

EXHIBIT 3.1. Legal intersections.

Topic	Dworkin: Relationship of Law and Professional Interests
Law and politics	Law and politics work together. Politics directs the standard of health care, protecting society from perceived harms, while law preserves and enforces the status quo.
Law and legal processes	Law operates through legal processes. Once legislated, law is subject to administration and adjudication, including civil, criminal, and constitutional courts.
Law and ethics	Ethics weighs variables to determine the good, the right, or the duty, but law is not the ethic. According to Dworkin, law embodies ethics by serving the norm.
Law and science	The contrast grows in scale with science since it explores, observes, experiments, and postulates truths about physiology and the human anatomy, whereas law works from existing structures and is instructed before it is instructive.
Law and medicine	Human beings are the subjects and objects of both law and medicine, but biomedicine has few relevant rules. Both law and medicine use methods of observation, value judgments, prediction, and intervention, but medical techniques are frequently experimental and physically invasive. Law is not science, especially when it comes to legal implementation, because it uses threats, promises, and rewards. Medicine exists for human health. Every person is to be fully informed about his or her health situation and make decisions voluntarily-without sales inducements. Humanity is not to be used as an economic end.
Law and the Christian religion	Dworkin does not venture a discussion here.

In trying to stay in touch with human life situations, courts are aware that case histories are only just beginning to accumulate on conflicts stemming from new medical technologies. The lack of case studies is largely due to medicine's unwillingness to submit to legal venues that appear ignorant of medical practices. Interdisciplinary participation is inevitable if law and medicine are to build mutual respect.

Medicine also has areas it considers inappropriate for public inquiry, although governments have not always viewed it thus. Between physicians and patients, there are issues of confidentiality, as well as highly personalized matters, such as reproductive decisions. The abortion cases in the United States served to emancipate reproductive decisions from governmental guardianship, even though *physicians* exercised dominion over therapeutic abortion, regardless of the law. Legal suits dealing with wrongful birth, wrongful life, and experimentation are representative of biomedical decisions that the courts have been asked to make.

Experimentation

Casey v. Planned Parenthood (Penn., 1989) banned all nontherapeutical experiments on an unborn child (definition: individual human organism from time of conception), but, according to *Rust v. Sullivan* (500 US 173, 1991), *in utero* research was appropriate when it benefited the fetus with a minimum risk (45 C.F.R. Sec. 46.208.a and 46.209.a. 1 & 2, 1993).

The Current Rule

Research is legal so long as vital functions are not artificially maintained. Research may be conducted in order to obtain important biomedical information that is unobtainable in any other way as long as the experiment does not terminate the fetus' heartbeat or respiration.[75]

Wrongful Birth

Parents received compensation from doctors who failed to disclose dangers to the baby's health. The physicians were charged with negligent conduct (genetic practice would otherwise be immune against its own negligence) despite claims based on superior professional competence or allegiance to the Hippocratic Oath, whereby the disclosure of information could prompt a decision to harm the baby by interrupting the pregnancy.

Awards for emotional damage: *Viccarov v. Milunsky,* 551 NE 2d8 (Mass. 1990). *Schroeden v. Perkel* 432 A. 2d 834 (NJ 1981); *Becker v.*

Schwartz 386 NE 2d 807 (NY 1978); *Speck v. Feingold* 408 A 2d 496 (Pa Super 1979); and *Berman v. Allen* 404 A 2d 8 (NJ 1979).

No emotional damages: *Smith v. Cole* 513 A 2d 341 (NH '86) and *Howard v. Lecher* 366 NE 2d 64 (NY 1977).[76]

Wrongful Life

Until 1992, life was always considered good. The case was based on the precedent established after *Quinlan* 355 A 2d 647 (NJ 1976): persons have the right to die if continuing life is a burden, not a benefit.

Gleitman v. Cosgrove 227 A F. Supp 692 (E.D.PA 1967): Damages cannot be measured. Damages are intended to restore one to the same position as before the negligent act.

Turnpin v. Sortini 643 P 2d 954 (Cal 1982); *Procanik v. Cillo* 478 A 2d 755 (NJ '84); *Harbeson v. Parke-Davis, Inc.* 656 P 2d 483 (Wash '83). Parents realize the child will suffer but also recognize the challenges associated in raising a child with a tragic disease. Many diseases are incompatible with long life; therefore, the award passes to the baby's estate (i.e., parents).[77]

Justice is the goal of law and presumes equality. Dickens offered a basic rule for justice—treat similar cases alike. The case precedent remains the constant between cases that are alike and those differing. Differences must be acknowledged, otherwise injustice results from disproportionate values.[78] Since the subjects of biogenetics are human beings and not property, justice is not subject to dilution.

Evidence-only based decisions often lack the sensitivity that is required for cases involving babies, genetics, and disabilities. Justice can only be served by placing the situation into a holistic framework. *In vitro* fertilization and multiple ova cases indicate that it is difficult, if not impossible, for judges to appreciate the intrinsic and, indeed, unique value of a fertilized embryo when it is solely based on empirical evidence. Legal counselors admit that embryos need to be loved, and the source of love is the parents.

Embryo and Experiments

Davis v. Davis, 113 S. Ct. 1259 (1993): Divorced couple argued for control of frozen embryos. She wanted to give spare embryos away. He did not want to be the father, and the court chose to respect this. She was not permitted to give the embryos away.

Del Zio v. Columbia Pres. Med. Center, No. 74-3558 (1978): Damages awarded for destroyed embryos.

York v. Jones, 717 F. Supp. 421 (E.D.Va. 1989): Required a clinic to deliver genetically related embryo to couple.[79]

In addition, jurisprudence is troubled by complicated medical–science terminology and lack of experience. Judges with limited exposure to medical education can easily misapply case precedents. The continually changing technology makes it difficult to decide if cases are similar or dissimilar. Jasonoff's "science at the bar" concluded that judges without expertise in genetics ought not to rule in medical-science-related cases.[80] The *Chakrabarty* case is a first-class example of how a biomedical legal ruling took on a life of its own.

Patenting Life Forms

In *Diamond v. Chakrabarty,* 447 US 303 (1980), the US Supreme Court approved genetically engineered life forms when a General Electric scientist developed bacterium that would break down crude oil spills (cell fusion, not rDNA). The Patent Office Board of Appeals denied the patent, but the Court of Customs & Patent Appeals reversed the decision. The Supreme Court defined biologically manip ulated inventions as patentable, based on 35 USC, Sec. 1011, drafted by Thomas Jefferson. It only took four judges (the minimum necessary) to grant congressional authority for patenting *new life forms.* Chief Justice Burger applied the "hands-off" approach in his rationale, deciding in favor of scientists (keep your hands off them); Brennen sought restraint, thinking patent laws would influence scientific enquiry.[81]

The U.S. Patent and Trademark Office (PTO) transferred, in principle, the patent from bacteria engineered to cleanup an oil spill to a mammalian gene (the Harvard mouse with its cancer gene insert). That precedent was later applied to a human organ.

The University of California treated John Moore for leukemia, removed his spleen, and licensed its pharmaceutical properties. Moore sued for propriety rights to his own tissue, but the court refused.[82] Once an invention is patented, only the patent owner has access. This discourages others from pursuing further research and development.[83]

There are significant legal inconsistencies stemming from the genetic engineering cases that blurred legal boundaries between the species of bacteria, mice, embryos, and human organs. It does not appear that the courts or legislatures are fully prepared, academically or experientially, to maintain justice or protect individual rights and freedoms.

National and international laws about reproduction become even more complicated than patent laws. When an English woman, Mrs. Blood, wanted to take her (deceased) husband's sperm to Belgium (where insemination was legal), the British government interpreted this as circumventing British law—her case became a challenge to British legal sovereignty over its citizens. The Crown would not license the transfer of embryos to Belgium, where the procedure was legal. In the *Dianne Blood* case, the British Human Fertilization and Embryology Authority (HFEA) bound an English citizen to English law.[84] This was inconsistent with the European Union's act allowing freedom of movement and employment, whereby a physician may practice medicine in Belgium or England, but the British patient could only receive therapy in her country of citizenship (except if injured while traveling). It was ironic.

In both the *Moore* case and the *Blood* case, individual rights were sacrificed. The arbitrators favored the University doctors in the *Moore* case and the British government in the *Blood* case. Juridical inexperience and sovereignty issues contributed to the confusion of purposes and goals; however, if the pattern continues, then systems, such as pharmaceutical ventures, will override constitutional principles. Human rights have the opportunity to influence the overall legal effort to guarantee new protections for the dignity of each person.

THE INTERNATIONAL LEGAL ARCHITECTURE
FOR BIOMEDICINE

Thesis: International rights and entitlements provide a vessel for uniform, transgeographical protections and justice.

Former civilizations operated with greater solidarity and less individualism than present societies. "Customary law" actually grew out of community life, and it had the ability to point beyond itself. "Constitutional law" also emerged from community life as a national, secular vehicle that addressed equity and justice in a universalized form while extending its application to the personal rights and protections of citizens—the nationalized version of a universal family. National constituents became members of a broader world community and desired to protect their interests in foreign domains. Roman law provided the common grounds for a discussion about international law.

Review of Legal Development

A simple review of the development of Roman law reveals that Rome contained a wide cross section of moral and religious values since it dominated several cultures. Roman law respected the customs of others. Historically, Roman law grew out of daily life. It provided a practical collection of living, general laws that set forth principles conducive to a harmonious and just society. Robert Morgan provided a good picture of how Roman law and religious law fortified "rights." For the Apostle Paul, living rightly and Law meant the same thing—his right descended from God. Roman citizens had rights as a matter of law and were entitled to live life according to the values of their forefathers—rights were legal entitlements. Romano–Germanic judges were ordinary lay citizens called by nonlawyer magistrates. Judgments required no rationale, nor were the hearings preserved. Popular politics loosely followed the Aristotelian concept that justice proceeds from virtuous people.[85] People followed the exemplary lifestyles of their leaders from the days of Plato and Aristotle to Abraham and Moses, with Jesus and the Apostles buttressing values in Christendom and the West. The wisdom of these men and others pointed past humanity to the Giver of Wisdom and to a Higher Source of knowledge—the Giver the Law. Modern codified law stems from the Justinian Empire, where it had been interpolated with Christian principles.[86] Dickens explained codified law as "behavior granted by express right or duty." Codified law guided behavior, but it did not prescribe it.

Demythologizing Legal Terminology

The law had both an evolutionary and a revolutionary character, which wrestled it away from religious control.[87] After the English, American, and French revolutions, Higher Law consisted of principles of justice framed by constitutional democratic systems. Principles were not subject to changing political values as witnessed by the American *Bill of Rights* (1789) and the French *Rights of Man* (1789)— citizens were endowed with inalienable rights of freedom, property, security, and a right to resist oppression. Réne coined principles, legal tender, rather than moral currency. Principles were expressed in solemn documents, which made them observable, and, therefore, scientific.[88]

Hegel perceived rights as principles connected to freedom (free will). Hegel's philosophy was about the "science of rights," but perhaps it would have been more appropriately entitled a "science of freedoms." Hegel believed people examined their choices intellectually and then they selected the option with the highest satisfaction. Theoretically, the decision was pure and objective because all the avenues had been thoroughly reviewed. Will was self-determined, in touch with its concept and was genuinely a choice—with freedom as its absolute goal. Responsibility was endemic to free choice. The duty to do what was right, while seeking the welfare of others and oneself, had a universal application. The duty itself came from a higher sphere, internal to the human mind.[89] Good conscience was essential to freedom.

Interpreting human rights and freedoms was an observable science that had a very broad reception. Gradually, the world formed a single interdependent market, uniting science, technology, medicine, sports, and tourism (respecting disciplinary boundaries, but losing national and geographical frontiers).[90] If the goals of law were to provide security for international relations, ensure justice, and protect human dignity from infringement and prejudice, the law had to take on a transnational consciousness—which is exactly what it began to do in 1948.[91]

"All human beings are born free and equal in dignity and rights. They are endowed with reason and conscience and should act towards one another in a spirit of brotherhood" (Art. 1, United Nations Declaration of Human Rights, 1948). Herein, reason, based in natural law, passed through to natural rights, but the political world was careful to distance itself from religious intonations.[92] All references to inspired or transcendent properties were termed as conscience and human consciousness, which were little understood, but undeniably important to being human. Roger Dworkin understood and explained this uniqueness in scientific secular terms. He said human life is inviolable because of "the processes invested in human creation." This thought, though of secular utterance, did not lose the sense of wonder that a religious person would express.[93] Wherever human dignity was exemplified in rights language, there also existed a respect that transcended national, ethnic, and religious ideologies. The winds of time blended similar streams of thought with new terminology. Much of the discussion focused on areas where religious principles merged into secular reasoning, even though the original ideology was preserved.

Freedom of conscience contains both religious and political concepts, which does not hide the differing rationale. For example, secular decisions are frequently "self-regarding," while the church will explain the same goal as "God-given." The scientists look to objectivity, but philosophers recognize that there is truth in experience and emotion. Consequences may be sweet or bitter.[94] Governments tend to control people by giving ultimatums (fear-based). This does not work in international law because enforcement mechanisms reside in persuasion.

The road forward needs to be paved in mutual cooperation, respecting the rights of all people to maximize their life—even Ultimate issues. Human life is indeed inviolable—with a mind, a neuromuscular system (body), emotions, experience, and genetic traits that extend for generations. Suffice it to say that law in the area of biomedicine has entered the threshold of deeply invasive considerations—both of mind and body. This is especially true when dealing with reproduction, genetic heritage, and future generations. Respect for human life has to be maintained because there are also those who wish to commercialize human properties—this commodification of human bodies introduces a plethora of dangerous ethical dilemmas.

TODAY'S INTERNATIONAL LEGAL BASKET FOR BIOETHICS: A WHOLE NEW FIELD

Throughout these pages, jurisprudence has worn different coats, but they all belong to the same body. The progression of legal history was dominated by stages of law, which formed from within the human narrative—as society acknowledged that humanity was one and the same race, rightfully entitled to respect.[95] At the same time, law was necessary and capable of balancing the wealth and challenge of human diversity. Communities do change, and law had to live and breathe. In the international forum, as in a multicultural community, the leaders agreed to promulgate human rights. Legal rights and elasticity acknowledge the constantly changing information system of a mobile society. They are particularly germane to the highly technical and controversial area of bioethics, especially in the field of reproductive medicine and genetic diagnosis.

Human Rights law is the best anchor for biomedical regulations when it comes down to the basic philosophy of government and its duty to provide, at least, minimal protections for citizens and for those who have no voice. Similarly, reproductive technologies affect women, children, unborn fetuses, disabled, and those with serious heritable diseases. (The church has always claimed a duty to protect the weak and vulnerable.)

When genetic diagnosis developed, the international community cautiously evaluated how human rights could be applied in the new genetic sciences. Every discipline and profession sent representatives to conferences and legislative sessions to inform international lawmakers. At first, documents were written in broad terms and, later, as technology intensified, instructions for molecular medical issues were detailed in international conventions, declarations, and treaties. In formulating the contents of the Universal Declaration on the Human Genome and Human Rights, UNESCO took into account over 100 international instruments affirming principles dedicated to the dignity, equality, and mutual respect of humankind.[96] Principles reflected:

(A) Human Dignity and the Human Genome (Art. 1-4)—Unity of human family; imperatives not to reduce individuals to their genetic characteristics; respect for genetic mutations as natural process of differentiation; the genome, in its natural state, is not to be used for economic inducement.

(B) Rights of the Person Concerned (Art. 5-9)—Research, diagnosis, and treatment must be based on rigorous assessment of risks and benefits; all cases require free, informed consent of the person or his agent; right not to know test results; research protocols need approval prior to implementation; discrimination based on genetic characteristics is prohibited; confidentiality to be respected; just reparation in the event of injury or damage to a person's genome.

(C) Research on the Human Genome (Art. 10-12)—No research takes precedence over human rights; human cloning prohibition (as contrary to dignity); universal availability of benefits and advances of genomic medicine; freedom of research for progress of knowledge is recognized as *freedom of thought*; and, research directed toward relief of suffering and health improvement for humankind.

(D) Conditions for the Exercise of Scientific Activity (Art. 13-16)—Scientific policy makers are responsible for intellectual honesty, integrity, caution, and utilization of their findings; states to protect free exercise of research (as long as used for peaceful purposes); states promote multidisciplinary and pluralistic ethics committees.

(E) Solidarity and International Cooperation (Art. 17-19)—State to guard population and family groups susceptible to genetic disabilities, fostering, *inter alia*, research to identify, prevent, and treat genetically based and influenced diseases, as well as rare and endemic diseases; states to work toward fostering scientific and cultural information exchange and cooperation, particularly between industrialized and developing countries; nations to encourage greater capacities of developing nations to realize benefits of biology, genetic medicine, and scientific knowledge.

(F) Promotion of the Principles Set Out in the Declaration (Art. 20-21)—States to promote education and training of bioethics in interdisciplinary fields; effective dissemination to raise level of social awareness of research in biology, genetics, medicine, and applications.

(G) Implementation of the Declaration (Art. 22-25)—States to promulgate this declaration and its understanding, organize appropriate consultations, and raise discussions about any evolution of questionable technologies and vulnerable groups; make recommendations in accordance with UNESCO's statutory procedures; *all interpretations must be consistent with human rights and fundamental freedoms.*[97]

The United Nations has a seasoned and respectable history, and the United Nations Educational, Scientific and Cultural Organization (UNESCO) houses a large assembly of experts from recognized universities worldwide. The UNESCO International Bioethics Committee (IBC) is the appropriate authority and structure for discussions pertaining to international bioethical legislation. It does, however, host a myriad of complicated socioeconomic imbalances among its members, which also must be dealt with in a just manner because discrimination, especially for health matters, is endemic to poverty. Each country is interested in promoting a healthy population. Genetic diagnosis and its technology can change the mortality rate—if it is affordable and accessible.

Jean Michaud, a former spokesman for the Bioethics Commission at Council of Europe (COE) and prominent UNESCO IBC consultant, believes the human genome holds great promise and would like to see equitable access to genetic technology as well as increased health literacy (c.f., competency for consent). The Council of Europe's research was the most aggressive in terms of biogenetic legislation, and the European Convention on Biomedicine provided a brilliant example of laws in terms of competency, counseling, and disclosure (i.e., the right not to know about untreatable diseases).[98] Amassing the funds to bring equitable distribution of genetic services to the public worldwide required cooperation from private industry. Governments worked with nongovernmental agencies to develop access and education, but these require huge amounts of capital.

The advent of genomics made biopolitics very challenging, according to Bertha Knoppers (HUGO) and Andrea Bonniksen. Bonniksen's research explained the inverse relationship that now exists between public and private interests. Private and public legal priorities shifted once the alchemy market cashed in on genomics. See Exhibit 3.2.

This juxtaposition makes a dramatic statement about the crossroads at which government and private interests meet. Money speaks loudly. Pharmaceutical representation was prominent at UNESCO IBC meetings. NGOs for the disabled, pediatricians, obstetricians, gynecologists, psychiatrists, and a multitude of humanitarian groups participated as well. Governmental representatives are concerned about national health care issues, protecting their populations from exploitation, and developing their economies to compete for greater

EXHIBIT 3.2. Private and public priorities.

Private Priorities

1. Research
2. Clinical
3. Professional Guidelines
4. Report/Research
5. Legislation
6. International Regulation

Public Priorities (Reverses Private Priorities)

1. International Principles and Laws
2. Legislation
3. Report/Research
4. Professional Guidelines
5. Clinical (Research Guidelines)
6. Research

Sources: Barbara Marie Knoppers, "The Internationalization of Norms in Genetic Medicine." Lecture at the International Conference on Genetic Diagnosis, Rennes, France, 1998. Also, Andrea Bonnicksen, "What Kind of Policy Formation Do We Need for Preimplant Diagnosis?" Lecture at the International Conference on Genetic Diagnosis, Rennes, France, 1998.

technological progress. One must still ask—who are the stockholders of international bioethical law?

The handling of scientific cases poses a number of challenges to the legislative and judicial setting that are only beginning to surface. Where medical science is involved, scientific jargon has to be interpreted to legislators and judicial officials by commissioned scientific professionals. This changes the representative nature of legislation. Science examines approaches to truths about the universe through observation and experimentation, but science's primary concern is science and its own academic freedom. Who funds medical and scientific research and development? Enormous grants are flowing into the universities from private interests. Science regulates science;

corporate and pharmaceutical grants enable scientists; and, in a deductive sense, scientific interests govern society in these regards.

Humanity is both the subject and object of scientific technology and is entitled to an intelligible account of the proposals being introduced by medical science—they are the holders of a priceless stock. Multidisciplinary committees at every level of the social stratum are trying to determine the best direction for health care in light of new technologies. One thing is clear: the subject matter makes it an international proposition since the operative parties—scientists, physicians, and corporations—are intensely mobile. Ordinary people throughout the world are presuming that their rights will be fairly protected. Citizens are relying on representative and professional expertise—and prudence.

Just law should embody ethics and serve public norms. Law needs to respond to the rapid advancements in medicine, technology, and biopolitics and maintain flexibility. Understanding "what molecular medicine is actually capable of" and "where it is headed" is a realistic approach to understanding what future legislation should look like in the area of genetic diagnosis. Being informed and taking a stand sustain democratic ideals—and validate freedom of conscience.

Chapter 4

Medical Experimentation
and Reproduction

INTRODUCTION

There has been considerable discussion about the paradigm shift from medicine to experimental science. In the first 150 years (1850-2000) of modern medicine it was practiced as an art. It showcased the two-way consultation between the patient and the physician. Now, physicians work closely with laboratory scientists to take advantage of new technology. Many doctor–patient relationships have evaporated into health management systems and laboratory diagnostics, but personal information has not. It is more accessible than ever before, due to electronically transferred statistical banks, supposedly blind, but probably not. Reproductive medicine converged with science in its use of oversimplified biochemical solutions, experimental trials, and statistics.[1]

In this chapter, the reader will travel the experimental highway as it develops and organizes information concerning new reproductive and genetic technologies that are used to assess solutions to difficult pregnancies. It will delineate what science can actually achieve—not the ideas presented to win grant money.

Unlike previous chapters in which religious precedents shaped the contents of theology, ethics, and law, this chapter follows more pragmatic lines. Medicine and science understand health in physical, palpable terms, and frequently relegate religion to philosophy following Cartesian dictums (i.e., God cannot be understood in physical measurements).

One will discover that the ideals of the Hippocratic Oath were slowly reconfigured by post-enlightenment individualization, the birth of the clinic, Darwin's theory of evolution, and scientific method. Doctors formed objective and dispassionate ways of dealing with patients' illnesses. In many ways, it numbed the practitioner's ability to identify with the patient's trauma.

At the height of the golden age of medicine, the Holocaust catastrophe demonstrated how easily good doctors were led into bad practices. Nazi racial ideology flashed warning signals for genetic abuse, gender selection, and discrimination against the disabled. After World War II, reproductive and genetic research intensified, sometimes cunningly, but its curators believed objective scientific strategies could protect against human mistakes while finding cures for disease, aging, and disabilities.

The interest in research quickly led to the mapping of the human genome, which allowed science to lay hold of a real hope for solving health problems, sometimes, by redesigning human embryos to alleviate heritable diseases. Genetics was credited with the potential to save future generations or destroy family lines. Collectively, medicine now considers practical techniques, scientific experiments, and clinical medicine.[2]

Some prefer not to gamble with natural processes. A reasonable and well-researched alternative is palliative care, which focuses on patient relationships. It values the dynamics of life and recognizes death as an important part of living. Palliative care provided a compassionate avenue for families to approach terminal diseases.

Regardless of one's methodology for treating or accepting illness, every member of society should be equipped to participate in his or her own health choices. Remembering that people are the *raison d'être,* physicians, nurses, counselors, and ministers who evaluate, advise, and counsel modern medical dilemmas need to be prepared to inform and empower decisions with up-to-the-minute resources, so patients can make and own their decisions.

MEANINGS OF HEALTH AND DISEASE

The well-known ethicist Leon Kass said the *aim* of medicine was to sustain health.[3] By health, Kass meant the absence of disease. One recognizes disease because it deviates away from normal, comfortable body functions.[4] But how does one identify normalcy when people have a rainbow of IQs, body shapes, sizes, and colors?

The clues to an individual's health were partially revealed in DNA. DNA presented an algorithm, a set of rules or instructions that repeated and, when properly translated, described a variety of physical irregularities. Dismantling a person's identity using DNA raises boundary issues because it is very personal. Genetic researchers also have been accused of playing God, but a good researcher will consider several courses of action, including issues affecting a person's faith, before making recommendations.[5]

TRADITIONAL MEDICINE

Definition: Traditional medicine honors a mutual exchange of information between doctor and patient. The patient describes irregular physical symptoms, and the doctor relates these to a particular ailment or organic dysfunction in order to determine the best treatment based on her or his professional education, training, and experience.

There is none as famous in all of medicine as the ancient Greek, Hippocrates. Through observation and prognosis, he laid the ground rules for practicing ethical medicine. Medical integrity consisted of: (1) do no harm; (2) no assisted suicide; (3) do not cause abortion, refer patients for specialist treatment when necessary; (4) do not abuse or compromise the patient–doctor relationship (by sexual intercourse); and (5) keep patients' confidences. As repayment for one's apprenticeship, the student was obliged to provide medical services for his teacher's family.[6] The Hippocratic Oath was respected across frontiers, cultures, and ages. It was linked to sacred arts and secular medicine.

E.H. Ackernecht's erudite text associated the incantations and healing practices of shamans and priests with the sacred. Autopsies were forbidden so as not to disturb the dead. Galen, an arrogant first-century physician, dissected a spinney-backed monkey and used its anatomy as a model for human beings. Typically, physicians watched for irregularities in blood, phlegm, and bile. Alchemy tricked and killed bodily diseases, while bloodletting was intended to drain disease out of the patient's veins. For many years, medicine was taught in Latin and only tonsured clerics understood it well enough to practice the healing arts. The bridge between science and medicine began in the seventeenth century. Anton von Leeuwenhoek opened-up the microscopic world with the discovery of red cells, protozoa, and bacteria in 1633. At Leiden, Hermann Boerhaave recorded patients' symptoms and created a bedside classroom and clinic.[7]

In *The Birth of a Clinic,* Michel Foucault spoke of the social and historical compilation of information that led to theories on disease. It contributed to a vast increase in knowledge. After the French Revolution, medicine changed dramatically, shifting the health profession from religious thinkers to the public domain. In just 50 years, it reorganized itself, the hospitals, and the patients' status. Doctors were compelled to drop Latin and speak so patients could understand the diagnosis. The popular scientific method replaced empathy with dispassionate objectivity. Disease was named and cataloged by symptoms. This enabled doctors to recognize a pathological disorder by the defective shape, size, or inflammation of organs, tissues, etc., until they discovered airborne bacteria and microbes linked it to contagion. The patient was no longer diseased, and death was no longer demonized. Physicians maintained a fidelity to discovering the cause and eliminating it.[8] Scientists performed autopsies and became more familiar with human anatomy.

Darwin's theory of evolution instigated a completely new chain of theories about cell development. Darwin observed the patterns in plant and animal genesis in *Origin of Species.* He compared human embryology with other species, which resulted in his very popular theories about recapitulation. He compared human babies gestating in fluids with tadpoles, which grew in water; both matured into air-breathing species. Darwin hypothesized a symbiotic relationship for the entire environment—with a random, indiscriminate coevolution that was not anthropologically centered. Humanity survived because it was fit and clever. Of course, Mendel's genetic experiments put Darwin's theories into perspective. John Maynard Smith attributed Darwin's lack of sophistication to the later exposition of detailed cell development and respective interdependencies.[9]

Scientific curiosity was prolific, education separated into disciplines, and medical curriculum developed. The first two years of medical training taught anatomy, physiology, central nervous system, biochemistry, pathology, and pharmacology. Then one studied the mechanisms of disease, controlled medical trials (observing therapies), diagnostics, and biostatistics. The old bedside school of signs and symptoms now had information about environmental effects, such as allergies, unclean water, and mosquitoes.[10] Embryology examined the health of developing cells and genetic principles. The golden age of medicine brought dark shadows with it.

THE PHILOSOPHY OF HOLOCAUST MEDICINE

Definition: Holocaust medicine was a eugenic philosophy based on Darwinian natural selection. The goal was to restabilize the German economy and create a utopian society—eliminating "unfit" individuals from Germany by compulsory sterilization, experimentation, and euthanasia.

The people in twentieth-century Germany believed that the doctors had disturbed God's plan for natural birth, life, and death. Hence, when the Nazi party took over, physicians were clandestinely assigned a role in social engineering. Some people dismiss the ensuing activities as too extreme to ever reoccur, but this dark discussion illustrates how different events, arising at the same time, fed superstitions that created a civil religion, a religion that, under the Nazi leadership, played upon the fallibility of the medical profession.

The Blurring of Myth and Scientific Theory

Daniel Jonah Goldhagen's book contended that the German *people* willingly participated in the atrocities of the *Shoah* (Holocaust). This was partially because the German subconscious still contained medieval premonitions about the curse of Jewish complicity in the death of Christ. Applying Darwin's evolutionary theory to the entire Jewish race implied the curse had to be excised before it spread like a cancer throughout society.[11] At the same time, Doctors B. Morel, W. Griesinger, E. Kraepelin and H. Maudsley published their research on the genetic basis for mental disease. Mental disease was considered a by-product of sin, a curse, in many circles. The boundary between myth and fact was blurred by superstition. At the same time, Count Arthur de Gobineau released his novel describing a fair-haired genetically superior breed of Aryans. Germans associated this book with their folk religion, which taught them that they were superhumans. The coevolution of genetics, mental illness, Darwin, de Gobineau, racial hygiene, and heredity was a mixture of fiction and science that tragically and erroneously led Germans to select-out people they referred to as useless and inferior people.[12]

Social Darwinism was well accepted among intellectuals and taught in German medical schools during the 1920s depression years. Its application bespoke: (1) a need for a biologically pure strain to maintain and preserve the state, (2) the implementation of the survival of the fittest theory, and (3) a popular desire to change laws that protected and catered to the biologically weak. Ironically, the University of Würzburg led the world in therapy for the mentally ill—preserving and regulating the most underdeveloped lives, both physically and mentally. People were out of work and hungry so they thought it was contentious that the government would use its money to assist "unfit" patients with mental and physical disorders.[13]

A German Civil Religion Emerges to Purify the German Genome

A civil religion emerged when the Third Reich initiated its new program in Germany. They designed a natural selection program to catch what nature missed and to end suffering. Genetics provided a reason for sterilizing women who might bear unhealthy offspring. Idealists sought to create a master race.[14]

The nation reinvented itself as a super quasi-human force. Several principles were extracted from classical texts, including Plato, Aristotle, Christian ideas, and the Monists—with a twist. From Plato's *Republic,* Deutschland was the good father, which was built from strong, superhuman Aryans. The stigma of Aristotle's unacceptable newborns fell upon babies who were diseased or crippled—they were drowned.[15] Monists, not Aristotle, taught that the spirit emerged in the human body, biologically, but Monist doctrine implied that the body had to be well suited. The Nazi Monists had manipulated the original theories of E. Haeckel and W. Ostwald, Nobel Peace Prize winner for chemistry. This scientific mysticism was intended to override unscientific religion. By it, the human spirit was naturalized and medicalized. Doctors were blamed for interrupting and tampering with natural selection. They were retrained to be "selectors" of good German stock.[16] Doctor–priests were supposed to purify the *Volk* (people) through genetic manipulation, eugenics, and mercy killing— congealing the Aryan myth.[17]

Hitler commissioned Joseph Mayer, a follower of H. Muckermann, S.J., a Roman Catholic, to detail religious points. He recommended Germans only marry other Germans. Premarital medical examinations were advised to avoid racial pollution. Practical eugenics and sterilization eliminated heritable diseases, physical impairments, low IQ, and criminal behaviors. Neither Mayer nor Muckermann had racist overtones, and Roman Catholics showed respect for handicapped individuals.[18]

The Third Reich borrowed theosophy from any source that benefited their designs. Luther had denounced certain illnesses as demonic, so the Protestant church suspected that mental deficiency came from sin. Venereal disease had symptoms of mental illness, too. Hence, it came to be that anyone with psychological disorders had to be exorcised before the whole nation fell into moral turpitude (c.f., Penitential manuals). One had to receive absolution before a Christian physician was allowed to treat him or her.[19] The misapplication of thirteenth-century literature to 1938 German laws required that only Jews treat Jews.[20]

Euthanasia was contrary to Church doctrine, and the 1930 *Casti Connubii* Roman Catholic canon forbade compulsory sterilization, but Mayer departed on this note and supported euthanasia. By approving it, he supplied the Nazis with a rationale for mass destruction. It created a political philosophy based on selecting and eradicating less-productive members of society. The Nazi bottom line was to build a utopia whose citizens were free from every sickness and anything that created social imbalance.[21]

National Eugenics: Sterilization, Euthanasia, and Experimentation

The Weimar Republic developed a philosophy of biological eugenics to solve its economic and political problems. They commandeered the medical profession to administer it. The law said, "respect completely everybody's will to live, even the most sick, tortured, or useless people . . . never breaking [someone's] will to live," but the law was secondary to national fitness. The methods, structure, and bureaucracy of institutions had, in important ways, buffered doctors from emotions. Patients were dehumanized and referred to as human *subjects*.[22]

Sterilization

Universities at Basil, Switzerland, and München, Germany, established sterilization as an undisputed solution in preventing defective births. Anyone considered genetically weak was a candidate for the program, including asocial types who were moody, insecure, or otherwise morally corrupt. The list included sex deviants, prostitutes, vagrants, and criminals. Sexual partners were mandated to conform to the Sterilization Law (July 14, 1933), and it was amended to allow abortions.[23] Eugenics covered prostitution, alcoholism, and juvenile delinquency. Interracial marriage was prohibited by the Nuremberg Laws (1935). Dr. A. Ploetz, founder of the Society for Racial Hygiene *(Gesellschaft für Rassenhygiene)*, believed that selection coalesced well with euthanasia. The idea assisted in obtaining hospital beds for injured soldiers and disoriented victims after bombing raids.[24]

Euthanasia

The children's euthanasia program was launched after Herrn Knauser appealed to the KdF to "put down" his retarded child. He received an authorization on Hitler's personal stationary. By August 1939, K. Brandt and P. Bouhler had formed the Agency for Children's Euthanasia (i.e., *Reichsausschuss zur wissenschaftlichen Erfassung von erb-und anlagebedingten schweren Leiden*). Departing from medical tradition, this committee of psychiatrists and pediatricians evaluated each and every request for children's euthanasia based on forms alone; there were no physical examinations given. Initially, only retarded children and epileptics were approved. Trainable children were sent to work camps. Physicians and midwives had a duty to report deformed births. The midwives were compensated for their trouble. People were intimidated if they raised retarded or abnormal children.[25] Even children caught stealing were given an IQ test. According to *Das Schwartz Korps,* SS Journal (March 18, 1937), mercy killing was in the best interest of the family.[26]

Hitler ordered the *Gnadentod* (October 1939). Its leaders, Bouhler and Brandt, named and appointed physicians to authorize mercy killing on all who were, in the doctor's judgment, incurably ill.[27] Individual welfare was based on social utility. Those who could be released from the burdens of their illness were *ballastsxistenzen.* Some perceived it as spiritual eugenics. Germans accepted the deaths of their own relatives, the mentally ill, the aged, homosexuals, people with surgical problems, residents of welfare institutions, and foreign workers.[28] This smaller genocide was carried out using poison gas, trained medical personnel, and organized institutional facilities. Students were trained to give lethal injections. Victor Brock declared: "The needle belongs in the hand of a doctor."[29]

In the 1930s, publications about euthanasia were abundant. In *Man, The Unknown* (1935), Alexis Carrel urged that the mentally ill and criminals be placed in euthanasia facilities and administered gas. Retarded children were called "nature's mistakes" in *The Journal of American Psychologists Association.* They said killing them was merciful. *American Scholar* and *Journal of the American Institute of Homeopathy* featured forcible euthanasia.[30]

K. Binding and A. Hoche set forth the boundaries in *Permission for the Destruction of Human Life, Its Extent and Form.* One could request an assisted death if the subject was (1) mentally competent, but terminally ill, (2) mentally retarded and without purpose, or (3) people who were brain-dead. The fate of the mentally ill came down to economic pressures (Section 716). Health care providers were the selectors. Heimrich Himmler saw no conflict between the Hippocratic Oath and mercy killing.[31] Human dignity was reduced to abstract reasoning.

Aktion T-4 launched Brandenburg's first euthanasia experiment in the shower room. It was classified as top secret. Institutions were systematically opened: Grafeneck (January 1940); Brandenburg (February 1940); Hartheim (May 1940); and Sonenstein (June 1940). Ironically, doctors used death to cure Germany's cancer of immorality. From September 1939 through July 1941, 70,000 mentally handicapped Jews were expunged with gas. With the establishment of concentration camps, Program *Action T4* became *14f13.* Translated, *f13* had three categories: (1) death by natural causes, (2) suicide, or (3) shoot escapees.[32]

Medical Experimentation

The 1931 experimentation guidelines, *Reichsrundschreiben,* Regulations of the Reich Health Department, were stricter than the Nuremberg Code and conformed to the Hippocratic Oath. They were in force throughout the Holocaust.[33] Himmler directed physicians to refine and purify the Nordic-German bloodlines. Experimentation was the natural outcome, and the existing eugenic operations made it easy. Doctors and psychologists volunteered for the euthanasia program. It was as if they had lost touch with what it meant to be human.[34]

Himmler and Brandt supplied human subjects for Dr. Rasher's experiments. They were informed, in advance, that the human "material" would die. The tests were supposedly to help soldiers. How long could one survive at high altitude before his lungs collapsed? If drowned in the English Channel, how long could one drink seawater or stay alive in the frozen sea? People were submerged in baths of ice water during the Polish winter. Prisoners were given live attenuated viruses, phosgene gas, and other experimental vaccines. Handicapped children were intoxicated, so they would urinate every 30 minutes, given insulin, scarlet fever, hepatitis, and Tuberculosis. Limb and bone transplants took place without anesthesia. Eyes were injected with dye when the eye had no circulation. Female menstrual cycles were deregulated by describing to the woman how she was going to be executed. Dr. Mengele even wrote letters to his wife that detailed his electroshock experiments on his prisoners.[35]

Dr. H. Spatz and J. Hallervorden at the Kaiser Wilhelm Institute ordered brains from postmortem children for dissection. Cleansing meant understanding the germ lines of the retarded. The Kaiser Wilhelm Institute focused on schizophrenia, feeble-mindedness, and epilepsy, as well as blood composition, physical chemistry of the brain, chromosomes, metabolic pathology, constitutional typology, and the chemistry of aging. After the experiments, researchers discarded the remains of their patients. Euthanasia deaths were indistinguishable from natural deaths.[36]

More than 150 medical journals were published during the Nazi reign. Many were edited following the Doctor's Trials. Dr. H. Voss wrote an anatomy textbook, which is still in use in some medical schools.[37]

The Aftermath: The Nuremberg Doctor's Trial and International Cooperation

The Nuremberg Doctor's Trials watched as doctors and officials justified medical experiments—presuming legal protection when there was none. Many physicians considered their profession superior to political and social forces, with noble, altruistic motives. After all, the Nazi government deemed them to be high priests of its own civil religion. The prevalent ideology remained that a people could be sacrificed for the greater good. Some pleaded wartime security or appealed to the empirical nature of medicine, claiming it had little to do with moral matters. Ironically, physicians argued that they did not have time to create conditions safe enough for the use of animals or nonprisoner volunteers. Some claimed wartime insanity or schizophrenia. Based on confiscated diaries, Götz strongly disagreed— medical regulations were loose before the war.[38]

The Nazi doctors violated laws of the Weimar Republic, international conventions, laws of customs and wars, as well as the basic morality of all civilized nations. Eugenic physicians became diagnosticians, slaves to forms, even forgetting the value of human life. S. Liebfried, K. Tennstadt, W. Wuttke-Groneberg, Mitscherlich, and Mielke dared, at great risk, to testify against F. Sauerbruch, W. Hueber, F. Reim, Brandt, Bloome, Brock, and Hoven at the Nuremberg Doctor's Trial. Some Nazi doctors committed suicide before their death sentences occurred, while others escaped with the assistance of prominent leaders such as Hans Harmsen, president of the Protestant Church Welfare Institute (a leading racial hygienist and supporter of sterilization), *Die Stille Helfe,* Vatican Bishop Alois Hudal, Surgeon Colonel H. Armstrong (U.S. 8th Air Force), presidents, prime ministers, and so on.[39]

Medical ethicists have worked diligently to prevent future abuses. International covenants include the Declarations of the World Medical Association, beginning with Geneva (1948), Helsinki (1964), and

Tokyo (1975).[40] Israel asked for the burial of the brain specimens preserved by Nazi doctors—they were laid to rest at Tübingen in 1986.[41]

Nazi cases were cited when G. Annas, Hastings Institute, and M. Grodin had to give evidence, so *Nancy Cruzan* could be taken off life support. They said it was a matter of "assisting a dying person to the end of her life with dignity."[42] They provided the U.S. Supreme Court with clear and convincing proof that Nancy herself would not want to be kept alive whereas, in Nazi Germany, people were executed against their will. Annas's Boston symposium redefined the ethics of euthanasia by differentiating murder from mercy.[43]

Nazi physicians' acceptance of eugenics, triage, euthanasia, human experimentation, and, finally, mass genocide, made them medical executioners. This was the penultimate slippery slope.

REPRODUCTIVE AND GENETIC MEDICINE

Definition: Molecular medicine uses modern reproductive technology and deoxyribonucleic acid (DNA) genetic science for therapeutic and forensic purposes.

The importance of genetics cannot be overstated. It is interactive with many causeways of human health. University medical schools now train molecular physicians. Most perinatal mortality and all cancers involve genetic mutations.[44] There are over 10,000 distinct genetic conditions. Many are rare.

James Watson and Francis Crick found DNA secretly hidden in the nucleus of every cell. Every living thing has a genetic history and identity. DNA consists of two strands of genes, on which is written information about each person's genetic code. DNA is invisible to the human eye. Therefore, researchers use confocal, light, epiflorescent microscopy and computerized microinjection—mixing chemical cocktails and thermodynamics. Scientists maintain an international network of data, but it changes very quickly.

The Architecture of DNA

Each DNA molecule is encoded by one of four chemicals: adenine, thiamine, cytosine, or guanine. These chemicals run along the entire DNA strand and are understood in sets of threes (i.e., ATT, CCG, etc.). (See Figures 4.1. and 4.2.) Geneticists say that three en-

DNA Structure and Replication

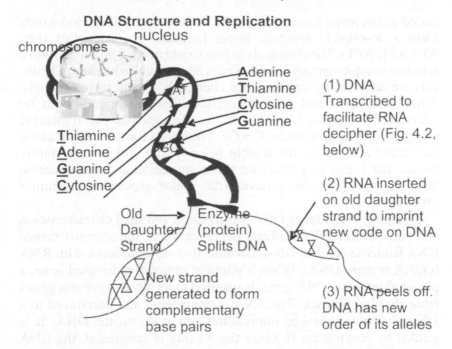

nucleus

chromosomes

Adenine
Thiamine
Cytosine
Guanine

Thiamine
Adenine
Guanine
Cytosine

Old → Enzyme
Daughter (protein)
Strand Splits DNA

New strand
generated to form
complementary
base pairs

(1) DNA
Transcribed to
facilitate RNA
decipher (Fig. 4.2,
below)

(2) RNA inserted
on old daughter
strand to imprint
new code on DNA

(3) RNA peels off.
DNA has new
order of its alleles

FIGURE 4.1. DNA structure. Protein added to split strands. Natural Replication (left): Daughter Strand makes encoding. Engineered DNA (right): (1) Transcription (Fig. 4.2). (2) RNA inserted to imprint its new code. (3) RNA copy peels off.

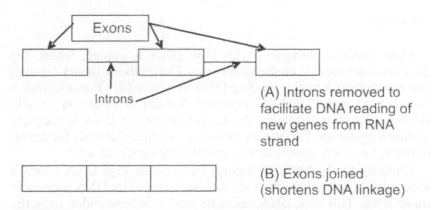

Exons

Introns

(A) Introns removed to
facilitate DNA reading of
new genes from RNA
strand

(B) Exons joined
(shortens DNA linkage)

FIGURE 4.2. Before attaching new RNA code information to daughter strand, the introns are excised, exons joined.

coded genes make a word (i.e., ATT, CCG, etc.), and several words form a descriptive sentence about heritable characteristics (i.e., ATT.ATT. ATT). The chemicals in one strand need to be paired with a separate complementary strand; it runs antiparallel to its mate. Chemicals are attracted by certain other chemicals to complete the algorithms that signal and issue instructions. Two hydrogen bonds tie adenine and thiamine (A=T) together. Cytosine pairs with guanine using three hydrogen bonds (C = G). The bonds form a catalyst along the strand and zip-up the double helix.[45] The coil is very tightly bound, but it can be penetrated for examination and manipulation through one of its two grooves (the major groove or the minor groove).

Changing the order of DNA words alters physical characteristics, and some believe DNA affects behavior. First, the scientist makes RNA from the original DNA, because it is easier to work with RNA (cDNA is copy-DNA). When a scientist removes a diseased gene, a placeholder gene, a "U" gene, is inserted in its place to prevent genes from slipping offtrack. The RNA is engineered and introduced to a DNA daughter strand to imprint the new code on the DNA. It is guided by polymerase II. Once the writing is completed, the RNA peels off. Mutations can occur when damaged DNA is replicated, but repaired enzymes destroy mistakes (a.k.a., aberrations). DNA replication is exceptionally accurate. Nature proofreads it using polymerase (Pol I and III).[46]

Variables

Other theories disagreed with how DNA is copied, where the chemicals are located on the strand, etc. The textbook theory (above) teaches that RNA begins reading DNA at *minus 30*. TF-transcription factors bind at the TATATA sequence. Similar to a train on a track, RNA begins to travel along the strand, while the DNA is securely clamped upstream. This theory presumes a molecular basis for development, i.e., each gene instructs specific characteristics.[47]

Contrary to the textbook theory, Peter Cook says DNA forms a loop, like a lasso, and pulls the chromosomes to its DNA factory to make RNA. This way, DNA has to be read in reverse order, from the end to the beginning, using polymerase chain reactions (PCR). Cook's nontraditional theory changes the process of RNA production and how genes are read, which casts a shadow on how marking, splicing, and modification actually work.[48] Altering genes is not an observable process. The scientist relies on a formula wherein chemicals attract specific genes, laboratory measurements, exposure to warming or cooling routines, time elements, etc.

After DNA is modified, it needs to be reinserted into the nucleus. DNA is very long, so scientists may cut away a few introns, "junk DNA" between activators, to shorten the strand so it fits back into the nucleus, but shorter DNA meant a shorter life for the Dolly clone, which aged more quickly than the mother did, since the DNA was shorter. Confidence in genetic engineering will grow as accuracy reaches the 100 percent mark. Presently, it is slightly above 85 percent.

The U.S. Human Genome Project began making maps of the entire genetic system. The *linkage map* identified single-cell diseases (i.e., sickle cell, cystic fibrosis, etc.) and multifactorial disorders (heart disease, high blood pressure, mental disorders, etc.). *Physical maps* assist in predicting prenatal conditions. The *Sequence map* identifies each person's genes. The *YAC map* provides data for copying the genes (i.e., telemeric and centromeric statistics), and the *Hybrid map* describes the chromosomes and whole cells.[49]

Family DNA is shared by communities. Each parent contributes 23 chromosomes to the embryo, totaling 46 chromosomes; each grandparent contributes one-fourth to its grandchild, one-eighth to the great-grandchild, etc. In an isolated geographic situation, the same chromosomes were repeatedly distributed among relatives, creating long chains of repeated chemical words. It was these long repeats that resulted in ethnic diseases (sickle cell anemia or Tay Sachs), as well as interfamilial illnesses, such as hemophilia. As people migrated, the genetic infirmity moved to other geographical areas. Marital diversity created new genetic codes (a.k.a., mutations) and acted as a key factor in keeping the human species healthy.[50]

Genetic Screening: Preimplantation Diagnosis (PID) and Prenatal Diagnosis (PND)

Screening for heritable diseases is a diagnostic tool, not a treatment. Tests are advised for those with a strong family history of a particular inherited disease, parents from high-risk ethnic groups, and mothers over 38 years of age. Screening offers a statistical analysis about the probability of future illness; it is predictive. Presently, reproductive cells, germline cells, are not supposed to be altered, because the changes would be inherited by future generations, without their permission. Legally, a person can agree to change and take risks with his or her own body, which legitimizes somatic therapy.

Scientific method draws generalized conclusions about genetic outcomes, but each zygote has its own unique genetic code. Personalized readings can only be accomplished after the sperm has fertilized the egg with the individual's new DNA. Prenatal diagnosis (PND) analyzes the embryo's DNA while it is inside the mother's womb *(in vivo)*. Preimplantation diagnosis (PID) fertilizes the *ova* in a petri dish before implantation in the womb *(ex vivo)* and is recommended when both parents have severe genetic disorders. Parents may prefer PID for religious reasons, since the examination takes place outside the mother's body before the fertilized egg attaches to the uterus, avoiding abortion.

A eugenic reading may be viewed *positively,* focusing on enhancing a person's features, such as blue eyes, etc., or *negatively,* concerned with eliminating genetic disease. Treatment may not be available, but prenatal testing assists parents in planning for special medical and educational needs that their child might require. Professionals need to keep the goals of the patient in mind, offering results only about the disease in question. Decisions are subjective because human beings are unique.

Prenatal Diagnosis

PND looks at the fetus in the early stages of development inside the uterus using amniocentesis, fetoscopy, ultrasound, viral, or blood analysis. Over 280 fetal abnormalities are discernable. With amniocentesis, the doctor draws fluid from the mother's amniotic sac using a needle. There is enough fluid by the fourteenth week. The mother has very little risk other than the possibility of infection. The fetus has a low risk of injury from the needle (0.1 percent), a slightly greater risk of spontaneous abortion (<1 percent), and may suffer from infant respiratory distress syndrome. Experts are uncertain as to the recurrence of the problem. Concerned by any risk to the fetus, Paul

Ramsey recommended against amniocentesis. Ultrasound can detect Trisome 21, Mongoloid condition, in about two-thirds of the cases during the eighteenth to twenty-second week of pregnancy. DNA tests based on blood diagnostics alone often fail to distinguish maternal and fetal cells, missing many disorders. Amniocentesis, fetoscopy, ultrasound, and viral screening report a 75 percent rate of success in diagnosing heritable diseases.[51]

Preimplantation Diagnosis

PID is used in medically assisted reproduction, and the tests occur outside the mother's body. The procedure is stressful and uncomfortable. The mother-to-be takes drugs to hyperstimulate the production of eggs (oocytes). The drugs have very unpleasant side effects (nausea, vomiting, loss of appetite, sleeplessness, etc.). When the eggs are fertile, they are surgically removed (harvested) and fertilized. Analysis occurs at the four-to-eight-cell stage—before the cells become a human embryo (differentiation).

After a healthy assessment, doctors often implant several embryos to ensure pregnancy, resulting in too many fetuses, which endangers the health of the mother and the fetuses. The embryos can be washed from the uterus, but *this* does raise the abortion issue. PID will still require a PND analysis sometime down the road to monitor the healthy development of the embryo.

Differentiation

At the eight-cell stage, the zygote begins human development when it forms a top and bottom, its axis, and the cells initiate body-building by generating the mesoderm, the ectoderm, and the endoderm. Differentiation determines and discloses the purpose of the cells, (whether to become a liver, kidney, etc.). Fetal growth factors (Fgf and Fgf-R) signal action. Fgf-10 tells the *mesoderm* to manufacture blood, bone, and muscle. These are integrated with the skin and nervous system, *ectoderm,* by the Fgf-R2b signal. Once the protective, leakproof skin covering (by Fgf-8) wraps around the blood and bone building properties (from Fgf-10), these bind to the mesenchyme with Fgf-R2, so that the early buds can begin protrusions that generate limbs. Finally, the *endoderm* is responsible for developing specific organs, beginning with the mouth and moving south down the body.[52] (See Figure 1.11a,b,c, *supra* p. 45.)

The hedgehog genes issue secondary signals to produce healthy cells. A cell is competent when it responds with the right answer (i.e., to make bone rather than skin). The sonic hedgehog (SHH) instructs the teeth, tongue, brain, esophagus, lungs, and the entire alimentary track. It diminishes as it travels along a developing limb, which signals fingers or toes to grow. When SHH forms the spinal cord, the variance of proteins initiates the nerve cells to give sensation and movement. Sonic hedgehog sends the instructions for brain chemicals to activate, such as, dopamine, etc. Indian hedgehog (IHH) repairs cartilage, and desert hedgehog (DHH) regulates sperm production in males.[53]

Hundreds of cells and cell functions are constantly changing as the embryo develops. Not knowing about Fgf signaling, Darwin viewed differentiation through recapitulation, comparing human embryos to tadpoles, since the baby gastrulated in embryonic fluid, like a tadpole in water, and both now breathe air, like frogs. Geneticists studied Drosophilae (fly) eggs to learn about genetics, because the fly's egg is relatively easy to study. It has segments that can be moved from one side of the egg to another area within the same egg, and it will mutate the fly's body (i.e., two wings grow on the same side).[54] A human egg is not like a fly's egg, nor is a baby like a tadpole. Humans build from a tadpole-like stage, never entering the adult tadpole period. In fact, human gastrulation is the opposite of recapitulation because a human baby develops as a whole person inside the womb, with a skeleton and a skull. An embryo's ectoderm and endoderm evolve, but parts of the skull grow far more gradually. Family genetics affect the length of limbs and the body's shape, such as webbed toes or too many fingers. Evolution never commanded a new species with more toes or fingers. Each fetus inherits about 70,000 genes from a long line of historical persons, some altered by mutation, some stable, and some fast. Different episodes continually affect development. A gene may divert from its purpose or extinguish itself, some cells fuse, genes recombine themselves, and complex hierarchical systems change commands.[55] The embryo develops its body parts through genetic signaling, cell development, hormones, embryonic development, biology, the environment—and the emotional, psychological, and spiritual aspects of being human.[56] These create new matrixes. Biology plays a role in the overall fetal development, but it is not necessarily the cause *per se* of degenerative growth.

Multiple Genetic Repeats

A DNA with lengthy genetic repeats indicates disease. Consanguine marriages between relatives will generate long repetitive algorithms in the baby. For example, the mother's TTA sequence plus the father's TTA sequence equals TTA-TTA-TTA . . . repeatedly. If mother contributes 35 consecutive TTAs, plus (+) father contributes 40 consecutive TTAs, the baby is likely to inherit 75 consecutive TTAs. Scores of repeats are frequently associated with muscular and neural disorders. PID counts the chemical repeats to calculate the probability of inheriting the dysfunction. After the results of PID, the doctor and patient decide whether to transplant the fertilized cells into the mother's uterus.

The Search for Cures: Screening, Genetic Pharmaceuticals, Cloning Tissues and Organs, Stem Cell Therapy, and Xenotransplantation

Genetic research, medical technology, and the doctor's clinical skills are being stretched to maximum capacity to ensure a healthy future. Some genetic disorders can be detected by screening and, in some cases, genetic pharmaceuticals are available for treatment. Pharmaceutical expenditure is being focused on cancer treatment, since it is the most widespread illness.[57] Somatic, treatments to one's body, such as protein manufacturing, enzyme design, antibodies, and hormones, can alter and enhance human life without affecting future generations.

Screening and Cures

People will go for screening when treatment is available. See the example in Exhibit 4.1 Identifying carriers may save suffering in future generations. Tay-Sachs, sickle cell anemia, and β-thalassaemia are screened anonymously to protect against discrimination. Tests for Tay-

EXHIBIT 4.1. Curable diseases.

Disease	Detection
Breast cancer	Detectable in women with the *BRCA1* and *BRCA2* genes. One in five are carriers but do not contract the illness
Colon cancer	Can be surgically corrected
Prostate cancer	Early detection reveals mutated antigens

Sachs are frequently taken at Jewish schools. Carriers are informed if marriage with another carrier is planned. Screening β-thalassaemia is mandated in Sardinia and by the Greek Orthodox Church. If two partners are carriers, the marriage will be interrupted.[58]

Screening also detects genetic illnesses for which there are no ready solutions see Exhibit 4.2.

Genetic Pharmaceuticals

Genetic pharmaceuticals aim at overriding the disease by sending a large number of healthy cells into the infected area. It is done by injecting a normal gene into a delivery vehicle (vector) that can rapidly reproduce itself. The vessel is usually a virus, bacteria, or yeast. Of course, the person receiving treatment will have natural immunities to viruses and bacteria that also must be compensated for by adding counter-counter immunities, etc. Genetic pharmaceuticals provide some treatments see Exhibit 4.3.

Cloning Cells and Tissues

Cloning cells and tissues has sparked a good deal of hope. Libraries of cloned cells provide ample material for experiments. Blood cells can be cloned and administered to correct blood imbalances. Skin cells are multiplied to replace the skin of burn victims. Organs and tissues can be cloned from stem cells, but delivery is a big problem. How do the cells get to the right place and grow into a liver?

EXHIBIT 4.2. Detectable diseases without solutions.

Disease	Description
Cystic fibrosis (CF)	Over generations, CF has accumulated a wide range of diverse mutations. CF is a single-cell disease that causes fluids to accumulate in lung bronchi, but each family or population may have one of thousands of genetic causal variations. Identifying the mutation is complex and expensive and may affect reproductive cells. It has been identified in approximately 70 cases out of 500. Ameliorating and neutralizing genes could counter CF, and scientists are working to lessen the severity, but there are side effects.[a]
Parkinson's, lupus (basal ganglic), Parkinsonians (resembles Parkinson's), a kinetic rigid syndrome, supra nuclear palsy (PSP), and Parkinson's plus	The brain loses about 80 percent of its dopamine production-a chemical for smooth walk and lucid speech. Breast tumors, rigidity (leadlike, stooped posture), brady kinesia (slow, short steps), falling, and semifrozen eye muscles are not uncommon. Dopamine therapies have limited value: (1) Levodopa has latent effects after five to ten years; (2) brain surgery can remove the dopamine area; (3) anticholinergics block everything; (4) monoamine oxidase inhibitors (MAOIs); COMT inhibitors.
The chorea group, including tremors, myoclonas (epilepsy), dystonia, and tics (Tourette's)	Initiated by genetic repeats of CAG. Dementia and strokes are accompanied by excessive movement in the upper body and hands (actional/kinetic), and it inhibits tasks (e.g., typing, writing, playing music). Symptoms occur in the eyes (blepharospasm), the voice (oromandibular receptor), or the face (spasmodic). Botulinum toxin interrupts the nervous system, but is ineffective after ten years, and the condition worsens. Dopamine repressors have been used in treating some of the chorea symptoms.

Huntington's	No symptoms until later in life, and it has no cure. Half of those who have a parent with Huntington's disease are at risk.[b]

Notes: [a]Steve Jones, "Genetics in Medicine: Real Promises, Unreal Expectations-One Scientist's Advice to Policymakers in the United Kingdom and the United States," from the Millbank Memorial Fund Prospectus (New York: Millbank Memorial Fund, 2000), 12, 15. See Robert C. Stern, "The Diagnosis of Cystic Fibrosis," New England Journal of Medicine 336(7)(13 February 1997), 487, 490. See also, Biesecker, "Genetic Counseling: Practice of Genetic Counseling," in Encyclopedia of Bioethics, Vol. 2 (New York: Macmillan Library, 1995), 926.

[b]Jones, 12.

EXHIBIT 4.3. Genetic pharmaceutical applications.

Disease	Therapy
ADA enzyme immunodeficiency	The missing ADA enzyme causing a child's immunodeficiency can be supplied by using a vector injected with leukemia retrovirus. It invades and genetically alters the T cells. There is no rejection when using the child's own bone marrow T lymphocytes. Experiments have been conducted for numerous diseases and muscular disorders. Most therapies are still in the elementary stages of development.
Heart blockage	When the heart is clogged and has only about 25 percent use, enzymes can be injected into the heart that develop capillaries, multiply arterial openings, and boost ventricular circulation. This is still experimental and surgeons are highly cautious.[a]

(continued)

(continued)

Diabetes	Diabetes has two distinct illnesses with genetic and nongenetic forms. It may be caused by viruses, diet, or environmental instability. Heritable transmission is high. Diabetes mellitus creates an imbalance in blood sugar, which causes kidney function to deteriorate. In many cases, chemical insulin stabilizes the necessary sugars and carbohydrates. Engrafting fetal pancreatic tissue has provided remedies, but environmental factors play a large role.[b]
Duchenne muscular dystrophy	Some similarities between humans and mice with Duchenne muscular dystrophy (DMD) gene. A missing gene was identified as *Xp21* (stop codon at 5' end produces no dystrophin). It was removed and reinserted two generations later to verify that it was the exact protein that caused the disease. Research on an Mdx mouse revealed utrophin (on chromosome 6) matched dystrophin and was a sound replacement drug. The experiments also revealed similarities to Becker muscular dystrophy (BMD) and B-thalassaemia. The problem was that the viral delivery system required an antibody against the natural immune system. The DMD experiment and other neuromuscular disorders offer encouragement to sufferers and their families.[c]

Notes: [a]Steve Jones, "Genetics in Medicine: Real Promises, Unreal Expectations-One Scientist's Advice to Policymakers in the United Kingdom and the United States," from the Millbank Memorial Fund Prospectus (New York: Millbank Memorial Fund, 2000), 6f.

[b]Andrew Simons, "Brave New Harvest," Christianity Today (19 November 1990), 24f. Also see Jones, 9.

[c]Kay Davis, "Identification of Disease," lecture, University of Oxford, Oxford, UK, 1999.

Embryonic stem cells prevent rejection and come from surplus embryos. They are usually cryopreserved after artificial fertilization.[64]

Stem Cell Generation

Stem cell generation is known as ontogeny. It became popular after the discovery of the hedgehog genes that differentiate and signal the growth of blood, bones, limbs, tissues, and organs. For example, scientists would like to control sonic hedgehog signaling to create dopamine-producing neurons for Parkinson's disease. Once produced, researchers would still need to get the neurons into the brain and hook them onto the proper synapses to effect treatment. Delivery is a major issue. If this were possible, it would revolutionize treatment for the Parkinson's family of diseases. A similar hope exists for repairing bone. Indian hedgehog (IHH) repairs cartilage. Experiments are being conducted to try to grow cartilage that could resurface knee joints. The therapy for diabetes is the most compelling if scientists can generate pancreatic β-cells that secrete insulin.[65] The experiments are controversial, however, because scientists need to experiment on human fetuses, at some point, if the research is to be applied to human patients.

The ethical issues of stem cell experimentation abound. Some fear women will be exploited to get pregnant in order to make possible stem cell therapies for family members. Others may be induced to conceive, abort, and sell them for research. Renowned ethicist Arthur Caplan contends that it is unethical to have an abortion when the goal is for donation. On the other hand, with permission from sperm and egg donors, scientists could fertilize countless embryos in their laboratories. At the University of Texas, John Robertson stirred controversy by proposing that the aborted fetus was simply an organ donor, a cadaver, for a relative. The downside of matching the blood of relatives is consanguinity. It increases the risk of regenerating the heritable trait one is trying to overcome.

Robertson set aside abortion as a separate issue from fetal stem cell donation. He wished to point out that a spontaneous abortion is a legitimate donation for research.[66] (Abortion is addressed in later chapters.)

Most researchers consider cell research, whether stem cells or cord blood, as an extension of cell or tissue transplant therapy. The genetic blueprint contains a formula for encoding specific genes to become particular tissues and organs.[67] The currency of success with molecular and cellular regeneration resides in the manufacture of simple skin and cartilage replacements derived from basic scientific experiments on embryonic stem cells (ES). The unfulfilled demands for organ donors and transplants make stem cell research to regenerate body parts a more pressing issue.

Xenotransplantation

Medical schools use animals, such as pigs, to teach students about the human body, because the interior architecture is similar to humans. Normally, animal organs would not be transplanted into humans. Human antibodies attack pig cells because they are lined with a sugar, α-galactose.[68] William Velander countered the rejection by converting α-galactose into an enzyme compatible with human systems, H-transferase. He fertilized the sows' eggs with this inhibitor gene, and the piglets developed the disease known as Pig-23. The first xenotransplantation organ surgery was on baboons, and their bodies accepted the pig organs, but the remedy was short-lived and the Baboons died.[69]

The greatest argument against animal to human transplantations came out of the HIV/AIDS epidemic, since it started when a human received a deadly and uncontrollable infection from a monkey. Xenotransplantation is a high-risk proposition. At least one dangerous virus lives in the pig's kidney. Oddly, scientists are not troubled by the threat of this pathology since the virus does not reproduce easily in human cells.[70] Nonetheless, patients with diabetes mellitus who need pancreatic β-cells (from s pig's kidney transplant) may not be so easily calmed when he or she learns about the danger associated with the pig organ that he or she is about to receive.

The ideal molecular treatment is to remove all genetic pathologies from the DNA before the body takes on any detrimental characteristics. Still, emotional surprises or the environment could very easily reintroduce harmful elements back into any purified body. Medical scientists, genetic specialists, and laboratory technicians are very good at what they know, but holistic approaches need the patient's input to reveal all the areas that are affected by the decision.

The Conciliation of the Physician's Goals and the Scientist's Values

Originally, a doctor's goal was to restore the patient's health. Are the patient's best interests compromised when the physician places the scientific aspects of medicine on a pedestal? Hippocrates's medical techniques were interpersonal. Science is a systematic search for knowledge. Funding the quest for knowledge comes from impressing grant sponsors who consider the scientist's success ratio, lauds, patents, copyrights, and trademarks on intellectual property.[71] Healing is the doctor's hallmark. Does the scientist value humankind in the same way?

David Morley believes that rewarding outstanding achievements, economically and professionally, encourages research and improves medicine for everyone. He argues that there is an inherent morality in the educational process. Science and medical students are encouraged to be (1) truthful, (2) avoid self-aggrandizement at the expense of fellow scientists, (3) defend freedom of inquiry and opinion, and (4) communicate findings through primary publications, synthesis, and instruction. Publication also invites disputation. In fact, a scientist has a special duty to bring the knowledge back to the community, which established the educational system that prepared him or her.[72]

Respecting the system and the patient are important parts of being a professional. While respecting the patient's right to make an autonomous decision, the expert is still responsible for teaching and guiding an informed choice. Doctors are acutely aware that parents are faced with the consequences of their decisions. Other children and family members will be affected by any change in lifestyle. When treating a genetic illness, the doctor and the patient are committed to a long-term relationship. A parent may even reject a sick child. Time also has to be allocated to civic responsibilities—to families and children who are dependent on institutional care. They have clinical and special education needs, too. Together, the patient, the doctor, and the community have to consider the way decisions are made and by whom.[73]

Doctors provide a communication bridge between the lab and the patient, especially with genetic screening.

Doctors wish to eliminate suffering and death. Science is diligently working on innovations and creating more pharmaceuticals. The use of ontogeny and ES cell research in cloning blood and cartilage are realized advancements for medicine. Reengineered DNA that increases heart circulation is amazing. The doctor's goals and scientific progress work well together until funding creates competition between scientists so fierce that they exaggerate progress to win the capital. If a pharmaceutical company is hosting the funds, the company awards areas that are marketable to the exclusion of many lesser, but still serious ailments. Humans should not be marginalized for profit, cloned for the sale of their body parts, or aborted for fluids that are rejection-free. How does the child-person who is being sacrificed feel? Human experimentation for social welfare occurred during the Holocaust, and it was disastrous. The ethical way is for a person, in the course of therapy, to agree to the release of medical information for social good. When signed, it constitutes voluntary, informed consent. Animals cannot give consent, and animal experimentation is important to medical advancement, but animals deserve proper treatment and, likewise, human recipients of xenotransplantation should be apprised of all the risks. All lives need to be respected—all creatures and human beings, even those too little to understand.

Patients may also elect to ignore genetic and reproductive services altogether.

PALLIATIVE CARE: CARING FOR PATIENTS WITH TERMINAL ILLNESSES

Definition: Palliative care is for the terminally ill. It provides patient-centered care nurtured by valued relationships. The dying are encouraged to make health care decisions as long as possible, show an interest in personal appearance, and express creativity. Psychological and spiritual values provide enrichment as death draws near. Active euthanasia is not a part.

Palliative care provides treatment for patients suffering from an illness for which there is no known cure and death is inevitable. Palliative care recognizes dying is a part of living, but it is opposed to active euthanasia. The goals are to:

- Relieve pain and other distressing symptoms
- Help patients and their families come to terms with terminal illness and death by providing psychological and spiritual care
- Promote living as active a life as possible, before death occurs
- Provide a supportive environment so the patient and his or her family can cope with the illness and bereavement[74]

Accepting the inevitability of death releases doctors, nurses, and patients from the tyranny of cure. Cure, according to Halina Bortnowska, presses one to be victorious over the enemy—that is, death. Similarly, William May labeled the physician as a fighter who battles with death through intelligent diagnostic procedural devices. In other words, saving life using all possible means is, potentially, *iatrogenic,* damaging the body to save it. Many prefer dignity and quality of life above the length of days. The death of a patient does not have to mean failure.

Respect and compassion for the terminally ill drew attention to palliative care facilities. England's foremost expert, Robert Twycross, claimed that the technology revolution was responsible for alternative treatment centers due to its sometimes unreal and insensitive expectations. Palliative care is patient-centered treatment, shifting the focus from death to life and empowering the patient to make health decisions for as long as possible. Science is used in service of love, and not vice versa.[75] Driven by compassion, relationships are a key element.

The Original Theme of Palliative Care Was Hospitality

Palliative care began as hospitality when, in the fourth century, a *hospis* (c.f., *hospitium*) was a rest stop and meeting place for travelers. In Latin, *pallium* means covering. Monasteries and convents frequently provided lodging while caring for the poor, the ill, and the dying. As part of their vocation, the religious comforted those dying in their quarters and at hospices.

In twentieth-century England, Cicely Saunders changed her life and the future of some hospitals after she encountered the wasting effects of cancer. She studied medicine, practiced nursing, and learned about strong opiods, such as morphine and diamorphine, which relieved cancer victims of their suffering. Cicely became a doctor. While working at St. Joseph's Hospice, she began to administer drugs 24 hours a day, rather than "as required," and this round-the-clock care attracted attention.

Later, palliative care units were opened for the increasing number of AIDS patients as well as end-stage respiratory, cardiac, and renal disease sufferers. There were independent hospices, government-supported care units, home care teams, and hospital palliative care teams. Since children had needs different from older patients, separate houses were created for them. Many children suffered from degenerative neurological diseases associated with congenital metabolic disorders (i.e., DMD, etc.). In contrast to hospitals, these medical facilities made arrangements for family members to stay at the houses with the ill.[76]

The Hospice Encounters Advanced Cultures and Culture Clashes

Doctors and hospitals showed little support for hospices. There was no financial incentive for medical professionals to do so, especially since insurance did not cover hospice stays, and they were arrogant about the science and technology that hospitals provided. Hospices seemed amateur, offering community-based staff that were, mostly, nurses and volunteers. In recent years, hospice care was made compulsory for insurance providers, and now there are more than 2000 individual hospice programs affiliated with the American Hospice Organization.[77]

Palliative care became a solution for many health care providers around the world. When the communist government demoted its senior doctors, the doctors opened hospice groups and asked the Roman Catholic Church for protection. Jan Stjernsward developed comprehensive hospice programs for the early detection of cancer, pain relief, and palliative care on behalf of the World Health Organization (WHO). He described cancer management with inexpensive drugs, including morphine in *Cancer Pain Relief* and published it in 20 languages.[78]

The best a doctor can do for end-of-life patients is to relieve suffering—preserving life becomes increasingly impossible. Patients are encouraged to make quality-of-life decisions in light of aggressive treatment, such as cancer surgery, radiotherapy, chemotherapy, AIDS therapy, and motor neuron treatments (amyotrophic lateral sclerosis), while, simultaneously, recognizing the burden of these treatments on their family members, both psychologically and economically.[79]

Doctors relieve symptoms because it moves the patient toward rehabilitation—both physiologically and psychologically. Short-term improvement can mean five extra years of life with bone secondaries for breast cancer patients, and hormone therapy radically changes prostatic cancer.

In a hospital and at a hospice, knowing when to withdraw treatment mediates compassion and suffering. Artificial respiration by nasogastric tubes, intravenous infusions, antibiotics, and cardiac resuscitation assists a patient through the initial crisis toward recovery of health, but when patients are close to death and do not expect to return to health, technology is of little help. Most doctors agree that it is not unethical to discontinue life support when to do so is the most humane and comfortable treatment for the patient. Professionals often invite the patient or his or her closest relative to decide the time—out of respect for the dignity of the patient or simply to avoid legal incidents.[80] There are guiding points in deciding the appropriate time to let someone go, based on:

- The biological prospects for the patient's recovery or relief
- The therapeutic aim and benefits of each treatment
- The adverse effects of treatment
- The need not to prescribe a lingering death[81]

Hospices take a nurturing attitude toward the dying patient. Some recommend his or her discharge into a home environment, while others wish to provide a sanctuary for the dying. As a patient comes closer to death, hope remains—it is just refocused on *being*. Being valued, being creative, being in relationships with others, and being in a relationship with a Higher Being—God, the Creator, Redeemer, and Sustainer. Palliative care means companionship as well as having a professional available to explain the symptoms that cause fear.

This is different from mainstream medicine, where doctors use distancing behaviors. Medical professionals have some knowledge of treating the psychological and emotional aspects of dying patients, but have little time to follow through. Spiritual needs are left to the family or hospital chaplains.

For Twycross, the hospice environment needs to embrace the human spirit, reflecting upon experiences that give rise to theological reflection, religious responses, and ethical beliefs. Hospice life offers acceptance, affirmation, beauty, and creativity. For those nearing the end of life, there is often a need for forgiveness, reconciliation, and righting relationships. The doctor and the hospice caregiver are not practicing Christian ministry, but experience has shown that people who are dying experience acute guilt, anxiety, incessant fear-based babble, tremendous fear, and perpetual screaming. Like Cicely's experience, drugs alleviate the trauma and provide a sympathetic and spiritual answer, sometimes inducing sleep until death. Those serving in hospices see patients and their families in very stressful situations and have little reason to believe that clergy can calm someone more effectively than drugs.[82] Medical and hospice personnel do not have the same goals as church ministers and may not be aware of this.

The pastor's goal is to assist the dying in making choices about Ultimate issues by mediating a clear conscience, counseling, and praying with the dying patient—often taking advantage of doctor's prescriptions for tempering pain. A professional minister is trained to *be with* a dying person. She reflects with the patient about life, reconciliation, death and resurrection—primarily, in a nonmedical, but compassionate way.[83] Religious people have a "way of living" and a "way of dying."[84]

A physician and a clergyperson are educated in particular fields to deal with specific and very different dimensions of living and dying. The patient benefits most when they respect one another's professional abilities.

Palliative Care: A Model for Living with Congenital Diseases

The hospice is exemplary for those giving health care to patients with congenital diseases. It teaches that life has great value, especially when one is confronted with overwhelming heritable, physical, and mental infirmities. The value of any life is defined by how much someone cares for the person—a patient's health is relationship centered. Professionals from many backgrounds are called upon to work with friends and relatives to create a balanced environment.

Physicians, mental health experts, counselors, nurses, social workers, and ministers are among those who contribute experience and educational resources. Licensed physicians and nurses understand human physiology and the effect of drugs in treating symptoms. Professionals and volunteers can recommend support organizations for emotional issues, medical options, and special educational needs. Care providers are trained in reinforcing positive attitudes, behavior, social acceptance, and nice physical appearances. People who choose hospice appreciate and respect the physically and mentally challenged—knowing and valuing each person for who they are.

Helping a person to refocus on life and personal worth rather than death and losses has a number of effects, including a desire to be fulfilled through activities, decisions, and relationships. It is a time to reconcile differences, to soothe guilt and matters of conscience—to ask forgiveness.[85] Being in the midst of a palliative approach reminds one that he or she may also assist others through organ and tissue donation.

"THE AIM OF MEDICINE IS HEALTH . . .":
DOES MEDICAL SCIENCE MEET IT'S GOAL?

Life is expressed in a physical body, and when the body is healthy, it enhances human flourishing. Medicine means sharing information that builds health. It is about a relationship between the doctor and the patient where they discuss the signs and symptoms of the patient's health by observing the body, recording changes in health, tracking causation, and creating records for the benefit of the greater population.

Understanding the physiology of human health began slowly because the Church feared that interfering with human bodies could damage the soul. Galen gained insight about human anatomy by observing the physiological processes in a spinney-back monkey, but it was Leonardo Da Vinci who dared to dissect human cadavers in the Church's basement. He wrote about the findings and illustrated his discoveries.

People have always been interested in personal health but, as Foucault explained, during the Middle Ages, medical knowledge was in Latin, and it took the French Revolution to extract medical literature from monastic settings and make the information public currency. Opening the channels of information brought about important understandings in treating ailments and living healthier lives. Keeping medical diaries illustrated irregularities in organs, tissues, skeletal structures, and circulatory systems, so surgeons and laboratories could develop treatments. During the industrial age, crowded living conditions, increased stress, lack of sanitation, pollution, and epidemics in the water raised people's awareness of public health issues. Industry also pumped smoke into the air, causing environmental changes that altered human bodies. Observing patients with contagious diseases initiated investigations into bacteria and virology, suggesting that both isolation and sterilization techniques contributed solutions to public health matters. Advances in hygiene and sterilization equipment opened a new way of thinking about disease and contagion.

Medical scientists continue to explore techniques that could remedy the myriad of genetic diseases that have resulted from aggressive scientific and economic policies, such as environmental pollution, nuclear radiation from war and industry, hazardous waste chemicals, and water contamination. Researchers hope to reverse cycles that endanger the health of future generations.[86] The discovery of DNA revealed one of nature's little-understood marvels, and research into its potential provides hope to parents and relatives who suffer from genetic aberrations, whether inherited or environmentally conceived.[87]

What medicine does not want to do is to create an illusion that genetic engineering is the final answer either by solving social ills or physiological dysfunctions. Myth and science became strange bedfellows in the 1930s and 40s, when racial and genetic theories were used to promote an ideology for a healthy, utopian society by purging and purifying Germany's genome—it resulted in the Holocaust. Human diversity was dishonored, and whole families were destroyed, along with their gene pools in a bloodstained history. The warnings contained in the discussion on the philosophy of Holocaust medicine are shadows of present medical ethical issues, such as medicalized reproduction, sterility, abortion, infanticide, euthanasia, genetic enhancement, and engineering. Not all progress has been beneficial, such as nuclear fallout, radiation, etc. Medical science also has a duty to try to alleviate some of the tragedy that resulted from poor science by creating interventions, verifying that a treatment is stable while calculating risks and benefits.

Palliative care is a valid alternative and is receiving more public attention. When the boundaries of life and death are laid bare, disabilities seem less important and life more valuable. This approach to illness lifts up relationships and recognizes the importance of personhood. Dying patients have been subjected to expensive medical technology, but Susan Collins' Gallup Poll on end-of-life care indicated that many Americans would prefer palliative care and pain management in the comfort of their own home. Health care is personal, and decisions reside with patients, their families, and physicians. Age, language, and cultural background affect attitudes toward pain. Some prefer self-administered medications to relieve chronic pain in life-threatening illnesses. Lack of control contributes to depression and anxiety.

Community leaders, such as those associated with DOEA (Department of Elderly Affairs), have been working toward individualized and independent value systems so that patients with differing values are honored. California medical school curricula require classes in pain management and end-of-life care. Hospitals and nursing homes have added a fifth vital sign, pain assessment, to the traditional four (i.e., pulse, temperature, respiration, and blood pressure).[87] Medical professionals are being reminded through legislation, periodicals, and cultural vehicles that decisions about ways of living and ways of dying involve more than opinions from physicians. There are many pathways.[88]

PART II:
APPLYING THE INFORMATION
TO ISSUES IN REPRODUCTION

Chapter 5

Issues Faced
by the Expectant Mother

INTRODUCTION

Motherhood is at the heart of this discussion because it remains at the center of humanity. People in every field of study are interested in understanding how new reproductive technologies and genetics affect mothers and babies, because it changes lives in their own families and communities.

Indeed, theologians, ethicists, lawyers, politicians, physicians, scientists, nurses, sociologists, and scholars have a duty to learn how genetics impacts their area of expertise and to communicate it to the community.[1] The theologian interprets and nurtures the relationship between God and humanity *(imago Dei)*. Ethicists reflect on and communicate the standard of care people owe to one another. The public official is required to negotiate and establish laws that guard the values the community has determined. Physicians and nurses provide health care, while medical technicians analyze the tests and interpret them for the physician who, in turn, discusses alternatives with his or her patient. Scientists detail the chemical algorithms in DNA to describe genetically transferred characteristics, including diseases, from the parents to their offspring. Pregnancy is a very special time in the life of a woman, so genetic screening can provide expectant mothers with the scientific data to guide and reassure them about their reproductive health.

Counseling Pregnancy, Politics, and Biomedicine
© 2007 by The Haworth Press, Inc. All rights reserved.
doi:10.1300/5697_06

Chapter 1 through Chapter 4 presented information related to modern assisted reproduction from the standpoint of theology, ethics, law, and politics, as well as medical experimentation. Clearly, many intellectuals pondered these things, so the woman who faces difficult choices about her pregnancy knows she is not alone. In her search for answers to difficult queries, she receives moral and material support from great men and women.

Chapter 5 (pregnant women) and Chapter 6 (embryos/infants) integrate and elucidate the information from Chapter 1 through Chapter 4. Reflection and application are the new foci.

In this chapter about the dilemmas that women face, theological and ethical reflections pair up to defend against those who challenge women's abilities to make decisions because of their gender. It is not prescriptive, but explains how to apply the previous information to resolve the dilemma. For example, God hardwired women in God's own image, which endowed her with the natural capacity to think and act ethically. This theory moves into the ethical realities of the twenty-first century, embracing the fact that women and men do not process information the same way and do not always agree on what is reasonable and what is not. Each woman needs to take this to a personal level, considering the issues and identifying the information that best resonates with her understanding and the way it affects others. It is to be expected that the reader may understand some theories, but not relate to others.

This chapter will advance women's self-determination, propose changing the masculine clinical model to a more feminine one, present the sociopolitical dynamics of abortion—in court. Furthermore, it will consider the science and industry side of reproduction, and look toward converging Christian principles with legal practices. This section offers encouragement, information, and examples for people to think about, but it does not provide answers. The reader decides. It is of great importance that ministers, partners, and society support women in making independent decisions about difficult pregnancies, so they own their resolutions.

The twenty-first-century woman has been legally emancipated from peculiar myths. The 1948 United Nations Declarations of Human Rights supported gender equality as well as freedom of conscience. Discoveries in human anatomy and biochemistry provided scientific explanations for gender differences, which adequately dismissed biological hierarchy. Nonetheless, the overall tenor of society has been to practice the traditional male orientations.

THE EXPECTANT MOTHER:
ADVANCING SELF-DETERMINATION

Theological and Ethical Reflection and Application: Women were made in the image of God and are naturally equipped to be self-determining. Employing one's mental capabilities in search of the best solution is ethical consciousness. It provides the resolve and fortitude to put the plan into action. Contemplating what is ethical enables moral behavior.

Women make major decisions every day, but pregnant women are often treated as if they are too delicate, clumsy, childlike, and overly emotional to be independent thinkers. Women do have hormonal responses, but they also possess natural wisdom and the capacity to make sound decisions because God created women in the divine image. It is her birthright. Women are natural mothers because they are sensitive, nurturing, relational, and caring. For millennia, women have simultaneously practiced motherhood with a profession and many other activities.

The fact that each person was endowed with a conscience and the ability to reason supports the proposition that the Creator intended women, as well as men, to be self-determining, but early hunter–gatherer myths deemed men biologically superior due to their physical strength.[2] Women were not invited to plan combat strategy. Conquests were attributed to tribal gods; hence, women, as noncombatants, missed the religious teachings.[3] Even after education was systemized, male education was very firmly in place, and women were left outside the system. This hindered their ability to articulate preferences and to enact informed choices. Change was slow, and it was not until the mid-nineteenth century that women received voting privileges and were able to share in moral decision making. But women everywhere realized that it would take time to eradicate several thousand years of demeaning images.[4] In 1948, gender equality was signed into law, based on the premise that all people were created in the image of God: "male and female he [God] created them."[5]

Created in the Image of Christ Means She Is Ethically Conscious and Morally Attuned

In the natural, a healthy woman has the necessary intellect to make ethical decisions. She is cognizant of her thoughts in relation to her conscience. God's primitive ethic is not instant in anyone, but it is generated and shaped dynamically by experience and relationships. In a life-changing move, a woman asks the Holy Spirit of Jesus to dwell with her; she consciously integrates God's Spirit with her Soul-self. The interactivity with the Holy Spirit changes that person's understanding of birth, life, death, and resurrection. Being aware that the Holy Spirit is developing within herself creates an extraordinary understanding about the embryo growing inside of her own body.[6] Since the Holy Spirit is the penultimate ethical and creative being, it is not surprising that Phil Hefner called human beings "created co-creators" or that Richard Niebuhr and Albert Schweitzer envision the "responsible self" or "whole self" overcoming the dilemmas that befall one's body and soul.[7]

The image of Mary, mother of God *(Theotokos),* was a natural symbol for divine stewardship. She was physiologically pregnant with Jesus and, simultaneously, enveloping Holiness. It was the Being within the being.[8] A woman's life *is* moral responsibility. It is the height of embodied meaning because the womb provides the experience for interpersonal consciousness, caring, and the reality of possibly hurting another. A mother's standard of value is measured by her ability to actually care about *whatever* baby is born to her and the ability to displace her own self-centered reality in order to benefit this new person—it is genuine stewardship over God's creation.[9] Within the role of motherhood, a woman first identifies her own self by her ability to care from within that relationship—applying sensitivity and nurture as she shares her body.[10] She literally does for the other as she does for herself.[11]

Every pregnant woman is aware that she will experience enormous pain at the time the baby comes. When a woman carries a baby to full term, she accepts suffering and risks death herself in order to bring the baby into the world. Entering into suffering volitionally does not make a woman mentally deranged as some have labeled it. This is the nature and reality of maternity. Self-sacrifice for the sake of another was modeled by Jesus, the suffering servant, as the penultimate of Christian love and duty according to several very profound thinkers on these subjects, including August Compte, Stephen Pope, and Joseph Fletcher.[12] The labor of childbirth challenges both the mother and the baby.

Every pregnant mother also experiences anxiety about the health of the baby—she realizes that her baby may be born with special medical and educational needs that require an extraordinary sacrifice in her lifestyle—and from members of her community. The mother-child relationship is a sacred bond, not a human right.[13] A woman can love the child for who he or she is far more easily than a person (i.e., father, doctor, etc.) who has not invested his body in the baby's development.[14]

Prenatal Maternity Care Has Built-in Misunderstandings

A patient thinks about pregnancy differently than her doctors and medical technicians. Maternal intelligence is based on reason and instinct. A woman is vulnerable to the idea that medicine and science are superior, and it distracts her intuitive sensibility. When a woman has a prenatal consultation, she is interested in a healthy maternity so the baby will be healthy, and most women presume the doctor will listen to her observations. Paul Tillich warned of "a manipulative, destructive interpretation [of life]" if technical knowledge were to overpower intuitive reason.[15]

In fact, genetic screening has an element of emotional aloofness. The expectant mother finds herself in a sterile clinical setting with technical, unfamiliar language that can be intimidating and give the wrong impression. The technology relies on computer-generated biochemical sequences that are impersonal, i.e., strictly limited to data. Patient confidentiality requires that personal information be kept to a minimum. Rather than receiving a consultation, a patient is processed. Her pregnancy is depersonalized. In a clinical setting, most maternity patients cannot distinguish between research and treatment. Although many genetic procedures are experimental, it is frequently not clear when the patient is participating in a clinical trial. If it is a random trial, she could lose the right to select her preferred treatments.[16]

A maternity patient presumes that all medical professionals are licensed and knowledgeable about anatomy, but scientists are not licensed, and molecular medicine is too young to have many case references.[17] Genetic diagnosis is respected due to its association with science and computers, but it is only *predicting* what might happen.

The counseling environment or doctor's office needs to incorporate a little bedside manner, acknowledge the intimacy of pregnancy, recognize the mother's abilities, and educate her. The expectant mother has been equipped to make sound moral judgments about the screening in a way the technician cannot because, when free to do so, she allows her sensitive nature to interact with the diagnostic information. A professional who educates her patient stands on a solid ethical foundation because it equips the patient to make the best decision possible for all concerned.[18] Education functions in tandem with a woman's conscience in evaluating health matters. It buttresses her discernment capabilities. She is protectively conscious of the baby within her body. She also has a sense of social continuity and the values of society as a whole.[19] Women integrate "character and deed," "person and society," as well as "ends and means" in the interpretation of life, death, and the quality of life.[20] True morality requires liberty, which is a function of will and reason.[21] An expectant woman is rational, intuitive, informed, and reflects upon God's disclosure of God's self. A woman who chooses genetic screening presumes that the information will be handed to her knowledgably and ethically. She has done all she can do. She will be able to complete the process with an educated judgment that is particularized to her situation and goals.

EDUCATING AND COUNSELING MATERNITY IN A MEDICALIZED SETTING

Reflections on Reproductive Medicine and Sensible Applications: A pregnant woman needs to be equipped to make difficult technical decisions concerning two lives—hers and the coming baby's. Good decision making is enforced by a realistic education, which is personalized to suit her particular concerns. She will do best in a friendly environment with sound counseling.

Counseling and education maximize the maternity experience when serious problems are looming in the distance. A person can tackle more complicated issues when she knows how to navigate the terrain, including the types of professionals available to assist her. Doctors, nurses, and social workers are on call because trained genetic counselors are in short supply. Families will be taught how to care for disabilities and integrate special children with siblings. Counselors and support groups guide the emotional needs of women while integrating exercises about grieving, guilt, and self-forgiveness. Knowledge genuinely empowers pregnant women. The mother's rights are *liberty,* not license.[22] Understanding reproductive health and medical alternatives unquestionably give a woman primary agency. Several medical and community resources are available, including the Internet. Providing the information is an ethical responsibility.[23]

Genetic screening alerts women about how to plan education and meet the needs of other family members when genetic problems are suspected. It applies to women who desire to become pregnant or who are expecting and to those aged 38 years or older. It is also applicable to parents who have family histories that are replete with heritable illness, women who have been exposed to environmental hazards, or those who have, otherwise, had difficulties conceiving. Screening examines personal gene sets, ethnic variables, and possible environmental mutations. The physician or counselor should explain the different roles of experts. The doctor, counselor, professional, coach, and teacher can provide details about the technology, develop preferences for genetic engineering, preimplantation diagnosis (PID), prenatal diagnosis (PND), *in utero* surgery, and abortion—or a woman may exercise her right not to know.[24]

The patient must explain *her* goals. Did she come to check the health of the baby? Does she wish to be examined for a particular risk with the intention of eliminating it (if possible)? Is she seeking information about all the genetic potentialities or to consider enhancements? Health competency is only part of the screening process. Counseling adapts the information to personalized issues to sculpt the most suitable decisions.

It is not all genetics. Environmental and industrial hazards are an important part of wise family planning because accidents, such as the Chernobyl nuclear explosion or the Three Mile Island nuclear incident, were responsible for major illnesses affecting myriads of children in the twentieth century.[25] Families are highly mobile and women, especially those who are new to an area, need to be informed about environmental factors that could challenge reproductive health.

Considering the Most Effective Therapy: Finding the Best Place and the Right Professional for Patient-Directed Screening

Conceiving, carrying, and giving birth to a baby are intimate experiences, all of which could be more meaningful if clinics were designed to express the warmth of a family living room, but most are not. Technical equipment, steel furnishings, and colorless sterility bespeak a laboratory setting. Making a woman feel like an experiment is disrespectful of her humanity, as if she were an animal, and it is intimidating. Creating an intimate atmosphere is neither expensive nor difficult, and it confers a gentle, comfortable environment that affirms the value of life. Many hospitals now provide homelike birthing rooms and brightly clad play areas for children. A comfortable location for counseling, teaching reproductive options, and explaining genetic diagnosis encourages a receptive attitude.

Genetic consultants come from a variety of professions: pastoral counseling, primary care, general practitioners, molecular physicians, medical scientists, genetic counselors, psychologists, nurses, and medical assistants.[26] There are as many approaches as there are professionals.

Pastors and Ministers

Pastors and ministers work on issues: matters affecting the partnership or marriage, the helplessness of the couple, blame, resentfulness, social pressure from the family, the infant's personhood, and issues affecting siblings.[27] They pay close attention to those who have lost sight of the image of God in humanity. Clergy need to encourage a healthy mind through hope and the use of sacraments.[28]

Clinical Professionals

Clinical professionals look for: an infant's specialized medical needs; special education for infants and children if there is a mental disability; family support groups for the particular illness; pastoral mentoring and spiritual guidance; personal counseling for psychological adjustments; and adoption programs tailored to match families with disabled infants. Other children at home, economic pressures, and one's country of residence can create exaggerated symptoms. If, for any reason, the expectant woman believes she is physically, emotionally, or financially unable to meet the demands of a handicapped child, she may elect to interrupt the pregnancy.

Women's Issues

Margaret Farley considers embodiment, biorhythms, emotion, and nurture.[29]

Medical Practitioner

James Drane recognizes that some patients will never darken the doorstep of a clergyperson.[30] Therefore, the medical practitioner fills several roles: assistance (i.e., *adsistere*, stand alongside), diagnostic, therapeutic, conversation, truth telling (c.f., spiritual), volitional, affective decision making, builder of respect, and social justice.[31] These qualities mature with experience.

Recognizing Differences of Opinion

The trained physician does not receive the same education as a minister, and vice versa. This needs to be clarified. In addition, maternity patients should be aware that the hospital's review committee does not involve the patient in decision making.[32]

Medical Ethicists

Medical ethicists recommend that a counselor and physician work together. Counseling heritable illness will be emotional because Down's syndrome, cystic fibrosis, economic pressures, etc., can be overwhelming. The parties in a reproductive consultation have differing norms, formed from traditions and customs, family preferences, as well as one's own academic and spiritual background. Glenn McGee suggested that the counselor include her opinion in the discussion. A family will find it easier to release guilt if they know genetic health is affected by behavior, culture, environment, humidity, temperature, nutrition, smells, metabolism, sights, and sounds.[33] Human beings are continually being shaped in character and intelligence—and these attributes cannot be improved by genetic engineering.[34]

Every physician, counselor, and clergyperson needs to listen with sensitivity.[35] Ethical reasoning, interpreting skills, and mediating abilities enable reproductive confidence while conveying an understanding of technology with its risks and benefits.[36] Acceptance of reproductive resources depends on the type of information exchanged and the way it is communicated. Professional terminology and body language can disrupt or empower the learning curve.

Family histories are necessary for health consultations, and the stories engage all the parties as they explore the issues.[37] Using lay terminology places the expert and the patient on the same level, so the descriptions of therapy and its options are easily understood. Intimate ethical issues are encountered, such as nonmarriage, contraception, artificial insemination, elective abortion, gender selection, and infanticide. At some point, the patient expects the professional to explain the appropriate application of the facts. Monitoring the couple's emotions is wise since discussions such as these have resulted in depression and patient suicide. A patient may risk disease rather than terminate a pregnancy if informed that a treatment was available even though there was no cure. One patient sued because the gynecologist did not inform her that a Tay-Sachs pretest was available. New York state denied the action.

Withholding information is justifiable in certain cases. The "duty to warn" may not solicit the "right to know." Discretion is advised in cases such as a woman with XY sexual chromosome (not the XX), a patient with a chronic depressive condition, or the exposure of a non-biological parent. Professional confidentiality is a guarantee of privacy. Although genetic information affects the entire family, a minister or counselor would be wise to obtain consent before contacting any family members.[38] The patient must be allowed to evaluate the burden and suffering in light of the particular family situation.

Recognizing Basic Terminology

Screening provides reproductive confidence when the mother is reassured of being in the normal range. Challenges occur when the tests reveal genetic hazards. When the DNA is screened, the transcription will give a digital account of the biochemical repeats. Each parent's reproductive tissue may be tested separately, but the fertilized egg is the actual subject of the investigation. The discussion goes more smoothly with a common set of definitions, descriptions, and contexts.

Somatic Therapy

Somatic therapy delivers healthy cells to a particular area of a person's body. A sample is evaluated, transcribed, and then the diseased organ or tissue is injected with genetically modified bacteria, viral cells, or yeast to replace the damaged cells. Somatic corrections are performed on the individuals themselves. Somatic changes are not inherited.

Germ Line Therapy

Germ line therapy alters reproductive cells and the affects are inherited from that time forth. Eggs will be extracted from a woman's body and fertilized. The alleles will be altered to enhance the features of the baby or to eliminate the risk of disease. Germ line therapy has bans.

There are two types of screening: preimplantation diagnosis (PID) and prenatal diagnosis (PND).

Preimplantation Diagnosis (PID)

Pharmaceuticals hyperstimulate the production of eggs, i.e. oocytes, which are harvested for fertilization in the laboratory. The entire process is quite uncomfortable. When Tay-Sachs, Duchenne muscular dystrophy, Trisome X, males with an extra Y, etc., are suspected, the sperm are sorted by electrical charging.[39] Later, the healthiest embryos are implanted. Prenatal diagnosis (PND) monitors fetal development.

Prenatal Diagnosis (PND)

PND is invasive because it involves chorionic villus sampling (CVS) of the outer layers of the placenta, alpha-fetoprotein sampling

(AFP blood test or amino screening of blood cells), and amniocentesis.[40] Amniocentesis calls for the insertion of a needle into the abdomen to extract fluid from the amniotic sac. It occurs in the fourteenth week. The mother has a small risk of infection; the fetus has 0.1 percent chance of needle injury, less than 1 percent risk of a spontaneous abortion, and possible respiratory distress syndrome. Amino tests at 8 weeks reveal six times the number of abnormalities as compared to tests at 16 weeks. Early CVS and AFP sampling detect neural tube failure (*spina bifida*), encephally, hydrocephalus, kidney disorders, and congenital heart problems. A high AFT rating indicates neural tube defects, and a low AFT predicts Down's.[41]

In Utero *Surgery*

Surgery requires full consent of the mother, because it has a high risk factor for both mother and baby. The most celebrated success story arose in 2000 when surgeons in Los Angeles repaired a baby's *spina bifida,* a degenerative, painful disease that results in paralysis and death. *In utero* surgery is only recommended where there is no other alternative.[42]

Abortion

Spontaneous abortion frequently occurs in an unhealthy pregnancy, although many women choose to have an abortion rather than have a baby that will be born seriously ill.[43] Barbara Rothman believes early abortions are easier on a woman physically, emotionally, and intellectually. Therapeutic abortion has been selected for sex disorders, dysgenic chromosomes, or for the health of the mother. While compulsory screening has a dicey history, it is now volitional, except for β-thalassaemia.[44] Late abortion is sometimes called infanticide.[45]

The Child's Self-Determination

Given the limited number of therapies, Jean-Marie Mpendawatu voiced concerns about compromising the mother's conscience. Normally, two experts make recommendations. If an expert has reason to believe that there is a need for further research, withholding information may protect a woman's conscience. Mpendawatu suggested preserving the child's individual rights, whenever possible. He disliked subjecting a minor heterozygote to medical intervention and preferred to wait until the embryo became a consenting adult.[46]

The Principled Way Forward

Pregnancy is the only case where the body of one person is required to save the life of another. People do not want to live in a society that compels surgery or sacrifice of body parts. Justice Warren Burger explained that the right to refuse treatment is not limited to "sensible beliefs, valid thoughts, reasonable emotions, or well-founded sensations."[47] The circumstance in which a woman consents to screening and the slow road to adjusting to the decisions that follow is a highly personalized journey. The environment, messenger, teacher, physician, and counselor influence how reproductive technology will be received. No one will ever doubt the moral benefit of having a healthy, homelike environment that offers a team of compassionate experts. The mother-to-be has hard choices ahead that need to be informed and volitional.[48] Hans Jonas admonishes clinicians to remember that medical procedures are definitive actions in a real person's life and "not even the noblest purpose abrogates the obligations this involves."[49]

ABORTION AND THE U.S. CONSTITUTION

Legal reflection and application: Abortion is a legally protected, therapeutic procedure that evacuates the fetus from the mother's womb. A woman's pregnancy is interrupted to prevent physical and emotional suffering of either the mother or the baby, whether due to rape, an intractable illness, or no reason at all.

In the United States, abortion is a very controversial and the most frequently prescribed alternative to an unwanted pregnancy. Regardless of whether a woman decides to abort or to have a disabled baby, there is no easy outcome. The mother–child bond is so fragile a love, yet it requires tremendous courage. The mother who can see beyond the loss of her own dreams for her child and is able to find a child's special abilities while hoping for a cure in the future is indeed a rare case.

There are many reasons why a mother decides not to have a baby but, for most women, it is one that is very painful. When suspicions of a dangerous fetal disposition are confirmed, statistics indicate that she will probably terminate the pregnancy. The mother or father cannot be blamed for genetic aberrations, and not everyone has the resources, emotionally or materially, to provide for the additional educational, medical, or familial care necessary for a special child. After radioactivity blanketed the Chernobyl region, pregnant women aborted or the babies were born disfigured; fearful husbands abandoned the family; and the government was too poor to provide basic staples, much less the medical and educational resources the situation demanded. The bleak reality was painful and women did not want to bring seriously ill children into the world.

Abortion is a legally protected option. There is great moral value in having the choice, the right, to make a fully informed decision, without public or private intimidation. In lieu of trying to justify or denounce abortion, the following pages will present the legal history of abortion and allow the reader to review the reasoning, pros, and cons. Perhaps, after the woman has measured the issues in the legal debates, it will better inform her decision. Liberty of conscience was designed so that a woman could discern the lesser of the two evils. There is no "highest good," so abortion cannot be an ethical value. Nonetheless, abortion weighs life at its most fragile point.

Ethics experts Richard McCormick, Paul Ramsey, Stephen Pope, and Joseph Fletcher have a spectrum of views on the meaning of life, but all the ethical theories in the world are useless until a mother can articulate the reason to herself.[50] She needs to come to terms with the decision. The disappointed woman will try to rationalize and prioritize her choices or else blame herself. Blaming the mother, husband, or family for dysgenic DNA (dysfunctional genes) is not acceptable.

The highest court in the United States decided that its citizens were entitled to procreative choices—without intervention. Choice is at the heart of ethics, otherwise one could not be held responsible for his actions. The public as well as the church spoke for and against the choice. Those involved in the stalwart juridical struggle, both church and state, offer insights about the way public values worked through the issues. Someone facing this decision may find points of identification as well as conflicting values.

To begin with, it must be noted that both the church and the court respect individual freedom, as enshrined in the Bill of Rights. The United States Supreme Court inherited the abortion issue because the *principles* of some groups clashed with the *rights* of others and, eventually, erupted into violence.

Privatizing Maternity Issues

The Legal Activity

Roe v. Wade was the port for this explosively emotional topic.[51] Mrs. Roe wanted an abortion, but the Texas court concluded that the fetus was a person. The law sided with the fetus because it was unable to defend itself. The court said she could govern the affairs of her own body, as long as it did not interfere with the life of another. The decision hinged upon the court's definition of *the beginning of life* and *personhood*.

When the case went to the Supreme Court, the justices researched the definition for personhood, but found it was deeply embedded in religious doctrine.[52] This posed another dilemma because the U.S. Constitution required the courts to: (1) refrain from using religious doctrines that favored one faith over another (i.e., establishment of religion) and (2) protect each person's freedom of conscience (i.e., the free exercise of religion).

The court turned to history. Wanting to discover the Founding Father's original intent, they began with ancient Greek law, knowing that the authors of the Constitution had all studied classics. It did not regulate childbirth or abortion. The closest it came was in patrimonial issues, saying abortion without the father's consent deprived him of his heir and was a criminal offense.[53] Otherwise, Plato suggested abortion was a family management tool and ancient medical texts instructed on abortifacients.[54] In Greek law, the intentional death of a fetus was not a homicide although Hippocrates warned against it. The authors of the American Constitution presumed that human life had great value, and they had no need to define personhood. James Madison had enumerated only preeminent rights: trial by jury, freedom of speech, freedom of press, and liberty of conscience (religious worship and belief).[55] *State v. Winthrop* decided that the fetus, *in utero,* was part of the mother's physiology.[56] Mid-nineteenth-century law delegated childbearing to women.[57] After reviewing all the information, the justices concluded that one became a person *after* he or she was born.

Where the Texas court had decided that the fetus was a person entitled to the protection of the state, the Supreme Court decided that the baby was not a moral or constitutional person until she or he was viable, that is during the third trimester of gestation.[58] Presumably then, the state did not have an interest in the first six months of pregnancy, the time when most abortions occur. After six months, the government had a compelling interest to protect its citizen.[59] Could the state regulate abortion during the six-month period prior to the time it had a compelling interest?

In deciding the *Roe* case, the Supreme Court took into account *Griswold v. Connecticut,* which prohibited government interference in the reproductive life of couples (i.e., regulating contraceptives).[60] As long as the woman gave her consent, the couple could decide to have a baby—or not. It was the mother's decision because, according to *Roe,* the mother may suffer mental and physical injuries if forced to carry a baby to full term against her will; rearing children changes a woman's career and income. There is also a stigma associated with unwed motherhood.[61]

Those opposed to the Court's ruling, such as Tara Kelly, argued that privacy was not a valid reason. She said this devalued the life of the unborn.[62] David Smolin objected to the *Roe* decision because it weakened public morality and confused the mother's responsibility to her unborn child.[63]

As citizens, women were entitled to equality and privacy, according to Anita Allen's view of *Roe.* Just as racial equality was established under the Fourteenth Amendment and the 1964 Civil Rights Act, gender equality deserved equal protection. For Allen, decisions about one's body included reproductive choices.[64]

Kelly, Smolin, and Allen disagreed about placing the fetal life above the mother's interests, but they affirmed the Court's decision to uphold woman's liberty of conscience and bodily integrity. Likewise, all agreed that the baby was entitled to protection, at some stage. For Kelly, Smolin, and the opponents to *Roe,* the Court dealt only with anatomical realities. It ignored consciousness, sentience, and the expectation that the fetus was a potentially rational being. The hands of the Supreme Court were restrained from philosophical and theological considerations, but an intelligent assessment needs a holistic approach, including religious contributions. The court gave both mother and fetus equal status (c.f., Amendments 5, 9, 14). Doctors were free from criminal prosecution if they performed an abortion.

Partitioning pregnancy into trimesters created other problems. Just as the Nazi doctors had to decide when a life was worth living, the state had to decide at what stage of gestation the fetus became a viable citizen, and why.

Planned Parenthood v. Casey (1992) modified *Roe's* trimester system (*Roe*), declaring the embryo was the same unborn human life throughout its evolution or gestation.[65] *Planned Parenthood* handed all maternity decisions over to the mother. The fetus was a whole, continuous, but unborn human life, which did not have constitutional rights above those of its mother. The Court recognized that the mother's conscience spoke for both of them. Decisions are costly in many ways, especially medical ones—they can be very expensive.

Manipulating Financial Resources to Control Abortion

The Legal Activity

For many years, financial aid was available for prenatal care, but opponents of the *Roe* decision did not want to fund abortion, as a matter of principle. *Beal v. Doe, Maher v. Doe,* and *Poelker v. Doe* came before the court because these women were refused aid for abortions, both nontherapeutic and therapeutic.[66] Medicaid was disallowed in *Beal* and *Maher*. A municipal hospital turned down *Poelker.*[67]

Most of the people who needed state aid for abortion were married, underrepresented minorities in low socioeconomic groups; they had other children and were unable to manage another child. When a minority requested aid to end a pregnancy, it was refused because it looked like racial profiling (i.e., compulsory racial discrimination).[68] Biskin explained that refusing aid violated a woman's free exercise of conscience and forced her to have the baby against her will. However, "free exercise" pertained to religion, and the state raised the neutrality flag—it had to take a nonpartisan stand between religion and nonreligion.[69] The most singularly quoted justification against abortion was religious. The Catholic coalition joined the Missouri state officials in drafting and legislating the Hyde Amendment. It prohibited public funding of abortions—except where the mother's life was threatened.[70]

McRae v. Califano alleged that the Hyde Amendment was unconstitutional because it showed favoritism to the Catholic denomination's definition of life.[71] Based on *Epperson v. Arkansas,* McRae argued that the Hyde document violated the "no establishment of religion" clause of the Constitution. It was not facially neutral, lacked secular purpose, and was, in fact, religiously motivated.[72] The lower court disagreed with Mrs. McRae, saying that the law could hold a parallel view with a religious organization and that it did not establish a religion. By the same token, no one would interfere with a legislator who was motivated by religious belief for promoting a law. The statesperson also has free-exercise rights. The Hyde Amendment was deemed religiously neutral.[73] The Court said: "poor women . . . have a right to an abortion, [but] Congress does not have to finance the exercise of that right."[74] No public monies were approved for abortion, not even for the poor.[75]

Restricting Public Aid

The Hyde Amendment used legislative tools and economic sanctions. They were aimed at the poor to curb on-demand abortion. This stirred a wasp's nest for abortions related to heritable diseases. The distribution of resources raised numerous ethical issues.

Freedom of Conscience

Lack of financial resources sets limits on a woman's choices. A mother who is unable to attain medical assistance for an abortion is forced to bring a baby into the world, believing that the child will endure lifelong suffering that abortion could have alleviated. Separation of church and state was intended to prevent statespersons from dictating religious opinions. It was also intended to curb the use of power by religious leaders. A legislature acting as a religious watchdog lacks constitutional acumen. In fact, accidents that create fear for pregnant women occur in the environment, such as the Chernobyl nuclear explosion, water pollution, etc. Denying financial aid for medical services to pregnant women with financial difficulties is highly problematic, constitutionally and morally.

Health for the Financially Privileged

Providing medical assistance only to those who can afford to pay for it discriminates against the poor. Health becomes a matter of privilege. Sometimes, prenatal care requires underwriting travel costs. A family without financial resources has to pay for extraordinary medical care, special education, and training for their special child.

Taking Part in an Experiment in Exchange for Services

University and corporate labs have asked financially disadvantaged patients to participate in experiments in exchange for medical services. In cases of economic necessity, consent may not be volitional. Ironically, public money funds embryo research, but denies abortions.[76]

Observations

The allocation and distribution of resources is ethically challenging. Many countries consider health care an entitlement right. Financial and professional provisions are guaranteed. The United States has not made this commitment, but it is ethically imperative that Americans pioneer medical cooperation to cover the cost of technology as well as rising health and insurance costs. Educational programs can also teach individuals how to participate in their own health goals.

The Use of Sex Education to Justify Withholding Abortion Funding

The Legal Activity

In the years following the Hyde Amendment, Congress made Title XX funds available to all educational facilities to teach responsible premarital sex using a preset government program. Teachers came from both secular and religious backgrounds. It was called the Adolescent Family Life Act (AFLA, 1981).[77] Plaintiffs, including clergy, the American Jewish Council, and taxpayers challenged the AFLA.

Bowen v. Kendrick alleged a conflict of interest and a violation of the Establishment Clause, because the grants only permitted the government's viewpoint; religious leaders were forced to use secular venues.[78] Justices Blackmun, Brennan, Marshall, and Stevens did not think religious groups should participate because the people attending the programs were not looking for religious values.[79] On the other hand, Title XX funds were community oriented and invited qualified teachers, regardless of faith.[80] They simply had to refrain from having discussions involving religious ideas. Patients were provided with medical pamphlets. Information that might prejudice a young woman against abortion was omitted. For example, women were not told that scar tissue from abortions, in many cases, prevents future pregnancies. That is, she might never be able to have another baby.[81]

Concerned groups set up sidewalk counseling centers near abortion facilities. They were determined to give patients the downside of abortion, hoping to persuade them not to abort.

The AFLA had provided classes about responsible sex, but the problems were much deeper—cultural, employment, bad living conditions, etc. Women who were already pregnant received sex education when they couldn't afford the cost of the children they already had.[82] The state was trying to control opinion that differed from its own. In an attempt to balance secular and religious opinions, a "no counseling" caveat was instated.

Counseling Was Part of the Human Fertilization and Embryology Act (1990), But Was Omitted from the Abortion Act[83]

Patients participating in genetic screening realized that abortion might be the only option to prevent the painful life and death of a child. In order to be self-determining, patients who have reproductive screening need to be educated and counseled about the technology and its options—in lay language. In addition, abortion is often approached as if it were a plumbing procedure. Eliminate the fetus and the problem is solved. Health is not mechanical, nor is it value neutral. Disease is a biological dysfunction, which causes symptoms in one's personal life. There is a physical threat that is accompanied by loss of self-esteem, loss of hair, lack of artistic ability, and loss of independence due to dependence on medical treatments. Bodily disabilities change a person's activities, the lives of the family, even the unconscious mind as well as hope for the future. A human being is greater than a biological organ and must be treated as a whole person, because health affects behavior and behavior affects Ultimate issues. A healthy physical equilibrium is not value neutral.[84]

Most women having amino screening have never experienced grief from the loss of a baby. This needs attention and sympathy; tragedy should not be privatized. The baby cannot be replaced like mechanical parts—it remains a traumatic experience.[85] Not permitting doctors who performed abortions to give counseling may have been well advised. The sidewalk counseling was likely to have been unprofessional, but the decision to refuse comprehensive counseling sessions altogether was not a patient-oriented decision—it was political and financial.

What Were the Goals of the Lawmakers?
Did They Abandon Constitutional Principles
for Monied and Professional Interests?

The Legal Activities

Madsen v. Women's Health Center changed attitudes toward fundamental liberties and health services. The goals of both constitutional law and medicine had lost touch with principles by the time *National Organization for Women v. Scheidler* entered the abortion bullring.[86] On the surface, many thought *Madsen* was a contest between politics and religion, but, as the plot unfolded, it revealed a clandestine elitism—the glorification of medicine, educated professionals, and monied interests. *Madsen* began by enforcing rights that protected women's access to abortion services.[87] The law sided with medical professionals, who were annoyed by sidewalk counselors. To them, the counselors were antiabortion activists and religious radicals. On the contrary, the protestors thought the risks needed to be explained to the women before they committed themselves to the procedure.[88]

Florida's Legal Action

The *Freedom of Access to Clinic Entrances Act of 1993* (FACE) ordered a 36-foot buffer zone. This allowed an area in which patients could continue to pass through for abortions while conscientious objectors stood on the sidelines saying what was on their minds.[89]

Challenge to State

Activists demanded an explanation. Sidewalk counselors believed their constitutional freedoms were violated by preventing them access to the patients, saying patients should be protected from "undue governmental influence," not from persons with different viewpoints. They wanted proof that the state had a compelling interest that justified barring the free exercise of religion, freedom of speech, freedom of assembly, etc.

Florida Responds

The court dismissed the challenge, saying the act was neutral to religion and that it did not need to show any compelling state interest.[90]

Allegations Against the Court

The citizens asserted censorship.[91] Hubbell enumerated the infringement of rights and freedoms that required the state to show cause.[92] The religious protestors claimed it was a fundamental right to persuade others to act, based on *Cantwell* and *Schneider.*[93]

The Court Justified Its Legal Position

Griggs agreed with the court's decision in this case, saying freedom of speech was not an absolute right.[94] Kelly joined several legal analysts with the opinion that "any right must yield to the rights of others." Herein, the protesters' right to free speech did not supersede privacy and safety. Ergo, the government had an interest in protecting the women's medical care.[95] Kelly quoted Justice Oliver Wendell Holmes: genuine freedom of expression requires "not free thought for those who agree with us, but freedom for the thought we hate."[96]

Justice Scalia disagreed with the rest of the court. He did not believe protecting abortion rights was a compelling interest for the state, and he was riveted by the suspension of the aforementioned constitutional issues. The government's interest, according to the O'Brien case, was to further the first amendment freedoms.[97] The FACE act was one-sided.[98]

Violators to Be Prosecuted As Criminals

The litigation criminalized all protests at abortion clinics. Local and federal law agencies and the FBI enforced fines and imprisonment. When it appeared that there might be an interstate campaign of violence toward clinic activities, the Department of Justice got involved.[99]

Suspending Constitutional Rights

With criminal sanctions imposed against sidewalk counselors, a *chill* fell on free speech.[100]

The Supreme Court Defended the Business of Abortion

National Organization for Women v. Scheidler criminalized protests at abortion clinics under the Racketeer Influenced Corrupt Organizations Act (RICO).[101] RICO quashed *Clairbourne's* decision supporting freedom of assembly and radically free speech.[102] Protestors were no longer conscientious objectors, according to *Scheidler,* but federal felons.[103]

Law Was Intended to Serve Human Interests

Law interprets the will and norms of the culture. The court had a responsibility to preserve and protect the very foundations of the U.S. Constitution and its original intent (Mesoethics). The early Supreme Court rulings made family matters private. With the woman's consent, couples decided to use birth control, have a baby, or interrupt a pregnancy. These were individual human rights. With the abortion cases, federal aid, and public sex education, the family issues of underprivileged people became public matters. Irreligion was preferred to religion. In fact, irreligion was a type of religion; it was a secular religion. Scalia's scathing dissent highlighted the corruption of basic First Amendment liberties, but the Supreme Court also failed women. It never provided abortion patients with the information that scar tissue could prevent future pregnanices and it omitted disclosure of the full scope of the risks and benefits of abortions.

The Tangled Web of Law and Technology

The Supreme Court justices in the *Roe* case were not aware that their definition of personhood would be used for genetic manipulation, nor were they privy to this understanding of *imago Dei*. Nonetheless, the judicial conclusions expressly communicated that the unborn fetus was an evolving human life and that the mother had the nearest understanding of what was best for that life. Procreative issues were not to be infringed upon.

Church communities respect human life because people were made in the image of God. Christian denominations have differing explanations, but scripture tells the reader that the human body was made to be God's activity in the world. Those arguing against abortion did not anticipate that abortion might be a realistic and compassionate answer for couples wishing to prevent serious, painful, debilitating diseases in their offspring. Those concerned about reproductive ethics wanted to protect the value of being human and worried that human life might be devalued by on-demand abortion or through experiments on human tissue.

When the technology revolution changed reproductive medicine, ethical ideals fell like dominos. Researchers were licensed to imitate nature, fertilizing eggs and inventing new genetic constructions. The time for manipulating fertilized eggs was originally set before the cells began to take on human characteristics at differentiation, but that changed, too.

Today, the embryo's "continuous, unborn human life," faces human cloning, stem cell research, cryopreservation, and destruction when an embryo is not implanted. The liberty guaranteed by the U.S. Constitution still has an uphill battle.

Human Cloning

Some argued that human cloning violated the "right to life, liberty, and property without due process of law" because the clone was denied a natural gestation. No sperm was needed so it was asexual reproduction. No one knew how it would affect the ensuing life, but a fully-grown embryo will never have its own DNA since its genes are identical to its sponsor. His or her DNA, the very fabric of its nucleus, was from someone else's property.[104]

Stem Cell Research

Embryonic stem cell (ES) research manipulates the embryo in order to harvest specific cells for making bones, tissues, and organs. The woman is given drugs to hyperstimulate her egg production. Her body is debilitated in this process. When the eggs containing the stem cells are harvested, she, literally, becomes like a human test tube. If the woman did this because she needed money, it was not a free choice, but one of economic necessity. The fetus was also a mere instrument of science; it was made to be killed. Were an experimental embryo ever to reach maturity, he or she would be mutated. Human stem cells are often in the same petri dish with other animal cells. If the animal cells had viruses, these could be fatal if transferred to humans (c.f., HIV/AIDS). At one time, it was illegal to combine human DNA with other species, but now it is part of the genomics plan.[105]

Cryopreservation

It is uncertain how this affects the health of an embryo.

Destruction of Embryos

The owners of embryos must give directions about the future use or destruction of the embryos.[106]

Commerce of Human Tissues, Organs, and Bodies

Scientists recouped the cost of experimental fertilization by accepting grant money from the government and private corporations; reproductive services were sold to anyone who could pay, including the buying and selling of frozen embryos. After General Electric won its patent for a genetically engineered bacterium, reproductive engineering became patentable and, therefore, its properties were subject to ownership. This made life forms a saleable commodity and warranted genes-for-profit.[107]

Legislators can debate morality, and judges can issue decisions. Whether or not the laws are just remains subject to review.

MOTIVATING ETHICS VIS-À-VIS LEGISLATING PROCREATIVE TECHNOLOGY

Locating a fulcrum and taking responsibility: Procreative choices are private. In the United States, there are no laws protecting women from unethical practices or errors that occur as a result of reproductive innovation and technology, except "assault and battery."

This discussion presents ethical dilemmas that are meshed into the fabric of reproductive science and technology, as well as the practical responses of political experts who also know science. In the U.S., objections to legislating genetics have come from several directions—research scientists, biomedical and scientific corporations, lawyers, and the public. Academics deplore any restriction of intellectual research; corporations want to patent the genius they employ for the cash harvest. If it is legislated, the victims will have to go to court to get remedies, and most courts are ill-prepared to adjudicate reproductive technology and are unaware that they are underqualified to do so or do not think it is relevant. The rules of evidence are inadequate for the task and tend to favor professionals and monied interests. In addition, procedural law is too insensitive for such intimate subject matter. So, how does society protect itself from exploitive and abusive situations? In order to protect women who can only get pregnant with a doctor's help, there will need to be legislation. Positing laws is the way society functions. The Europeans and international legal societies have contributed a respectable body of law, even considering that science is light years ahead of bureaucracy. Due to the way legal structures evolved, many laws are in general agreement with Christian tenants. Some of those principles will be addressed in the following.

Educating the users about the technology bridges the gaps where the law has not yet made an impression. Just as moral behavior can be taught to men and women of science, reproductive techniques can be explained to the maternity patients who use these. Women who are expecting babies in this day and age need on-site education, because it was not available to most of them in school. This is where experience and education work well in favor of Christian principles.

There are several professionals who are knowledgeable about reproductive matters, despite the insufficient number of genetic counselors. Many clergypersons study medical ethics in seminary. Religious professionals prefer to equip people to be self-determining, because it shapes the ethical soul. Ministers are ideally suited to counsel difficult pregnancies and walk through the grief that strikes those faced with serious illness or the death of a baby. Doctors' legal liability decreases when their patients make their own decisions. In a democratic society where education is mandatory and litigation proliferates, it makes more sense to teach patients about state-of-the-art medical techniques and practice ethical medicine than it does to legislate morality. Otherwise, law schools will have to develop curriculum on biomedicine, and judicial procedures will need to be civilized to include compassion and the etiquette necessary to deal with sensitive issues.

Scientific Knowledge and Responsibility

Government Grants

Genetic scientists encountered an increase in public scrutiny due to the flood of press surrounding DNA, some of whom could not resist the use of inflammatory insinuations (monster babies). The National Institutes of Health (NIH) made government grants conditional on conforming to specific guidelines because medically assisted procreation is mostly experimental. In light of genetic diagnosis, there is much to consider. Weighing the values poses real challenges.

Doctors and Families

Doctors admit that they do not have all the answers, but try to balance medical ethics somewhere between happiness and pain. David Morley finds nothing wrong with this utilitarian approach as long as physicians hold fast to the rights of the individual. Patient rights provide a corrective to purely utilitarian attitudes.[108]

The social, emotional, and financial consequences affect parents, siblings, and the community. Special children may be rejected by their own families. Institutional care is crowded and expensive. Morley reminds people facing tough decisions that unavoidable temporary consequences are not necessarily final solutions. Who decides? The doctor–patient relationship fosters a learning experience, so parents can be involved in the diagnosis from the beginning. They have to balance the tension between preserving life and preventing suffering.

Edward Slater argued that the prevention of suffering comes before the preservation of life. He suggested what had previously been unthinkable—that it was merciful not to preserve the life of a seriously disabled infant. After delivery, the physician usually attends to the child, parents, and hospital staff, that is, the nurses and other care givers who have been affected by the birth of a baby with a serious disorder. He also has to bear in mind the distribution of limited medical, institutional, and special education resources. Staying focused on locating the highest good in difficult situations is in keeping with the superior value system that most Christians hope to find.[109]

The Pros and Cons of Science Professionals

There are rich pools of experience for empowering and equipping decisions for a difficult pregnancy. Science may be seen positively as a fountain of knowledge that creates the technical means to promote health and the sanctity of life. *Sciencia* means knowledge in Latin. It is a systematic search for truth and not intended for self-aggrandizement, although that does sometimes happen. It requires freedom of inquiry, but the findings are published and taught. Publishers must report responsibly and are expected to disclose risks and benefits.[110]

It is satisfying to know that the research environment has structural guidelines and controls. Professional societies regulate grant monies. In hospitals, there are human subject review committees (HSRB, a.k.a. IRB) with professional and lay participants. Opinions from the research subjects as well as scientific colleagues are part of the process. Ethics committees have an obligation to respect the religious values of families, although it poses a formidable challenge.

There are also gaping holes for scientific endeavors to go astray. It is impractical to license scientific experimentation because discovery is incalculable. The scientist is the only one who understands the experiment and when normal conventions are inadequate, she or he is responsible for weighing the principles, values, and consequences. Philosophical ethics were not part of most scientists' training. Institutional safeguards set the standards; they are not necessarily consistent with the values of the surrounding community. Problematic issues are not reported to employers, but to professional societies. This is less effective, yet avoids job conflicts.[111]

Baruch Brody researched ways in which scientific integrity might be preserved by having specific policies about disclosure. What type of disclosures should institutions require? To name a few challenges, there are conflicts of interest, ethical compromises, commercial incentives, grants, free laboratory equipment, money, finder's fees, equity (stock), patents, copyrights, trademarks, royalties, etc. Monitoring and managing compromised values means taking one of four courses of action: eliminating all financial incentives, divesting interests, a complete withdrawal from the study, or asking one to step down as principal investigator (PI), but stay on the project. Penalties include oral reprimands, written reprimands, modified compensation, less office or lab space, fewer assistants, salary reduction, fines, restraints on publication, probational disqualification from research, or permanent suspension from employment.[112]

Can the Public Determine Ethical Codes for Scientists?

Most ethical constraints come from within the scientific industry, because the federal government cannot legally interfere with state policies or private businesses. Brody's suggestions were aimed at internal institutional regulation. If corporations imposed sanctions, secrecy would ensue. Researchers and corporations can go underground or move to a new location. A corporation is a legal person—without a conscience. Medicine has nearly entirely been incorporated by management companies (HMOs), government health administrators (NHS), etc. Stockholders are concerned with the bottom line, and they fund public officials. Court authorities are among these. In fact, the courts did chill the public conscience for what appeared to be monetary interests. Scientific freedom is great news for the academy and commerce, but is it good news for expectant women—the subjects of the new reproductive techniques? Many bioethicists would like to concretize standards in reproductive medicine.

Ethical Laws and Guidelines that Correspond with Christian Church Positions for the Legislation of Genetic Diagnosis

Bioethics is about respecting human life, male and female, rich and poor—in all of our wonderful diversity. Organized religion has a very substantial interest in having its congregations healthy and protected by law. The church is concerned that the God-human relationship be enhanced—beginning with the anthropological and psychological, because these feed its theological goals.

Individual human beings do not need any more restrictions, but they do need to be protected from being used as means either for scientific experiments or for corporate profit. One way to protect communicants is to educate every man and women to participate in their own health decisions. This means people inside and outside the faith community. Another protection is to bring businesses and professionals under the legal umbrella.

Over the years, several legal, medical, scientific, and religious experts from around the world have collaborated in writing legislation on health, human rights and modern reproductive technology. Treaties include the European Convention on Human Rights (1950), the Treaty of Rome (1957), the United Nations Convention on the Rights of the Child (1989), the European Convention on Human Rights and Biomedicine (1997), as well as declarations from UNESCO's International Bioethics Committee. Where rules are absent, it does not mean that there is an abuse of the law. Making laws is simply a precaution.

The global community is in various stages of understanding procreative issues, because it needs to consider cultural precepts as well as the gradual nature of human understanding, acceptance, and consent. The material discussed below uses broad definitions and has standards that allow soft, medium, and hard applications because community values and fears of abuse vary. All of the contributors used the following definitions with sliding degrees of application:

National Decisions About Preimplantation Diagnosis (PID)

Artificial reproductive technology (ART) is used for avoiding the transmission of serious inherited disorders. PID requires consent and is legal in private clinics in the US and Canada. Due to the increased potential for eugenic application, discrimination, and abuse, the Scandinavian consensus recommends PID only for serious cases. Canada restricts sex selection to serious gender-related illnesses.

National Decisions About Prenatal Diagnosis (PND)

PND is used to evaluate embryos for heritable or other disorders. PND requires informed consent and is legal in public and private medical facilities (United States, Canada, Scandinavia, etc.). Commercialization of PND kits marginalizes the poor.

National Decisions About Genetic Testing

Genetic testing requires consent in Australia. Testing for maternity and paternity is universally accepted as a valid form of identification. Restrictions: young children are excluded so as not to burden them with difficult decisions (Scandinavia); presymptomatic testing only for diseases where therapy is available (Scandinavia); prohibition of adolescent testing for adult cumulative diseases (Canada). Parents who failed to be tested for genetically-passed illnesses have been subjected to suits for wrongful life by children who now suffer from detectable diseases (Canada). There can be no uniform standard defining normal DNA.

National Decisions About Information Dissemination

The release of personal genetic information requires patient approval, generally speaking, before the doctor can divulge information, which is wrong, in principle, in cases where family and community members could otherwise avoid tragedy. Some countries consider genetic information family property, so there are degrees of responsibility as to who has access to genetic information. Disclosure to family members is required when there is a high probability of irreversible or fatal harm (Canada). Carriers of heritable diseases must be identified and, in Australia, family dysgenic information is obligatory. Genetic predispositions have the potential to threaten employment opportunities as well as health and life insurance.

Academic Freedom

Scholarship and academic research will remain open, but professional misconduct cannot be tolerated among doctors, hospitals, universities, professional labs and institutions, and licensing authorities.

Eugenics

Eugenics has received minimal attention in this book because it reaches into things like plastic surgery, but there is strong opposition to any alterations in the genetic line when these could be inherited. It poses a generational injustice because offspring are affected by genetic engineering, but are not yet alive to give consent. The expense of eugenics marginalizes people of lower economic groups.[113]

Practical Steps the Government Can Take

- Fund facilities to train genetic diagnosis teachers and counselors
- Create grants, scholarships, and benefits to encourage growth of the profession
- Pass laws to institute education and provide counseling as well as teaching services at prenatal facilities, genetic diagnosis centers, and clinics
- Pass laws with heavy sanctions for any person who does not behave professionally, respecting all human life and other living creatures

Guillod's Recommendations

Professor O. Guillod, Institute of Health Law, showcased Swiss solutions to reproductive issues. These have much in common with Christian interests. He recommended:

- The pre-embryo be accorded the status of a regular human being
- A series of sanctions, including prohibitions on germline therapy, hybrids, chimeras, freezing embryos, and sex selection
- The child has a right to his or her natural genes (no eugenic surgery)
- Permission to trace parentage using DNA fingerprints for health reasons
- Parents act as representatives for their minor children
- All information remain strictly confidential, unless specific consent is given to release it
- Nondiscrimination[114]

Feuillet-Le Minitier Recommendations

Mrs. B. Feuillet-Le Minitier came to alternative conclusions in view of diverse religious attitudes and the rights of women, sperm, and egg donors as well as people with differing abilities:

- Identify legal personality at birth. Currently, it contradicts existing inheritance laws, since a fetus can inherit property while still *in utero*
- Protect physical integrity by enforcing privacy, informed consent, equality before the law, and eliminating frivolous human research
- Be aware that genetic diagnosis and abortion marginalize the handicapped; note that character based on social being, endangers biological being
- Weigh the importance of disclosing biological parents compared to the responsibility owed to anonymous, altruistic donor parents[115]

Of course, self-determination is the correct ethic. One thinks, deliberates, rationalizes, decides, and acts upon one's own choices, all of which yields true moral responsibility. The ultimate goal is to value humanity so highly that there is no need for law enforcement, because each possesses a well-developed ethic that comes naturally.[116] It is within human capacity to make ethical decisions without laws. Indeed, it is the very goal of *imago Dei* to prosper in the fullness of ethical expression, but precautions need to be enacted to protect against corporate abuse of people's health needs, especially the activity surrounding the human genome and the lives of expectant mothers.

Chapter 6

The Moral Status of the Embryo

INTRODUCTION

The discovery of DNA overwhelmed the world of health science as explorations into nanospace took on great significance. The task so far has been to explore how this marvelous discovery impacted procreative choices. Prenatal diagnosis (PND) and preimplantation diagnosis (PID) developed an avenue for tackling heritable diseases but, is the embryo itself compromised by recent trends in experimentation? Reproductive technology aspires to generate medical miracles—some of which are yet to come into existence. To date, the bottom line for a troubled pregnancy has been to interrupt it, which contradicts the Hippocratic Oath tradition that bid doctors not to abort the fetus. Most Western countries permit therapeutic and elective abortion. The previous chapter dealt with some of the discomforts and dilemmas women encounter as a result of reproductive technology, and it looked at how Western law systems dealt with these.

This chapter takes a fresh look at the fetus, the child-to-be who is immediately and physically affected by state-of-the-art medicine. The philosophical task at hand is to develop a compelling, defensible, and appropriate bioethic toward the human fetus. Bioethics, by definition, respects the human body and promotes its ethical treatment. Chapter 6 integrates and elucidates the information from Chapter 1 through Chapter 4 as it considers issues affecting the moral status of the embryo, which is already more difficult than issues concerning the mother, since the embryo is in the process of maturing, physically and consciously. The embryo expresses its awareness with its whole

Counseling Pregnancy, Politics, and Biomedicine
© 2007 by The Haworth Press, Inc. All rights reserved.
doi:10.1300/5697_07

body. For example, if the mother takes a drink of an alcoholic beverage, the baby shifts position in the mother's womb. Therefore, ascribing value and meaning involves some level of physical consideration— science intersects theology, ethics, and law. To decide whether or not there is a convincing case for the moral status of the embryo, the reader needs to take this to a personal level and consider how the information is relevant to the issues. The discussion is uncomfortable and emotionally charged, so expect to wrestle with it. One immediately discovers that reproductive science has become immensely complex.

When researchers discovered that blood and stem cells from the fetal cords of aborted fetuses could be used therapeutically for other patients, the picture became strange indeed. The aborted fetus became the treatment, an object of pharmacology, and scientists wanted more fetuses with which to experiment. With fetal stem cell research, a utilitarian standard was placed on human fetal life. In modern reproductive medicine, a fertilized embryo has become a tradable commodity. Commercial interests are increasing. DNA engineering, fetal stem cell research, a market-driven economy, and competing interests suggest the devaluation of human life and a need for stronger movement toward restraints.

Hence, it is appropriate to consider what the fetus *is*. What is its moral and physical status as a developing person? These pages will begin by discussing fetal life as a *potential person*. The discussion follows the chronology of experimentation, since the earliest assistance to an endangered fetus used ultrasonography and *in utero* surgery. Its subject was a 22-week-old embryo, which made the fetus a patient, together with its mother.

It was not until much later that scientists learned how to change human gametes (fertilized embryos), even though they were invisible to the human eye. These miniscule cells responded to the brightness of the light when placed under light microscopy. They were alive, had the potential to become human beings, and were worth saving. Experimentation lasted up to but not after human characteristics developed, i.e., differentiation.

Fetal research grew from there, and medical reproductive technology (MRT) specialists wanted to create and use the *sui generis* human fetuses for testing their theories. Hence, the zygote offers technical value to the medical community. There are alternatives however. With the denaturing of fetal cells, those performing the experiments began to dehumanize the fetus. Its material value entered genomic research, which seeks to increase health resources and, with it reap financial gain. In order to justify the experiments, the genetic data must be collected, stored, and evaluated. Were personal information to become public, it has the potential to stigmatize families. It also creates a genetic underclass of those who cannot afford the technology. Society and the Church have grave concerns about devaluing the human fetus in favor of its instrumental value. While many countries created regulations for reproductive and genetic experimentation, the United States had no laws governing private practices, making it easy for abuses to occur.

When human rights experts authored the Declaration of Universal Norms for Bioethics, it contained enduring values. During its drafting, governments representing whole populations and faith traditions alike agreed that human beings must never become objects used for research. There is something wrong when people who were created in the image of God become instruments of scientific research. At the end of the chapter, a brief but impressive case makes the point that drives home the point.

REFLECTIONS ON THE STATUS OF THE FETUS

Thesis: In an age of technology, theological reflections on the embryo need to think about God as a relationship.

The interdependency of the mother and fetus has been distinguished in myth and religion as a sacred state of being. Fetal gestation was revered as the fountain of human life. Fertility was a religion. Later, the relationship of the mother and child was deified in Christianity. Times have changed. Becoming pregnant and caring for the *in utero* life of the baby has been medicalized.

This chapter reflects on the fetus as a second patient not in competition with its mother but as a separate entity. The fetus is a human life, a gift that deserves care, nurture, good health, and every opportunity to fulfill his or her potential. From the womb of time, God had a design for every life and desired to see it flourish. In certain cases, man's negligence and miscalculated experiments have corrupted the natural environment, affecting genetic health and generating other unhealthy states, preventing some fetuses from reaching maturity.

The Desire to Save and Enhance Human Life During Gestation

Michael Harrison began to experiment with *in utero* treatments on lambs in 1978 to learn surgical techniques that would help save human lives. The size and physiology of a gestating lamb resembled that of a human fetus. By 1985, he was able to remove a 23-week-old human fetus from its mother's womb to unblock its urinary track; the fetus was later returned to the mother's uterus. Mitchell was born nine weeks later through a second cesarean section.[1]

In cases of difficult pregnancies, the options, according to Professor Steinbock, were surgery or termination. In rare cases, life-threatening respiratory and renal problems could be repaired between 20 and 30 weeks *in utero*; then, the fetus develops as normal. The baby could be delivered early for an operation, either by inducing labor or by cesarean section, or the baby could go full term and then receive surgery.[2]

In Mitchell's case, bed rest and drugs prevented labor and miscarriage; he was placed on ventilatory support for four weeks and monitored until he was six years of age.[3] Mitchell's heart and nervous system were especially at risk,[4] which brought severe criticism down on Dr. Harrison.

Criticism about his experiments and the moral duty owed to an embryo prompted discussions as to how much *suffering* the fetus actually endures during medical intervention. Does a fetus know pain when under the surgical knife? Do abortion techniques cause the fetus to suffer? Early speculation led to the conclusion that embryos in early gestation were not conscious and did not experience pain until 22 weeks because of an underdeveloped nervous system. Without consciousness or the ability to feel, the fetus had no moral status up to, at least—22 weeks. Similarly, an encephalic infant or those in a permanent vegetative state (PVS) had no moral status. Babies and the elderly had a stage when they were unable to articulate pain or pleasure, but their lives were valued. Society would not allow experiments on a patient in PVS unless it would clearly benefit the person. No one desired suffering, but when the risk of pain and death were very high, everyone agreed that the species mattered. Humans were not the same as other animals. The human fetus could become a living sentient, conscious person and, given a lifespan, had the potential to change the world.[5]

Measuring the Boundaries of Fetal Life

The moral status of the fetus meant reflecting upon the boundaries of life, especially the beginning of life. When a baby is only an *idea,* its value lives in the imagination of its parents. Living in hope and ex- pectation of having a family is not a palpable calculation, but human beings have a natural proclivity to reproduce and, for millennia, have understood that intercourse leads to progeny. Emotional concepts in- clude physical realities, but the wish or desire to have children differs significantly from an intellectual approach to the study of human life. Today, religion, social relationships, natural evolution, and scientific data shape most worldviews about what a fetus *is*. The meaning is dependent on the context of contemplation.

Very astute scientific thinkers rightly argued against a scientist's ability to be emotionally neutral and objective, since all analyses were influenced by the analyzer's upbringing, cultural background, school- ing, etc. Nonetheless, observable, positive (physical) measurements are still part of the public education process of describing human life. There is no going back on this.

Technically, a new life begins when the sperm fertilizes the egg and a unique DNA is created. By the four- or eight-cell stage, prenatal diagnosis or preimplantation diagnosis can forecast reproductive confidence or genetic problems. Ethically, fetal therapy is intended to benefit the fetus itself. Any diversion from this norm leads to various grades of dehumanization. When unhealthy cells or supernumerous embryos are about to be discarded, a technician may consider these merely as primitive cells and turn toward their pharmaceutical uses, such as medical treatment for others. For H. Edgar, it was ethical to use an embryo for transplant surgery and experimentation when it would have been discarded anyway.

Typically, science universalizes concepts. If it is ethical to use dis- cardable cells in surgery, human or animal, it would be ethical and of great utility to create embryos in the lab for experimental purposes.[6] After it was discovered that blood from the umbilical cord had no rejection properties, scientists hypothesized that fetal cells had the same high adaptability to nearly every human blood and tissue phenotype. Its experimental attraction became enormous. Empirically speaking, the closer the embryo was to its primitive nature, the less it resembled a human being and appeared lower on the hierarchical scale of evolution. With limited functional maturity, the embryo was treated with a sliding degree of respect.[7]

There is a need for social reflection when science earmarks a fetus as a therapeutic marvel. It is arguable that there is a moral obligation to a not-yet-born fetus—as an endangered species.[8] Mentally and physically, fertilization gives rise to a human life.

The following statements consider the zygote in a literal fashion and, simultaneously, portray it with meaning and connections, which go beyond the natural to awe and wonder.

- The embryo is a continual link to humanness—and, arguably, to God.
- Ova and sperm are components of a zygote; a zygote becomes an embryo; an embryo becomes a fetus. There are differing levels of respect—ova and sperm are not accorded the same respect as the fertilized zygote; an *in vitro* zygote does *not* have the potential to become a human being unless it is implanted.[9] Note: Asexual reproduction, such as used for cloning, does not suit this definition.
- When the sperm fertilizes the egg, it creates a new DNA that constitutes a personal monograph and generates a chemical basis for lineage, while still of its same heritage.
- The zygote is the stage after fertilization and before the primitive streak when it will twin and differentiate.[10]
- A zygote is willfully conceived in a procreative effort to produce a baby, *in vivo* or *in vitro*. It has the capacity to develop into a person, i.e., it is alive.
- One biologist marked individualization at the thirteenth day of embryonic development.[11]
- The embryo lacks the capacity to experience features of life, which are essential to a meaningful existence, such as the full use of its five senses.
- The fetal body is a vessel containing life that, unhindered, will develop into a complex organism, evolving in size and form.

- The embryo is preconscious. Consciousness is material in evaluating personhood. Experiments on embryos in the uterus indicate that the environment and the mother's behavior affect the fetus; when it is born as a human baby, a complex personality has already begun, and the child's cultural environment will enhance what was already a plenipotent human life.[12]

Indeed, people are communal beings from the time of fertilization. The coming together of sperm and egg is a communal function. Together, they form a new DNA. The multiplication of cells bearing the new identity develops into a zygote, fetus, infant, child, and adult. What was once a community of cells forms a person who becomes part of a larger community, endowed with the capacity to contribute to those relationships. The ongoing process of education and experience changes his or her awareness.[13] Each stage contributes to a fuller person. Consciousness, intertwined with culture, has particular social attributes, such as intentionality.[14]

A baby is conscious, but not necessarily intentional; a mentally disabled adult can lack intentionality and still be a member of the community. Society recognizes the human worth of both a baby and a disabled person. It also shows respect for the dead. One born into a free, democratic, and constitutional environment is entitled to life, liberty, and property. One also has the right to conscious choices that will enrich the divine-human personality. The person has the right to explore faith to the end, so that he or she may do what is right and be ethically responsible. Members of society are not to be used as a means to an end because the person is the end.[15] A person is defined by his or her community, identifies with the society, and faithfully communicates community values from generation to generation. This takes love and cohesion, and a vision for the future. Responsibility is a high moral calling.

One human life can perpetuate generations. Although different groups cannot agree when life starts or what exactly life is, holistic views tend to be pragmatic. For Roman Catholics, fertilization begins life; for Jews it is the fortieth day; and materialists mark the primitive streak or implantation as life's beginning. Others, such as Steinbock, revere sentience and consciousness as the seat of being fully human. Joseph Schenker defines life by defining death as an irreversible loss of that life.[16]

ETHICAL REFLECTIONS ON THE MORALITY
OF USING A FETUS FOR HUMAN HEALTH

Thesis: The value of a fetus' life depends on the ability of those closest to it to love it. The moral status of a fetus is based on family relationships, and when defined by his or her social utility, this detracts from its value.

The results of genetic diagnosis often yield death, not life, since there is no therapy for most genetic insufficiencies. The fetus loses its intrinsic value with a prediction of bad genetic health, and this encourages abortion. A strange twist occurs when the embryo can be used for stem cell therapy; it develops an external value and becomes means to a happier end for someone else. George Boer and John Robertson insist that abortion and the use of the fetal remains are separate issues. Abortion has been the subject of endless controversy in the United States, and experts believe that the motivation for interrupting a pregnancy determines its ethical tone. The moral outcome for fetal cell research relies on the separation of abortion from the practical utility of a dysgenic zygote.[17]

In the case of a spontaneous abortion, the use of fetal tissue has no ethical problems in itself. If the fetus were expelled due to contamination, introducing diseased cells into stem cell therapy might be a different moral issue, but using a nonviable fetus (i.e., loss of heartbeat or breath) does not pose moral problems if consent was obtained in advance. There are also no problems with administering transfusions and performing therapy using postpartum cord blood, except that blood has a short shelf life.[18]

The real problems arise when one conceives a fetus for the sake of stem cell research or therapy. There are important ethical cautions against stem cell research.

- Creating embryos for research increases the risk of consanguine donors and related diseases, such as hemophilia.[19]
- Research to patent genetic treatments pays its human subjects, mostly women, for their reproductive tissues. George Annas denounced conception-for-profit because it demeaned women as fetal-containers.[20]
- Assigning a monetary value to a human fetus devalues its life.[21]

Justice Michael Kirby confirmed that despite the nobility of research for health projects, respect toward human beings declined and moral practices diminished with each utilitarian application. Economically poor individuals form a new underclass, since they are unable to afford the treatments, but can receive them in exchange for experimental rights—donors were set up for adverse psychological effects. Corporate grants for university experiments are often conditional on the companies obtaining patent rights. Kirby and Yang found that, sadly, the product was often part of the human community and the providers were commercially exploited.[22] In many cases, moral acceptability was and is crafted by its market value. If someone wants to purchase something, it is worth investigating. When monetary gain sculpts morality, greed turns morality on its head.

Good intention is not forlorn. Those arguing in favor of fetal research hope to invent and provide new treatments, but their arguments necessarily depersonify the fetus in order to justify its use. Zygotes, fetuses, and embryos are referred to as cells, tissues, organs, etc. Following the Holocaust, moral accountability and civil controls became critical. For this reason, laboratory investigators prefer to privatize decisions; therefore, parents became responsible for granting permission to experiment on aborted fetuses.[23]

Schenker and Boer drew the moral road map concerning fetal tissue transplant (FTTR).[24]

- Informed consent was valid if donation was not coerced and there was sufficient time for consideration between the abortion and its medicalization.
- In emergencies, even with consent, FTTR is morally unacceptable because the mother does not have enough time to consider the decision.
- Consent is not valid if it lacks specific purpose.
- There are legal conflicts between protecting vulnerable donors and protecting rights of privacy.[25]
- Donation is defensible when the mother has an abortion to protect her health.
- FTTR is morally troubling when the life of a fetus is terminated by withholding treatment (i.e., encephalic, without cranium or cerebral hemispheres).

- FTTR is moral and uncompromised if the donor does not designate the recipient.
- Donation is morally sound when there is no financial gain.
- Morally, the physician should not benefit from the subsequent use of the gift.[26]

Currently, based on the above arguments, Kirby, Yang, Boer, and Schenker do not favor the use of a human fetus for research. Creating embryos for general research and donating aborted fetuses for fetal tissue transplant (FTTR) are riddled with dignity issues.

The majority of moral commentaries on science projects considered the advent and growth of a fetus into a person as something reserved for the particular fetus itself, not for society. The information, overall, attributes a genuine moral status to each developing human life by linking the material fetus to its potential, so that every human being has the opportunity to develop—even the God-human relationship. The evidence of conflicting practices justifies some type of formal regulation or restriction.

ZYGOTE RESEARCH

Thesis: The fetus bears a unique life passing through several developmental cycles as it fills out its humanness. Each level is part of the whole, and the fetus remains whole at each stage of life.

Curiosity cannot be arrested and science has always encouraged research. From a scientific perspective, zygote research and fetal therapy are exciting. New DNA cells are vivacious with life and potential. Since stem cells differentiate into cells and tissues of all kinds, they have a wide potential for neural and blood applications. Rapid generation proffers libraries of tissues for researchers.[27] Scientists cannot resist performing clinical trials using human fetuses, although genetic screening was intended to benefit the fetus itself. The problem is that a zygote can become a live person who is connected to the community—even members of the scientific community prefer alternative sources.[28]

Trials exploring alternative resources, such as stem cell research, take time and are funded by grants from pharmaceutical companies, private firms, and governmental health agencies. Companies develop new products to replace those that are expiring and always need new markets to sustain and increase profitability. Businesspersons offering grants to researchers want an attractive product and a quick return on their investment.

Scientists, government health services, and corporations were overwhelmed when they discovered umbilical cord blood could contravene problems of matching tissue and blood types. The mother was on one end of the umbilical cord and the fetus at the other. Deductively, fetal cells were presumed to provide the answer to alleviating rejection factors. This changed the aims of clinical trials, methods, quality control, and the ethical climate governing the scientific environment.

There are three types of stem cells. Embryonic *totipotent* cells develop into any tissue, and, if implanted in the uterus, they become a baby. *Pluripotent* cells are derived from embryos for tissue formation and, once removed, can be kept alive in an artificial medium, proliferating almost endlessly with no chance of ever becoming a living person. Scientists manipulate *multipotent* cells into a limited number of tissue types.[29]

This means that there are alternatives to using fetal stem cells by replacing them with (1) adult stem cells, (2) transferring DNA to denatured cells, or (3) performing experiments with animal tissues. Adult stem cells supply bone marrow, liver, lung, cardiac, or neural cells that form neurons, astrocytes, and oligodendrocytes. Adult stem cells are reasonably adaptable, but lose potency as they age.[30] When the patient's own DNA or that of a close relative is used to cultivate tissues for the transplant, rejection is diminished. It requires time to prepare, and some people do not have that luxury.

Therapeutic cloning, transferring DNA to other cells, reprograms the nucleus of embryo cells to match the recipient's blood or tissue type. These totipotent cells avoid immunity and rejection, but the patient runs the risk of uncontrolled proliferation of the transplanted cells, as well as the transmission of infectious diseases. This is less likely with embryo cells than adult cells.[31]

The third avenue is animal experimentation and xenotransplantation. It practices its art by transferring DNA to a denatured cell of another species *via* ectogenesis, parthenogenesis, the fusion of female gametes and crossing species using various cloning techniques. After HIV erupted like Mount Vesuvius as a result of mixing the body fluids of monkeys with humans, crossing animal species raised red flags. Since it generated immune deficiencies and other rejections, xeno-transplantation and animal experiments continued cautiously.

As a result, reproductive technology learned about stabilizing multi-zygote pregnancies by observing this in animals. Removing embry-onic stem cells (ES) from mice demonstrated the generation of cardiac muscle cells, hematopoietic (blood) cells, pancreatic cells, neural cells, etc. Investigating the DNA of primates contributed to the therapy used for Parkinson's disease. Although these experiments were valu-able, animal processes do not automatically transfer to human situa-tions.[32]

Alternative research in all these areas made great strides forward. Infant mortality has been reduced, and infertility treatments have been discovered. Microinjection of sperm into the *zona pellicula*, the egg's outer membrane, revealed when the gamete was ready to be transferred into the uterus to maximize healthy fertilization and avoid/reduce multiple fetuses. Zygote freezing, storage, and thawing tech-niques improved. Understanding the metabolism inside the uterus revealed ways in which antigen immunities could be used for contra-ception.[33] Reproductive and fertility trials have come a long way, but these need to be distinguished from fetal stem cell research. The rea-son is important. After an embryo was disconnected from its human-ness, one scientist was totally unable to distinguish between fertility studies and stem cell research.[34]

Knowing what science can and cannot do matters. Reproductive issues exist in the present, and stem cell therapy is still an art in prog-ress. Scientists hope that stem cells will treat neurological disorders, heart blockages, bone diseases, cancer, immune deficiency, and dia-betes. Pickel and McCall Smith forecast repairing damage to the myelin sheath and improving Parkinson's, Alzheimer's, and multiple sclerosis.[35] Sadly, there was no evidence behind the miraculous re-covery of a Parkinson's patient who received a transplant of six fe-tuses at a clinic in Mexico. The publication sought approval to detach the fetus's intrinsic value as a continuing human life by exonerating its noble sacrifice to treat a disease—or was the fetus just a jumble of molecules? Today, people hope fetal cells will be able to repair or replace every human property that anyone could ever need, even reinventing one's own body for spare parts when the other one's are worn out. Professionals have classified every combination with a potential for curing major health problems.[36]

Gathering Ethical Perspectives into One Basket

The fact is, medical experimentation progressed so rapidly that the public voice has been chilled, which means it has no audible conscience. Questioning or criticizing science often results in an insult about one's intelligence, but science has ethical and moral contradictions.

Respect for Human Dignity and Reverence for Life

Respect for human dignity and reverence for life are overarching principles. These terms were used by Albert Schweitzer and Gandhi in addition to Christian ethicists. Human zygotes have the potential to be fully human despite being confused with property. Life, the *bios*, is not a human invention and cannot be invented or patented. Humans do not reproduce asexually, so cloning violates the unborn person's right to be human. Such practices raise serious challenges to the Bill of Rights, as well as the sacred connotation of "right" as described in Pauline texts.

Freedom of Conscience

Freedom of conscience was based on ethics. Human subject research requires fully informed, volitional consent, as a matter of conscience. Conscience is inviolable and immaterial, so humanity cannot be defined solely in material terms—it contradicts the meaning of conscience.

Do No Malfeasance

Do no malfeasance was challenged when the 14-day/8-cell stage was extended to the 16-cell stage. The change from a zygote to a fetus, the sign of humanization, was no longer a serious boundary. Creating human embryos without intending implantation interrupts its human potential. Intentionally manipulating a fetus that carries mutations resulting from experimentation into childhood is malevolent behavior, exceeding child abuse. To create human embryos for FTTR research is not the same as donating an organ.

Every Human Life Is an End in Itself

Every human life is an end in itself, not a material means to someone else's end.[37]

Truthfulness

Truthfulness is offended when hypotheses are represented as material facts. Claiming discoveries before the fact to obtain research grants does not make them real.

There Is a Moral Responsibility to Communicate Scientific Information to the Community

Patents hinder this duty because researchers cease investigating projects, publication ends, and the information line dies. Patents are thought to contradict the duty to share knowledge.

Justice

Justice involves equal opportunity. An underclass is created when reproductive health care services do not benefit all women or subordinates the poor to serve the experimental needs of others. Discrimination is an issue when resources are too expensive or inaccessible.

Autonomy

Autonomy is jilted when researchers entice someone to sell eggs, sperm, womb, etc., by exchanging money or medical services for human procreation. Note that the sale of human organs was prohibited to preserve the dignity of the whole person.

Being Born into the Human Family Generates Rights Greater than other Species

When something is not permissible for animals, it is difficult to justify the procedure on fetuses.

These are but a few general observations, but they are sufficient to show that ethics are sliding. This problem compels the public to demand a broadly based lay forum to regulate reproductive ethics, genetics, and fetal experimentation. John Robertson scoffed at lay participation, saying the lay community was not astute enough to write ethics, nor were they necessary for licensing research.[38] The fact remains that reproductive and molecular medicine developed an unhealthy branch, one that has dehumanized and denatured the very life they were proposing to save.

Public opinion has prompted international representatives to draft resolutions.[39] Numerous experts carefully examined the risks and benefits of reproductive therapy, the ethical use of diagnostic procedures, technology relating to human fetuses, as well as the consequences of privatizing and disseminating personal genetic information. Members of the church community also provided well-informed comments about reproductive science and theology to legislative forums.

SUMMONING ETHICAL PRINCIPLES INTO LEGAL PERSPECTIVES

Thesis: Law is a reflection of the public conscience from the culture in which it is made. In a world in which business and science are transnational, law becomes a global responsibility.

There is, indeed, value and necessity in exchanging cross-cultural information, because most Western nations are populated by citizens from a variety of cultures and religions. The high mobility of scientists and corporations also provides an incentive for nations to form alliances for the enforcement of reproductive values.[40] Cultural diversity is a rich part of human heritage, and it validates minorities whose individual rights need to be protected by human rights legislation.

Among those deserving of protection are the weak, the vulnerable, and some who have differing abilities. Handicapped individuals are extremely hurt and offended by a culture that treats disabilities, ones they live with daily, on the same level as disease.[41] This comes from the terminology inherent to DNA. The genetic alphabet, short as it is, calls irregularities "spelling errors," suggesting that disabled people are [spelling] mistakes, but everyone has differing abilities and disabled persons do not consider themselves "spelling errors." In that regard, all human life needs to be mined for its unseen potential, especially human beings created by a God who is invisible, but whose work is manifestly expressed in human lives and is extended to a variety of cultures.

The Self in Self-Determination

Philosophers argue that within every human personality there is a higher self, which is entitled to self-determination, as a personal right, i.e., a human right. This ideal drove Immanuel Kant, J. S. Mill, and John Locke. From the *Magna Carta* to the U.S. Bill of Rights, constitutional principles defend life, liberty, and the pursuit of happiness. The right to a healthy existence was presumed. Both God and governments wanted humankind to care for one another. From a government perspective, unborn babies were future citizens of the country; St. Paul considered babes in Christian faith as future citizens of heaven.[42] Generations yet to be born have much to be concerned about in the wake of biotechnology. Indeed, important genetic decisions that pass to unborn children could be made, without consent. Hence, there is a necessity to establish bioethical rules.

Working Toward Broad Sociocultural Moral Agreement

International politicians have been in the process of mediating and harmonizing medical practices and cultural rights. The broad range of views cultivated a compromise between prohibitions and permissions. Some wanted strict controls that specified what, if any, exceptions applied to embryo research. The lack of boundaries has not worked.[43] As with many bioethicists, stem cell expert McCall Smith prefers guidelines recognizing sociocultural values and encouragement for new discoveries.[44]

Government Overreaching

Americans hesitate about legislating bioethics for fear of government overreaching, but federalism exists. When the U.S. government allocated public funds for research, reproductive medicine entered the federal jurisdiction; family issues remained at the state level. The separation of powers has its own fallacies extending to federal, state, judicial, executive, and legislative branches. Separation does not prohibit agencies from interpreting laws to suit their needs. One branch can undo another.

Market-Driven Economy and Procreative Tourism

Legislation is advisable in a market-driven economy such as the United States, and also where procreative tourism exists. That usually occurs when a person goes to a place that permits what another nation prohibits. Although science is completely external to law, economic activity is directly applicable to law.

Discovery and *invention* need to be defined due to biopatenting and intellectual property rights. Justice Robinson, The Hague court, defined them. *Discovery* applies to things in or about nature. *Invention* applies to that which is made by human hands.[45] When human beings are the center of discovery and a market exists, such as for fetal tissue transplants, laws are necessary. Business professionals make administrative decisions, but they do not contemplate and write ethical policies.

The Human Embryo, Research, and Zones of Respect

Revel and McCall Smith, UNESCO, presented the basics about humanly engineered fetuses.[46] Embryos created by *in vitro* fertilization (IVF) can be implanted *in utero*. Three-quarters of the embryos that are fertilized but not implanted go to stem cell research because they were unacceptable for implantation or would be destroyed. Therapeutic cloning occurs when the nucleus of a donor is transferred to a denucleated egg, oocyte, and it can also be used to grow stem cells for research, but not for implantation.

In light of the above formulas for making embryos, McCall Smith and Revel presented the following observations and recommendations.[47]

- An embryo with the potential to develop into a person should not be the subject of research; it has a human status and is entitled to respect.

- Low-quality embryos should not be implanted and, therefore, lack human potential. As long as there are no commercial motives, these are suitable for stem cell research.
- Creating embryos for stem cell research creates a separate class of embryos. Nonetheless, they deserve equal respect before the law and protection from discrimination.
- Therapeutic cloning is objectionable because it is one step away from reproductive cloning.

Informed Consent and Fetal Experimentation

Informed consent is especially important in the collection of sperm, eggs, and tissues for experimentation. Donors need to know the purpose of the research, its methods, and the specific ways the egg or sperm will be used. Samples are only to be used for that purpose. Consent must be expressed, free, voluntary, and fully informed. Each new trial requires new consent. The donor needs to be given the right to withdraw consent at any time. Embryo donation is not advised as a commercial transaction, property, an object of barter, or for a profitable venture because no human being can own another human being, or even a zygote who will "be." The principal investigators need to verify the accuracy of all representations and that every experiment involving a fetus is therapeutically beneficial to humankind. Independent evaluators need to oversee embryo trials and make sure that experimental zygotes are never implanted.

Genetic Data and Privacy

The information used for scientific trials is personal. Privacy and confidentiality need to be protected in all cases. Information that might harm an individual is not to go outside of the research because circulating personal information leads to a new genetic underclass that could suffer prejudices in health, education, insurance, and employment. Appointing independent observers assists in maintaining nonbiased conclusions, but all those involved in fetal and genetic experimentation need to be reminded that genetic data is personal. Canadian George Radwanski argued that storing data compels its abuse.[48]

The UNESCO Genetic Data document details information germane to reproductive screening as it respects fetal life, autonomy, privacy, property, equality, nondiscrimination, justice, and solidarity.[49] It also covers counseling, informed consent, withdrawal of consent, reproductive education, confidentiality, anonymity, use of postmortem samples, and the rights of children.

Both secular and ecclesiastical viewpoints uphold the value of fetal life. The U.S. Supreme Court affirmed the embryo as a whole, continuous person, while religious law was committed to protecting ethical values centered on humanity created in the image of God. The secular bridge between constitutional law and Divine law, which provides a vehicle for moral continuity, comes from ensuring liberty of conscience.

Freedom of Conscience

Terminating a pregnancy affects the conscience of the expectant woman, the father, the nurses, doctors, etc. The conscience is very fragile, and every person that makes a decision to interrupt a pregnancy deserves the time and opportunity to reflect on what is best for the future of the fetus. It is intimidating and unkind to burden a woman who has just learned that her fetus is extremely ill by asking her to decide whether or not she intends to donate her baby to medical research, organ transplants, etc. Investigators must also live with their conscience, so it is best not to create a situation in which someone has to depend on the tragedy of genetic aberrations and abortion to obtain grants and fulfill their research goals. The Hippocratic Oath and the no-malfeasance rule serve the consciences of physicians, scientists, and the patients. Profiting from the disappointment and misfortune of others weakens the conscience. The goal of medicine is human health, not performing moral acrobatics with an individual who is grieving. The business of genetic diagnosis, reproductive technology, and alternative research methodologies has been to improve infant mortality. Creating human embryos for experimentation, with the express intent of destroying them later, has a bipolar element to it and a great potential for abuse. Likewise, the conscience is conflicted by altering human germ cells, creating an underclass of embryos, experimenting on fetuses and whole-cloned embryos—even when it may potentially avert severe heritable diseases (i.e., Tay Sachs, etc.). In addition, cloning disrupts the entire cytoplasmic structure of a cell, altering its properties such as the mitochondria, etc. It begs the question as to whether there can even be a healthy regeneration of reproductive cells. If cloned embryos did mature, the telomere problem remains (e.g., animal experiments cannot guarantee that humans are exempt), along with the eventuality of accidentally creating someone with disabilities. These are things that we simply cannot know.

After scrutinizing and weighing ethical principles concerning fetal research, a business' motivation to create a product, and realize therapeutic achievements, a need is indicated for additional moral balancing. There are a myriad of concerns involving not only fetal stem cells, but the parties to the research (i.e., parents, scientists, corporate stockholders, etc.). As it presently stands, respect for human life needs a *bonafide* way of doing science; one which does not pretend that life is no more than a jumble of cells. Human cells are highly adaptable, growing at amazing rates, but human life itself is also a profound mystery. The church, by its very nature, stands hand in hand with disabled individuals, and it recognizes that the status of the fetus is more about "being alive" than it is about genetics.

WHAT SCIENCE CANNOT KNOW

The Ball Case

As case studies are a common practice, it is appropriate to reflect upon the case of Marshall Stewart Ball.[50] It challenges human ability to determine the value of life at any stage of growth, based on visual and physical evidence alone. Although a body can be isolated for examination, God is creative and instills that gift into his creation, which is expressed in the subtle and the miraculous (see Exhibit 6.1).

In Conclusion

To wit, science has plenty to learn about life and about consciousness, even at the at the microcellular level. At present, the scientist cannot look at what appears to be a jumble of cells and simply deduce that the life form has no value. Scientific method requires that the truth of each experiment be challenged, tested, retested, and falsified— yet fetal experimentation ends in the death of the only thing that could falsify it. The test of knowledge must take place before conclusions can be published. There is much to be learned about fetal life.

EXHIBIT 6.1. The Marshall Stewart Ball case.

Marshall Stewart Ball was born with a perfectly normal phenotype, or so it appeared to the physicians and his family. Mrs. Ball began to notice that he was not developing like the other toddlers; his neuromuscular system did not mature, grand mal seizures began, his stare was blank, and his face recorded no emotion or expression. At the age of three, Marshall had no muscular control; he could not talk, crawl, or play. He could not return his parents' love in any external way, but they continued to speak to him and teach him.

In a moment of excitement while hearing a story with animal sounds, Marshall moved one finger. This signaled to his mother that "someone was in there." His mother taught him how to use his finger to tap out letters on a board. His very first message was a lovely poem that explained who God was for him, and it gave his mother incredible hope for her son. She contacted Dr. Lawrence Becker, who worked with prodigies and savants but not, unfortunately, with disabled children. Dr. Becker watched as Marshall tapped out a few words on his minikeyboard: "Even though my individuality finds knowing perfection, I listen for the answers to wishes from above."

Some time later, Marshall wrote a book of collected poems for his father's birthday present. The introduction was strangely beautiful: "Questions nicely want good answers. . . . I hope to gather thinkers, to give them my thoughts and love." This boy sits perfectly still and stares blankly into space, yet out of the depths of silence poetry awakened— there was life in his personal universe that science could not have predicted—and probably would have extinguished. Although he completely lacked communication skills, Marshall's book sold more than 195,000 copies. This is more than what most authors achieve today. Marshall's life was his words. His struggle became a story of valor, which entered and touched many lives. He was alive and, therefore, free to meet his potential.

Sources: Troylyn Ball, "The Mystery of Marshall," *Guideposts* 55(11) (January 2001), 56-60. Marshall Ball, *Kiss of God: The Wisdom of a Silent Child* (Austin, TX: n.p., n.d.)

It is possible to create a "flesh-made 'word'" using applied genetics, but how could science even come close to imitating the sensitivity and beauty that springs to life in the "'Word-made' flesh"? Humankind was made in God's image because God desired to sovereignly create and sculpt human beings into *logoi* who will live within God's Eternal Being. It is a great, incalculable mystery!

Appendix

Legal Documents and Cases

GOVERNMENT DOCUMENTS

Charters

Charter of Paris for a New Europe, Paris, 21 November 1990.
African Charter. 1981. *Human and People's Rights.*

Constitutions (See National Documents: Constitutions)

Covenants

United Nations Secretariat. 1966. *Covenant on Civil and Political Rights.*
United Nations Secretariat. 1966. *Covenant on Economic, Social, and Cultural Rights.*
United Nations Secretariat. 1996. *International Covenant on Civil and Political Rights.*

Conventions

Organization of American States. 1969. *American Convention on Human Rights.*
Council of Europe. 1997. *Convention on Human Rights and Biomedicine.*
Council of Europe. 1998. *Additional Protocol to the Convention for the Protection of Human Rights and Dignity of the Human Being with Regard to the Application of Biology and Medicine, on the Prohibition of Cloning Human Beings.*
European Union. 2000. *Convention, Charter of Fundamental Rights of the European.*
United Nations Secretariat. 1992. *Convention on Biological Diversity.*

United Nations Secretariat. 1965. *Convention on the Elimination of All Forms of Racial Discrimination.*

United Nations Secretariat. 1948. *Convention on the Prevention and Punishment of the Crime of Genocide.*

United Nations Secretariat. 1971. *Convention on the Prohibition of the Development, Production and Stockpiling of Bacteriological (Biological) and Toxin Weapons and on their Destruction.*

United Nations Secretariat. 1997. *Convention for the Protection of Human Rights and the Dignity of the Human Being with Regard to the Application of Biology and Medicine.*

United Nations Secretariat. 1985. *Convention on the Rights of the Child.*

United Nations Secretariat. Department of Education, Science, and Cultural Organization (UNESCO). *Convention against Discrimination in Education. 1960.*

Conventions concerning Intellectual Property. *Bern Convention for the Protection of Literary and Artistic Works.* 1886.

Conventions concerning Intellectual Property. *Budapest Treaty of the WIPO on International Recognition of the Deposit of Microorganisms for the Purposes of Patent Procedures.* 1977.

Conventions concerning Intellectual Property. *Paris Convention for the Protection of Industrial Property.* 1883. (Revised 14 July 1967).

Conventions concerning Intellectual Property. *Trade Related Aspects of Intellectual Property Rights Agreement (TRIPs) annexed to the Agreement establishing the World Trade Organization.* 1995.

Conventions concerning Intellectual Property. United Nations Secretariat. Department of Education, Science, and Cultural Organization (UNESCO). *Universal Copyright Convention.* 1952. (Revision 24 July 1971).

Declarations

Counsel of Europe. Parliamentary Assembly. *Written Declaration No. 247.* Strasbourg, France, 26 April 1996.

United Nations Secretariat. 1985. *Declaration on Basic Principles of Justice on Victims of Crimes and Abuse of Power.*

United Nations Secretariat. 1979. *Declaration on the Elimination of All Forms of Discrimination against Women.*

United Nations Secretariat. 1971. *Declaration on the Rights of Mentally Retarded Persons.*

United Nations Secretariat. 1975. *Declaration on the Rights of Disabled Persons.*

United Nations Secretariat. 1948. *Universal Declaration of Human Rights.*

United Nations Secretariat. Department of Education, Science, and Cultural Organization (UNESCO). *Declaration on Race and Racial Prejudice.* 1978.

United Nations Secretariat. 1989. *Rights of the Child.* Arts. 8, 29.

United Nations Secretariat. Department of Education, Science, and Cultural Organization (UNESCO)—Bioethics Committee (IBC). 1997. *Universal Declaration on the Human Genome and Human Rights.*

United Nations Secretariat. Department of Education, Science, and Cultural Organization (UNESCO). *Declaration of the Principles of International Cultural Co-operation.* 1966.

Recommendations

United Nations Secretariat. Department of Education, Science, and Cultural Organization (UNESCO). *Recommendation on the Status of Scientific Researchers.* 1974.

Resolutions

Council of Europe. 2000. *Resolution on Human Cloning on the European Parliament of 7 September 2000.*

Intellectual Property. In accordance with *Preamble to the Universal Declaration of Human Rights.* 22 C/Resolution 13.1, 23 C/Resolution 13.1, 24 C/Resolution 13.1, 25 C/Resolutions 5.2 and 7.3, 27 C/Resolution 5.15 and 28 C/Resolutions 1.12, 2.1 and 2.2.

Rules, Guidelines

United Nations Secretariat. 1993. *Standard Rules on the Equalization of Opportunities for Persons with Disabilities.*

United Nations Secretariat. Department of the International Labor Organization. *Convention (No. 111) Concerning Discrimination in Respect of Employment and Occupation.* 1958.

United Nations Secretariat. Department of the International Labor Organization. *Convention (No. 169) Concerning Indigenous and tribal Peoples in Independent Countries.* 1989.

NATIONAL DOCUMENTS

Constitutions

Right of Association
Belgium, Art. 20 Constitution. *Right of Association.*
Denmark. Art. 78-1 Const. Act. *Right of Association.*

Germany. 1964. Art. 9 Basic Law, Art. 30. *Right of Association.* (Prussian Constitution 1850).
Greece. 1975. Art. 12-1. Constitution. *Right of Association.*
Italy. 1991. Art. 2 Const. Charter. *Right of Association.*
Luxembourg. 1928. Art. 26. *Right of Association.* (Const. 17 Oct. 1868).
Netherlands. 1848 Constitution. *Right of Association.*
Portugal. 1976. Sec. 41. *Right of Association*
Spain. Act of 24 Dec. 1964 (Sec. 3, para. 1). *Right of Association* amended 1987 Const.
Switzerland. 1974. Art. 56. Fed. Constitution. *Right of Association.*
Reproductive Technology
Ecuador. 5 June 1998. *Constitution.*
Ireland. 1 July 1937 (amended 7 October 1983). *Constitution.*
Switzerland. 18 April 1999. *Constitution.*

Legislation

Australia. 2001. *Gene Technology Act 2000.*
Austria. 1992. Law no. 275 on reproductive medicine.
Brazil. Law no. 8974/95 of 5 January 1995 on genetic engineering.
Costa Rica. Law no. 7739 of 1998 *Code of Childhood and Adolescence.*
Finland. 1999. Statute no. 488/1999. *Medical Research Act.*
France. 1994. Law no. 94-654. *On the donation and use of elements and products of the human body, medically assisted procreation and prenatal diagnosis.*
Germany. 1990. *Federal Embryo Protection Law.*
Hungary. 1992. Law no. LXXIX. *On protection of the life of the embryo.*
Japan. 2000. *Law concerning regulation relating to the techniques of human cloning and on the similar techniques.*
Norway. 1997. Law no. 29. *On the medical use of biotechnology.* (Amendment of Law no. 56, 1994).
Peru. Law no. 26.842. *General Law of Public Health/Law;* no. 27.337 *Code of Childhood and Adolescence.*
Poland. 1996. *On family planning, protection of the human fetus and the admissibility conditions for the artificial termination of pregnancy.* (Amendment of Law, 1993).
Spain. 1988. Law no. 35. *On assisted reproduction procedures.*
Sweden. 1991. Law no. 115. *On measures relating to the use of human fertilized oocytes for research or therapeutic purposes.*
United Kingdom. 2001. *Human Fertilization and Embryology Act/Law.* (Amendment of the *Human Fertilization and Embryology Act,* 1 November 1990).

Bills

Belgium. Senate. *Protection of embryos.*
France. Draft of the revised "Bioethics Law," presented by the Prime Minister on 28 November 2000.
Italy. Bill no. 4048. *On the discipline of medically assisted procreation.*
Netherlands. *Rules relating to the use of gametes and embryos* (a.k.a., *Embryos Bill*).
Pontificia Academia Pro Vita. August 2000. *Declaration on the Production and the Scientific and Therapeutic Use of Human Embryonic Stem Cells.*
United States of America. National Bioethics Advisory Commission (under President Clinton, now disbanded). *Ethical Issues in Human Stem Cell Research.*
United States of America. National Institutes of Health. 2000. *Guidelines for Research Using Human Pluripotent Stem Cells.* (Amendment of 1999 Guidelines).

STATES SUPREME COURT CASES

Allegheny v. ACLU, 109 S. Ct. 3036 (1989).
Beal v. Doe, 432 U.S. 438 (1977).
Bradfield v. Roberts, 175 U.S. 291 (1899).
Bowen v. Kendrick, 487 U. S. 589 (1988).
Bray v. Alexandria Women's Health Clinic, 113 S. Ct. 753 (1993).
Califano v. Yamasaki, 442 U.S. 682 (1979).
Cantwell v. Connecticut, 310 U.S. 296 (1940).
Church of Lukumi Babalu Aye v. Hialeah, 113 S. Ct. 2217 (1993).
Commission for Public Education and Religious Liberty v. Nyquist, 413 U.S. (1973).
Committee for Public Education v. Regan, 444 U.S. 646 (1980).
Diamond v. Chakrabarty, 447 U.S. 303 (1980).
Employment Division v. Smith, 494 U.S. 872 (1990).
Epperson v. Arkansas, 393 U.S. 97 (1968).
Everson v. Board of Education, 330 U.S. 1 (1947).
Grand Rapids v. Ball, 473 U.S. 373 (1985).
Griswold v. Connecticut, 381 U.S. 479 (1965).
Halushka v. University of Sashkatchewan (1965) 53 DLR 2d: 436.
Harris v. McRae, 448 U.S. 297 (1980).
Heffron v. International Society of Krishna Consciousness, 452 U.S. 640 (1981) at 647.
Lemon v. Kurtzman, 403 U.S. 602 (1971).

Madsen v. Women's Health Center, 114 S. Ct. 2516 (1994).
Maher v. Doe, 432 U.S. 519 (1977).
McDaniel v. Paty, 435 U.S. 618 (1978).
McGowan v. Maryland, 366 U.S. 420 (1961).
NAACP v. Clairbourne Hardware, 458 U.S. 886 (1982).
National Organization for Women v. Scheidler, 114 S. Ct. 798 (1994).
Planned Parenthood v. Casey, 112 S. Ct. 2791 (1992).
Poelker v. Doe, 432 U.S. 519 (1977).
Reynolds v. U.S., 98 U.S. 145 (1878).
Roe v. Wade, 410 U.S. 113 (1973).
Rust v. Sullivan, 111 S. Ct. 1759 (1991).
Schneider v. New Jersey, 308 U.S. 147 (1939).
Shelton v. Tucker, 364 U.S. 479 (1960).
Skinner v. Oklahoma, 316 U.S. 535, 541.
Thornburgh v. American College of Obstetricians and Pediatricians, 106 S. Ct. 2169 (1986).
U.S. v. Grace, 461 U.S. 171 (1983) at 177-78.
United States v. O'Brien, 391 U.S. 367 (1968).
Wallace v. Jaffee, 472 U.S. 38 (1985).
Walz v. Tax Commission, 397 U.S. 602 (1971).
Ward v. Rock Against Racism, 491 U.S. 781 (1989).

LOWER COURT CASES

American Life League, 855 F. Supp @ 137.
Bartling v. Superior Court, 209 Cal. Reporter 70 (1984).
Bartling v. Glendale Adventist Medical Center, 229 Cal. Reporter 360 (1986).
Becker v. Schwartz, 386 NE 2d 807 (NY 1978).
Berman v. Allen, 404 A 2d 8 (NJ 1979).
Brock, 863 F. Supp. at 851.
Chrisman v. Sisters of St. Joseph of Peace, 506 F. 2d 308 (9th Cir. 1974).
Council for Life Coalition, 856 F. Supp. at 1922.
Custody of Minor, 393 N.E. 2d 836, 837-38 (Mass. 1979).
Davis v. Davis, 113 S. Ct. 1259 (1993).
Del Zio v. Columbia Pres. Med. Center, No. 74-3558 (1978).
Doe v. Bolton, 319 F. Supp. 1048 (1973).
Gleitman v. Cosgrove, 227 A F. Supp 692 (E.D.PA 1967).
Harbeson v. Parke-Davis, Inc. 656 P 2d 483 (Wash 1983).
Howard v. Lecher, 366 NE 2d 64 (NY 1977).

In re President and Directors of Georgetown College, 331 F. 2d 1010, 1017 (D.C.Cir). Certificate denied, 377 US 978 (1964).

Kass v. Kass, NJ, Case No. 7808640.

McRae v. Califano, 491 F. Supp. 630 (E.D. N.Y. 1980).

Northeaster Women's Center Inc. v. McMonagle, 665 F. Supp. 1147 (1987).

Procanik v. Cillo, 478 A 2d 755 (NJ 1984).

Quinlan, 355 A 2d 647 (NJ 1976).

Quinn v. Leatham, AC 495, 506 (1901).

Riely, 860 F. Supp. at 693.

Salgo v. Leland Stanford Jr. University Board of Trustees (1957).

Schroeden v. Perkel 432 A. 2d 834 (NJ 1981).

Smith v. Cole, 513 A 2d 341 (NH 1986).

Speck v. Feingold, 408 A 2d 496 (Pa Super 1979).

State v. Winthrop, 43 Iowa 519 (1876).

Turnpin v. Sortini, 643 P 2d 954 (Cal 1982).

Viccarov v. Milunsky, 551 NE 2d8 (Mass. 1990).

York v. Jones, 717 F. Supp. 421 (E.D.Va. 1989).

Notes

Chapter 1

1. Jn. 8:14 (NRSV) Italics added.
2. James M. Gustafson, *Intersections: Science, Theology, and Ethics* (Cleveland: The Pilgrim Press, 1996), 29.
3. John Hedley Brooke, *Science and Religion* (Cambridge: Cambridge University Press, 1998), 330, 334. See also, Ian Barbour, *Ethics in an Age of Technology* (London: SCM, 1992), 27.
4. Arthur Peacocke, *Theology for a Scientific Age* (London: SCM Ltd., 1996), introduction, 10, 12, 15, 17, 21-23. See Basil Mitchell, *The Justification of Religious Belief* (London: Macmillan, 1973). Ref., J. Leplin, "Introduction," in *Scientific Realism*, Ed. J. Leplin (Berkley: University of California Press, 1984).
5. 1 Tim 3:16 (NRSV).
6. George A. Maloney, "Introduction," in *Pseudo-Macarius*, edited and translated by George A. Maloney (New York: Paulist Press, 1992), 2-3. Ref., Kallistos Ware, *The Orthodox Church* (London: Penguin, 1993).
7. Jn. 1:1-4, 14 (NRSV).
8. Gen. 1:1, *Biblia Hebraica: Stuttgartensia*, Edited by K. Elliger and W. Rudolph (Stuttgart: Deutsche Bibelgesellschaft, 1990).
9. *Pentateuch with Targum Onkelos, Haphtaroth and Rashi's Commentary*, translated and annotated by M. Rosenbaum and A. Silbermann (New York: Hebrew Publishing Company, 1965), 2. See Franz Delitzsche, *New Commentary on Genesis*, translated by Sophia Taylor (Minneapolis: Klock and Klock Christian Publishers, 1978), 73. (Original by T & T Clarke, 1888.) Also, Samuel Driver, *The Book of Genesis* (London: Methuen and Co., 1904), 14. See Also, John Skinner, *The International Critical and Exegetical Commentary on the Holy Scriptures of the Old and New Testaments: On Genesis*, Ed. by Samuel Rolles Driver, Alfred Plummer, Charles Augustus Briggs (Edinburgh: T & T Clark, 1963), 3, 30-31. Ref. note, Gen. 1:1, 2 (NRSV).
10. John Polkinghorn, ed., *The Work of Love: Creation as Kenosis* (Grand Rapids, MI: Eerdmans, 2001).
11. Keith Ward, *God, Chance and Necessity* (Oxford: Oneworld, 1996), 37-38.
12. Jn. 1: 3-4 (NRSV). Ref., Arthur Peacocke, *Paths From Science toward God: The End of All our Exploring* (Oxford: One World, 2001).

Counseling Pregnancy, Politics, and Biomedicine
© 2007 by The Haworth Press, Inc. All rights reserved.
doi:10.1300/5697_09

13. Nancey Murphy and George Ellis, *On the Moral Nature of the Universe* (Minneapolis: Fortress Press, 1996), 47. Ref., Keith Ward, *Religion and Creation* (Oxford: Oxford University Press, 1996).

14. R. Stannard, *Science and Wonders* (London: Faber, 1996). See Tim Appenzellar, "Someplace Like Earth," *National Geographic: Searching the Stars for New Earths* (December 2004): 68, 82-84.

15. Ref., Keith Ward, *God, Chance and Necessity*, 19, 43, 57. Ref., John N. Jonsson, *Quantum God: The Infinite Within Life's Finite Uncertainties* (Waco, TX: Baylor University, March 2000). Ref., Niels Bohr, *The Theory of Spectra and Atomic Constitution* (Cambridge: Cambridge University Press, 1922). Also ref. Niels Bohr, *Atomic Theory and the Description of Nature* (Cambridge: Cambridge University Press, 1934). Additional ref., Niels Bohr, *Atomic Physics and Human Knowledge* (New York: Science Editions, 1958). Ref., B. Hoffman, *The Strange Story of the Quantum*, 2nd ed. (Mass.: Harmonsworth and Glouchester, 1963). Ref., Keith Ward, *God, Chance and Necessity*, 19, 43, 57.

16. Ward, *God, Chance and Necessity*, 57, 61. Ref. Pierre Teillard de Chardin, *The Phenomenon of Man* (New York: Harper, 1959).

17. Gen. 1:26-27, 3 (NRSV).

18. Delitzsche, 73. Skinner, 30-31. *Pentateuch with Targum Onkelos*, 2. *Midrash, Erub* 18a. For textual imagery Ps. 5:1, 3; Ps. 8:6; Sir. 17:2-4; 1 Cor. 11:7; Col. 3:10; Eph. 4:24, Ja. 3:9; Babylonian myth 120, 1:33.

19. *The Greek New Testament*, 4th ed. (Münster/Westphalia: Deutsche Bibelgesellschaft, 1993), 313.

20. Jn. 1:1-4 (NRSV).

21. Jn. 1:1 (NIV), note. See C.K. Barrett, *New Testament Documents*, 2nd ed. (London: SPCK, 1978).

22. Ref., Ruth Edwards, *Discovering John* (London: SPCK, 2003). Other influences: Prov. 8:22, Ecclus. 24:1ff; Wisdom 7:22-8:1).

23. Jn. 1:14, *The Greek New Testament*.

24. Jn. 1:14 (NRSV).

25. Jn. 1:17-18 (NRSV).

26. Col. 1:15-20 (NRSV).

27. Jn. 1:1, note (NRSV).

28. John Habgood, *Being a Person: Where Faith and Science Meet* (London: Hodder and Stoughton, 1998), 153-55.

29. Vladimir Loskey, *The Mystical Theology of the Eastern Church* (Cambridge: James Clarke, and Co., 1957), 69.

30. Augustine, *City of God*, (New York: Penguin Classics), Books 11,12. Also, Thomas Aquinas, *Summa Theologiae*, translation by Fathers of the English Dominican Province (New York: Benziger Bros., 1947), Part 1a, *questios* 44-46. Ref., Emil Brunner, *The Mediator* (London: Lutterworth Press, 1947). Also ref. Ward, *Religion and Creation*.

31. George Eldon Ladd, *A Theology for the New Testament* (Eerdmans, 1987), 241.

32. Rudolph Bultmann, "New Testament and Mythology," Vol. I (London: SCM, 1985), 19, 31, 34.

33. Ward, *God, Chance and Necessity,* 321f. Refer to Karl Barth, *Church Dogmatics,* Vol. I, trans. G.W. Bromiley (Edinburgh: T & T Clarke, 1975), 420, 433. See also, Habgood, 153-55, 226. Ref. David Brown, *The Divine Trinity* (London: Duckworth, 1985). See Jn. 1:1, 14, 13:34; Mt 5:44; Col. 2:9 (NRSV).

34. For more information see Polkinghorne, *The Works of Love.*

35. Ezek. 37:1a, 4-6, 11a (NRSV). Richard Leakey and Roger Lewen, *The Sixth Extinction: Biodiversity and its Survival* (London: Orion Books, Ltd., 1996), 14.

36. Lk. 2:7 (NRSV). Jesus' birth and infancy, Lk. 1:26-2:40, c.f., Mt. 1:18-23; Is. 7:14 (NRSV). See Is. 48:16 (NRSV).

37. Lk. 1:35 (NRSV). References: Gregory of Nazianzus, *Ep. Cled.* (St. Vladimir's Seminary Press, 1986), 101. Augustine, *On the Trinity,* Trans. and Ed., Desmond M. Matthews, Gareth B. Clarke (Cambridge: Cambridge University Press, 2002), 11:8.

38. Is. 7:14, 8:8,10; Ex. 3:12; Mt. 1:23; Lk. 1:31, 2:12 (c.f., Gen. 3:15, 21:22, 24:43) (NRSV). Karl Barth, I:486. See Gregory J. Riley, *One Jesus, Many Christs* (San Francisco: Harper Collins, 1989), 75.

39. Jn. 1:12-13 (NRSV).

40. Rom. 8:19 (NRSV).

41. Holmes Rolston, *Genes, Genesis and God: Values and Their Origins in Natural and Human History* (Cambridge: Cambridge University Press, 1999), 56-60.

42. Heb. 2:14 (a and b); 2:27 (NRSV).

43. Jesus' descent, Mt. 1:1-17, 22:41-45; Lk. 3:23-38; Rom. 1:3; Gal. 3:16. See also, Rom Harre, *The Philosophy of Science: An Introductory Survey* (Oxford: Oxford University Press, 1985), 255.

44. Is. 43:12 (NRSV).

45. Ezek. 37:11; Jn 6:48; Lk. 2:4, 2:11 (ref. 1 Sam 17:12, 20:6) (NRSV).

46. Lk 2:41-52 (NRSV).

47. E. O. Wilson, *Consilience—The Unity of Knowledge* (London: Little, Brown, 1998). Stephen J. Pope, *The Evolution of Altruism and the Ordering of Love* (Washington DC: Georgetown University Press, 1994), 6-8f, 19ff, 24.

48. Melvin Konner, *The Tangled Wing: Biological Constraints on the Human Spirit* (New York: Harper Colophon Books, 1982) 175, 230 and also, chapters 9-13.

49. Lk. 2:41, 46-47; Mt. 7:27; Ex. 23:15; Dt. 16:1-8; Lk. 22:8 (NRSV).

50. Ref. Gordon Mursell, *Out of the Deep: Prayers of Protest* (London: SCM, 1998).

51. DT 10:12 (NRSV). A. Hyman and J.J. Walsh, eds., *Philosophy of the Middle Ages: The Christian, Jewish and Islamic Tradition* (Indianapolis: Hackett Publishing Co., 1973), 438-449.

52. Jn. 14:10b; Mt. 5:17-20 (NRSV). Consider Lk. 17:21 (NIV Study Bible).

53. Arthur Peacocke, 108-109.

54. Patricia S. Churchland and T.J. Sejnowski, "Perspectives on Cognitive Neuroscience," *Science* 242 (1988), 741-745.

55. Reinhold Niebuhr, *The Nature and Destiny of Man* (New York: Charles Schribner's Sons, 1941), 57ff. See Habgood, 68f., 137.

56. Jn. 2:3-4; 7:4-5 (NRSV). Gustafson, *Intersections,* 136f.

57. Mt. 12:6 (NRSV). Also 1 Cor. 3:16; 6:19; 2 Cor. 6:16 (NRSV). Temple of God 1 Ki. 6:1,6:38, 8:10, 8:27; 2Ch. 36:19, 36:23; Ezra 6:14; Ps. 27:4; Is. 6:1; Eze. 10:4, 43:4; Hab. 2:20 (NRSV). See Steven Coakley, *Christ Without Absolutes* (Oxford: Clarendon, 1988), 114f.

58. For more information see Jürgen Moltmann, *Way of Jesus Christ* (London: SCM, 1990).

59. Hyman and Walsh, 438-49. See Etienne Gilson, *The Spirit of Medieval Philosophy* (Gifford Lectures 1931-32) (New York: Charles Scribner's Sons, 1936), 269f.

60. Athanasius, *Four Discourses Against the Arians*, (St. Vladimir's Seminary Press, 1989), Discourse 1, Sects. 47 and 48.

61. Mt. 3:13-17 (NRSV). C.f., Mk. 1:9-11; Lk. 3:21-22; Jn. 1:31-34 (NRSV).

62. Testimony/witness Jn. 1:34 (NRSV). Baptism in the Holy Spirit: Mt. 3: 16-17; Mk. 1:10-11; Lk. Jn 3:21-22 (NRSV).

63. Jn. 3:3ff. (NRSV).

64. M. Boden "Consciousness and Human Identity: An Interdisciplinary Perspective," in *Consciousness and Human Identity*, Ed. John Cornwell (Oxford: Oxford University Press, 1998), 1-5. Also, John Searle, "How to Study Consciousness Scientifically," in *Consciousness and Human Identity*, Ed. John Cornwall (Oxford: Oxford University Press, 1998), 23-35. See Habgood, 30.

65. Bernard Ballentine and Anthony Dickenson, "Consciousness—The Interface Between Effect and Cognition," in *Consciousness and Human Identity*, Ed. John Cornwell (Oxford: Oxford University Press, 1998), 64, 83. See S. Rose, "The Rise of Neurogenic Determinism," in *Consciousness and Human Identity*, Ed. John Cornwell (Oxford: Oxford University Press, 1998), 87, 94. Also, Frederick Olafson, *What is a Human Being?: A Heideggarian View* (Cambridge: Cambridge University Press, 1995), 64.

66. 1 Jn. 3:16 (NRSV).

67. C.f., Rom. 4:20 (NRSV). Habgood, 153-55. Also ref., Jürgen Moltmann, *Way of Jesus Christ*, trans. Margaret Kohl (London: SCM, 1990).

68. Ref. Laura Weed, "The Amygdala and the Autonomic Nervous System in religious Ecstasy and Post Traumatic Stress Disorder," lecture at MetaNexus Seminar (Philadelphia, PA: MetaNexus, 2002). Ref., Daniel G. Amen, *Images Into Human Behavior: A Brain SPEC Atlas* (Los Angeles: Mindworks Press, 1998), CD-ROM, *http://brain.com/atlas* and *http://amenclinics.com/bp/atlas*. Also ref., D. G. Amen, *Healing the Hardware of the Soul* (Los Angles: Mindworks Press, 2002).

69. Keith Ward, *God, Chance and Necessity,* 158. Also, Keith Ward, *God Faith and the New Millennium* (Oxford: Oneworld, 1998), 125, 127.

70. Bonaventure, *The Mind's Journey to God,* translated by Lawrence S. Cunningham (Chicago: Franciscan Herald Press, 1979), 10, 39-41, 55f.

71. Rom. 2:15 (NRSV). See Michael Baylor, *Action and Person: Conscience in Late Scholasticism and the Young Luther* (Leiden: Brill, 1977).

72. Mary Midgley, "Putting Ourselves Together Again," in *Consciousness and Human Identity*, Ed. John Cornwell (Oxford: Oxford University Press, 1998), 160ff.

73. Armand A. Mauer, *Medieval Philosophy,* Vol. 1, 2nd ed. (Toronto, Ontario: Pontifical Institute of Medieval Studies, 1982), 1:145-53, 230-60. Refer to, Efrem

Bettoni, *Duns Scotus: The Basic Principles of His Philosophy,* translated by Bonansea (Washington DC: Catholic University of America Press, 1961), 15, 73-76, 108f, 181f. Also, Austin Farrar, *Freedom of the Will* (London: A & C Black, 1958), 39.

74. Divine revelation: Jn. 1:1-14; 1 Cor. 11:7; Col. 3:1; Eph. 4:24; Jas. 3:9; Ecclus. 17:3ff, Wis. 2:23 (NRSV). See John Jonsson, *Mythology: The Entmythologisierung Controversy* (Charlotte, So. Carolina: Nilses Publications, 1979), 28-31.

75. John H. Brooke, *Science and Religion,* 134, 139, 141f.

76. Susan Greenfield, *Journey to the Center of the Mind: Toward a Science of Consciousness* (New York: W.H. Freeman and Co., 1995), 17, 135ff., 140f, 143-54. Also, Nancey Murphy and George Ellis, *On the Moral Nature of the Universe-Theology, Cosmology and Ethics* (Minneapolis: Fortress, 1996), 68. See A. Aertsen and G.L. Gerstein, "Dynamic Aspects of Neuronal Cooperativity: Fast Stimulus-Locked Modulation of Effective Cooperativity," in *Neuronal Cooperativity,* Ed. J. Kruger (New York: Springer-Verlag, 1991): 52-67. Also, G.K. Aghajanian, J.S. Sprouse, and K. Rasmussen, "Physiology of the Midbrain Serotonin System," in *Psychopharmacy,* Ed. H.Y. Meltzer (New York: Raven Press, 1987), 141-50. Additional reading, H.H. Jasper and J. Tessier, "Acetylcholine Liberation from Cerebral Cortex during Paradoxical (REM) Sleep," *Science,* 172 (1971): 601-602.

77. Nancey Murphy, "Mental Causation," www.st-edmunds.cam.ac.uk/cis/murphy. See also, Donald McKay, *Behind the Eye,* Gifford Lectures, Ed. Valerie MacKay (Oxford: Blackwell, 1991), 43-44.

78. Ref. Gen. 17:9; 22:8, 13-14 for God-self-maledictory covenant (NRSV); Jud. 13:20 (God entered the sacrificial fire) (NRSV).

79. Ref., Keith Ward, *God: A Guide for the Perplexed* (Oxford: Oneworld, 2002).

80. Karl Rahner, *Theological Investigations,* Vol. 4 (New York: Herder and Herder, 1972). Ref., W. Pannenberg, *Jesus—God and Man* (London: Westminster, 1968).

81. Acts 7:1b-53 (NRSV).

82. Moltmann, 53.

83. C.f., Is 29:18-19; 35:5-6; 61:1; Mt 11:5; Lk. 4:18-19; 7:22 (NRSV).

84. Mt. 17:2-3, *The Greek New Testament.*

85. Ward, *Religion and Creation,* 153. Dan. 11:33; Pr. 4:18; Mt. 13:43; Jn. 5:35; 1 Cor. 15:42; Phil. 2:15; Is. 7:14—the sign of Immanuel (NRSV).

86. John Jonsson, "The Transfiguration of Jesus" (Pietermaritzburg, S. Africa: U. of Natal, 1979). Jesus' light: Jn. 8:12-14. Also, Jn. 1:3c-5:9, 8:12ff., 12:46; c.f., Ex. 13:22; Is. 42:6; Zec. 14:8 (NRSV).

87. Mt. 17:2-3 (NRSV).

88. Mt. 17:4., 23:7; Mk. 9:5; Lk. 9:33 (NRSV).

89. Lk. 20:36, 38 (c.f., Jn. 1:12) (NRSV).

90. Jesus' transfiguration: Mt. 17:1-8; Mk. 9:2-8; Lk. 9:28-36; c.f., Jn. 9:1-41; Dan. 12:2 (NRSV).

91. Jn. 8:12 (NRSV). Jesus' Light, Jn. 1:3c-5:9, 8:12ff., 12:46; c.f., Ex. 13:22; Is. 42:6; Zec. 14:8 (c.f., Jn. 8:12-14) (NRSV). Less confidence, Jn. 5:31-33; 8:54 (NRSV).

92. Lk. 9:30, 31 *(The Greek New Testament).*

93. Lk. 9:30-31. Compare notes NRSV, NIV Study Bible, etc.

94. Lk. 9:30-31 (NRSV).

95. Jn. 3:8; 3:12 (NRSV).

96. Refs. for enosis, Irenaeus, *Adversus haereses,* 3.19.1. Also refer to Basil of Caesarea, *On the Holy Spirit,* Trans., David Taylor (Lovanii: Peeter), 1.2. See ref. Gregory of Nazianzus, *Funeral Oration for Basil* (SLG Press Fairacres Publications, 1986), PG:36 560A.

97. Mt. 4:1-11; Mk. 1:12-13; Lk. 4:1-13. Mt. 8:1-4; Mk. 1:40-45; Lk. 5:12-16. Mt. 9:1-8; Mk. 2:1-12; Lk. 5:17-26. Mt. 12:1-14n; Mk. 2:23-3:6; Lk. 6:1-11 (NRSV).

98. Jn. 10:11ff. (NRSV). Prophesies: Is. 40: 11, 42:13; Jer. 23:1-6; Ezek.34 (NRSV).

99. Suffering Servant Songs: Is. 41:8-11, 42:1-4, 49:1-6, 50:4-11, and 52:13-53:12 (NRSV). Also, 1 QH6, 11, 1 Enoch 85-90, 91-93, 4 Ezra 7:26-44 (c.f., Syr. Baruch 24-30). Also ref., R. Martin-Achard, *From Death to Life* (Edinburgh: Oliver and Boyd, 1960). See ref. G. Nickelsberg, *Resurrection, Immortality and Eternal Life* (Cambridge, Mass: Harvard University Press, 1972).

100. Jn. 18:31 (NRSV). Messianic claimant, Mk 15:26. Jn 19:19 (NRSV). Jesus predicts his death, Mt. 17:22-23; Mk. 9:30-32; Lk. 9:22, 43b-45; Lk. 18:31-33(NRSV).

101. Jn. 11:48 (NRSV).

102. Mt. 26:53, 62; 27:11-14; Mk. 15:2-5; 14:60; Lk. 23:2-5, 9; Jn. 18:29-19:6; 1 Tim :13 (NRSV).

103. Jürgen Moltmann, *The Crucified God: The Cross of Christ as the Foundation and Criticism of Christian Theology,* translation by R.A. Wilson and John Bowder (New York: Harper and Row, 1974), 4. See Wolfhardt Pannenberg, *The Apostle's Creed: In the Light of Today's Question* (Philadelphia: Westminster Press, 1972), 96. Also, Reinhold Niebuhr, *The Nature and Destiny of Man* (New York: Charles Schribner's Sons, 1941), 57ff.

104. Mk. 15:24, 37, 45-46; Mt. 27:59; Lk. 23:46; Jn. 19:38-42; Acts 13:29 (NRSV).

105. Jn. 19:33-35 (NRSV). 1 Cor. 1:23; 5:7; 8:11; Gal. 3:13; Rom. 5:6(NRSV).

106. Mk. 15:45b-46; Mt. 27:59; Lk. 23:52-53; Jn. 19:38; Acts 13:29 (NRSV).

107. Mt. 28:2-3, 9 *(The Greek New Testament).*

108. Mt. 28:2-3, 9 (NRSV).

109. Corporeal evidence: Jn. 20:27, 21:12ff. (NRSV).

110. Lk. 24:16; Jn. 20:15-16; Mt. 23:7 (NRSV).

111. 1 Cor. 15:5ff. (NRSV), εγειρω terminology (c.f., Dan) *(Greek New Testament).* ωφθη appearances: Mt. 17:3; Lk. 1:11, 22:43; Acts 2:3, 7:2, 7:30, 9:17 *(Greek New Testament).* Paul's conversion: Acts 13:31; 16:9; 26:16 (NRSV). Change of heart: 1 Cor. 15; Rom. 6:2ff. Col. 2:11 (NRSV). Groups—Acts 2:1ff. (c.f., Lk. 24:34) (NRSV).

112. Ref., R. Voorst, *Jesus Outside the New Testament* (Grand Rapids: Eerdmans, 2000). Also see, W. C. van Unnick, "The Newly Discovered Gnostic 'Epistle to Rheginos' on the Resurrection I," *JEH* 15 (1964), p. 141-144.

113. Laying down and raising up one's life: Jn. 10:11ff., 6:35; Is. 52:13 (NRSV). Bread of life: Jn. 6:48, 51-58, Mt. 8:20, 26:26, 28 (NRSV).

114. Resurrection and Vindication: Acts 2:23, 3:13ff., 5:30; Rev. 1.9; Mt. 26:64 (NRSV). Resurrection and Parousia: Acts 1:8; Jn. 14:15ff.; 1 Cor. 15:22; Col. 3:1, c.f., Mt. 18:20, 25:31ff; 28:20 (NRSV). Resurrection and exaltation: Jn. 3:13f; Phil 2.6ff.; Heb. 4:14ff, 6:29f; Gen. 5:24; 2 Kings 2:11 (NRSV).

115. Acts 9:3ff; 1 Cor. 9:1, 15:8 (NRSV).

116. C. J. deCataranzaro, *Sources chrétiennes [SC];* ET (New York: The Classics of W. Spirituality, 1980), Cat. 22, Hymn 45:6. Ref., John of the Cross's *Dark Night of the Soul,* Ed., Halcyon Backhouse (London: Hodder and Stroughton, 1988). Also ref., Hildegard of Bingen, *Scivias,* translation by Bruce Hozeski (Santa Fe, NM: Bear, 1986). See ref., Teresa of Avila, *Interior Castle,* Ed., Halcyon Backhouse (London: Hodder and Stroughton, 1988). Texts, Gen. 2:21—Adam; Gen. 15—Abram, etc.

117. Carolyn Franks Davies, *The Evidential Force of Religious Experience* (Oxford: Clarendon, 1989), 44. William James, *Varieties of Religious Experience* (New York: Modern Library, 1936), 385.

118. See article, "The Evangelical Doctrine of Theosis," *Journal of the Evangelical Society* (June 1997).

119. C.f., Habgood, 226. Also see, Pierre Teillard de Chardin, *Science and Christ,* trans by Rene Hague (New York: Harper and Row, 1968), 74f.

120. Moltmann, 293-94. See Keith Ward, *Religion and Creation,* 333. Ref., Plotinus, *The Ennead,* Trans., Stephen Mac Kenna (London: Faber, 1969), 69.

121. 1 Cor 15:46 (NRSV).

122. Gen. 1:31 (NRSV).

Chapter 2

1. Michael Walzer, *Spheres of Justice* (New York: Basic Books, 1983), preface. Also, Alasdair MacIntyre, *After Virtue* (Notre Dame: University of Notre Dame, 1981).

2. Michael J. Sandel, *Democracy's Discontent: America in Search of a Public Philosophy* (Cambridge, Mass.: The Belknap Press of Harvard University Press, 1996), 3f.

3. Ibid., 3f.

4. Tom L. Beauchamp, ed., *Philosophic Ethics: An Introduction of Moral Philosophy* (Washington DC: Georgetown University, 1982), 367. For Prescriptivism, see Rom M. Harre, *Language of Morals* (Oxford University Press, 1952), 69f.

5. Sheila Jasonoff, *Science at the Bar: Law, Science and Technology in America* (Cambridge, Mass.: Harvard University Press, 1995), 160f.

6. Henry Sidgwick, *Outlines of the History of Ethics* (London: Macmillan and Co., Ltd., 1960. Orig. 1886), 1.

7. Ibid., introduction.

8. Bernard Mayo, "Ethics and The Moral Life," in *Ethics and the Moral Life* (New York: Macmillan and Co., 1958) in *Philosophic Ethics: An Introduction of*

Moral Philosophy, Ed. Tom L. Beauchamp (Washington DC: Georgetown University, 1982), 155.

9. G.J. Warnock, "The Object of Morality," in *Object of Morality* (London: Methusa and Co., 1971) in *Philosophic Ethics: An Introduction of Moral Philosophy,* Ed. Tom L. Beauchamp (Washington DC: Georgetown University, 1982), 25.

10. Sidgwick, introduction, 12f.

11. David C. Lindberg, *The Beginnings of Western Science: The European Scientific Tradition in Philosophical, Religious, Institutional Context, 600 BC to AD 1450* (Chicago: University of Chicago, 1992), 21.

12. Sidgwick, 12-15.

13. Lindberg, 39.

14. Sidgwick, 25.

15. Ibid., 31-35.

16. Ibid., 36-37, 39, 41.

17. Ibid., 42-45, 53, 57, 63. Also, Lindberg, 48.

18. Joseph Fletcher, *Situation Ethics* (Philadelphia: The Westminster Press, 1966), 39, 54. See James M. Gustafson, *Ethics from a Theocentric Perspective,* vol. 2 *Ethics and Theology* (Chicago: University of Chicago, 1984), 124-128.

19. Sidgwick, 106-107.

20. Lk. 10:27 (c.f., Dt. 10:12) (NRSV).

21. Job 29:12-16, c.f., Ps. 68:5-6b and Is. 61:1-3 (NRSV).

22. 1 Cor. 15:46 (NRSV).

23. Mt. 5:3-12 (NRSV).

24. Lk. 6:20-26 (NRSV). See notes in NAB.

25. Lk. 6:27-31, 36-39 (NRSV).

26. 3 John and 1 Cor. 13:4-8.

27. 1 Cor. 13:4-8a (NRSV).

28. Jas. 2:8 (NRSV).

29. Fletcher, 120-35, 138-40, 152, 154.

30. 1 Jn. 3:23 (NRSV).

31. Stephen J. Pope, *The Evolution of Altruism and the Ordering of Love* (Washington DC: Georgetown University Press, 1994), 87.

32. Ref., Richard Dawkins, *The Selfish Gene* (Oxford: Oxford University Press, 1989).

33. Pope, Stephen, J., *The Evolution of Altruism and the Ordering of Love* (Washington D.C.: Georgetown University Press, 1994), introduction, 4, 19, 64, 67-70, 74ff., 78, 109ff., 140-44, 153-154.

34. Stanley Hauerwas, *The Peaceable Kingdom: A Primer in Christian Ethics* (Notre Dame; University of Notre Dame, 1983), 34, 40, 45, 69.

35. Sidgwick, 113.

36. Ibid., 128, 130-131.

37. 1 Cor. 13 (NRSV).

38. Sidgwick, 109f., 128, 131.

39. B. M. Dickens, "Law, Ethics, and Justice in Human Reproduction," in *Aspects éthiques de la reproduction humaine—Ethical aspects of human reproduction,*

Eds. Claude Sureau and Françoise Shenfield (Paris: John Libbey Eurotext, 1995), 21f.

40. Pierre Teillard de Chardin, *Science and Christ,* translation by Rene Hague (New York: Harper and Row, 1968), 35f.

41. Sidgwick, 141.

42. Chardin, *Science and Christ,* 37-40. See, Walter Kaufman and Forrest E. Baird, Ed. *Medieval Philosophy,* Vol. 2 (Englewood Cliffs, New Jersey: Prentice Hall, 1994), 328. Ref., Thomas Aquinas, *Summa Theologica* (London: Blackfriars with Egot Spottiswoode, © 1964-1981).

43. Sidgwick, 141.

44. Ralph Lerner and Muhsin Mahdi, *Medieval Political Philosophy: A Sourcebook* (Canada: Collier-Macmillan Limited, 1963), 297f. Ref., Aquinas, *Commentary on Politics,* translation by C.I. Litzinger (Chicago: Regnery, 1964).

45. Lerner and Mahdi, 272-90. Also, Kaufman and Baird, 2:390. See also, Thomas Aquinas, *Summa Theologica.* Ref., Aristotle, *Nicomachean Ethics and Politics* (CRW Publishing Limited Book Blocks, 2004), vi, 11.

46. Kaufman and Baird, 2:396.

47. Immanuel Kant, *Groundwork of the Metaphysic of Morals,* translator H.J. Paton (NY: Harper and Row, 1964), 13, 20.

48. Immanuel Kant, *Kant: Political Writings,* editor and translator Hans Reiss (Cambridge: Cambridge University Press, 1970), 1-17.

49. Ibid., 39-44, 51-52. Also, Beauchamp, 110. See Charles D. Broad, *Five Types of Ethical Theory* (London: Routledge & Kegan Paul, n/d.), Ch. 5.

50. Kant, *Groundwork of the Metaphysic of Morals,* 24-26.

51. Ibid., 52-57, 69-71, 79-81, 83.

52. Dickens, 23.

53. Sidgwick, 163, 237f., 240-42, 244-45. See Jeremy Bentham, *The Works of Jeremy Bentham,* Vol X [Life] (Continuum International Publishing Group Ltd., 1994), 560-61, 79. Also, Beauchamp, 97f.

54. Sidgwick, 247-48, 250, 252. See John Stuart Mills, *On Liberty and Considerations On Representative Government* (1859), Ed. R.B. McCallum (Oxford: Basil Blackwell, 1946), 5, 13f., 67, 95-96.

55. Beauchamp, 100-101.

56. Sidgwick, 299-301.

57. Ibid., 302. Ref., James Marineau, *Types of Ethical Theory* (1885).

58. Sidgwick, 303f.

59. See Alasdair MacIntyre, *After Virtue* (Notre Dame: Univ. of Notre Dame, 1981).

60. Lisa A. Cahill, "Within Shouting Distance: Paul Ramsey and Richard McCormick on Method," in *Cross-Cultural Perspectives in Medical Ethics: Readings,* Ed. Robert Veatch (Boston: Jones and Bartlett Publishers, 1989), 70-81. Recommended reading, Paul Ramsey, *Ethics at the Edges of Life* (New Haven: Yale University Press, 1978).

61. Dickens, 23-24.

62. John H. Brooke, *Science and Religion* (Cambridge: Cambridge University Press, 1998), 53.

63. John Hallowell, "The Liberal Expression of Individualism," in *Cross Cultural Perspectives in Medical Ethics: Readings*, Ed. Robert Veatch (Boston: Jones and Bartlett Publishers, 1989), 82-85.

64. Beauchamp, 214ff. See Ruth Maclin, "Moral Concerns and Appeals to Rights and Duties," *The Hastings Center Report* (October 1976), 31, 37-38.

65. Joseph F. Fletcher, "Four Indicators of Humanhood—The Enquiry Matures," in *On Moral Medicine: Theological Perspectives on Moral Medicine*, Ed. Stephen E. Lammers and Allen Verhey, 2nd ed. (Grand Rapids: William B. Eerdmans Publishing Co., 1998), 377-78. See Michael Tooley, "Abortion and Infanticide," *Philosophy and Public Affairs* 2 (Fall, 1972): 37-65. Also, Richard A. McCormick, "To Save or Let Die, The Dilemma of Modern Medicine," *Journal of the American Medical Association* 299 (8 July 1974): 172-76. See also, Robert H. Williams, *To Live and To Die* (New York: Springer-Verlag, 1974), 18.

66. William May, "The Morality of Abortion," *Catholic Medical Quarterly* 26 (1974): 116-128.

67. James E. Wood, Jr., Bruce Thompson, and Robert T. Miller, *Church and State in Scripture, History and Constitutional Law* (Waco, TX: JM Dawson Institute of Church State Studies, Baylor University Press, 1958), 140ff.

68. C.A. Pierce, *Conscience in the New Testament* (London: SCM Press, 1955), 13ff., 41, 50f., 77ff., 91ff., 99ff., 104f, 114. Ref. Rom 2:15; 1 Cor. 4:4; 1 Cor. 8; Heb. 9:9, 14; 10:2, 22; 13:18; 1 Tim. 3:9; 2 Tim. 1:3, 1:5; 1 Pet. 3:16, 21 (NRSV).

69. Michael G. Baylor, *Action and Person: Conscience in Late Scholasticism and the Young Luther* (Leiden: EJ Brill, 1977), 35ff., 44, 47, 53, 97, 101f., 143, 244f.

70. Pierce, 114f., 122f. Ref. J. B. Lightfoot, *St. Paul's Epistle to the Philippians, excursus: St. Paul and Seneca*. See Baylor, 254. Also, James E. Wood, Jr. and Derek Davis, eds., *Law and Morality* (Waco, TX: J.M. Dawson Institute, Baylor University Press, 1995). Ref., UN Universal Declaration of Human Rights, Art. 18.

71. R.S. Downie and Elizabeth Telfer, "Respect for Persons," from *Respect for Persons* (New York: Schocken Books, Inc., 1970), 23-29, in *Philosophic Ethics*, 130, 132,134. See John Hartland-Swann, *An Analysis of Morals* (London: George Allen and Unwin Ltd., 1960). Also, James Childress, "Autonomy," in *Cross-Cultural Perspectives in Medical Ethics: Readings*, Ed. Robert Veatch (Boston: Jones and Bartlett Publishers, 1989), 233.

72. Gerald Dworkin, "Moral Autonomy," from G. Dworkin, H. Tristram Engelhardt Jr., and David Callahan, eds., *Morals, Science, and Sociality* (Hastings-On-Hudson, NY: The Hastings Center, 1978), 156-71, in *Philosophic Ethics*, 135-140.

73. Hallowell, 82-85. See Beauchamp, 124-27. Also, W.D. Ross, "What Makes Right Acts Right," in *Cross-Cultural Perspectives in Medical Ethics: Readings*, Ed. Robert Veatch (Boston: Jones and Bartlett Publishers, 1989), 214.

74. Albert Jonsen, "Do no harm," in *Cross-Cultural Perspectives in Medical Ethics: Readings*, Ed. Robert Veatch (Boston: Jones and Bartlett Publishers, 1989), 204, 206.

75. Edmund D. Pelligrino and David C. Thomasma, *For the Patient's Good: The Restoration of Beneficence in Health Care* (Oxford: Oxford University Press, 1988), 54-55, 57. See M. Siegler, "Searching for Moral Certainty in Medicine: A Proposal for a New Model of the Doctor-Patient Encounter, *Bulletin of the New*

York Academy of Medicine, vol. 57, No. 1 (1981): 56-69. Also, S. Toulmin, "The Tyranny of Principles," *Hastings Center Report,* Vol. 11, No. 6 (1981): 31-39.

76. Pelligrino and Thomasma, 14-17, 195. See L.H. Newton, "The Patient as Responsible Adult: Derivations and Consequences of Revised Perspective," in *Proceedings of the Fifty-fifth Annual Meeting of the American Catholic Philosophical Association,* vol. LV, Eds. D.O. Dahlstrom, D.T. Ozar, and L. Sweeney (Washington DC: American Catholic Philosophical Association, 1981), 240-49. Also, *Bartling v. Superior Court,* 209 Cal. Reporter 70 (1984); *Bartling v. Glendale Adventist Medical Center,* 229 Cal. Reporter 360 (1986).

77. Pelligrino and Thomasma, 52-54. See, J. Katz, *The Silent World of Doctor and Patient* (New York: Free Press, 1984). Also, J. F. Childress, *Who Should Decide? Paternalism in Health Care* (New York: Oxford University Press, 1982). Ref., MacIntyre, *After Virtue.*

78. Pelligrino and Thomasma, Preface, vii, 34. Mayo, 151-54. Also, Joel Feinberg, "Obligations and Supererogation" from "Supererogation and Rules," *Ethics* 71 (1961) reprinted in Feinberg, *Doing and Deserving* (Princeton, New Jersey: Princeton University Press, 1970), 3-7, 16, in *Philosophic Ethics,* 175. Also see, Beauchamp, 164.

79. Robert Veatch, *Cross-Cultural Perspectives in Medical Ethics: Readings* (Boston: Jones and Bartlett Publishers, 1989), 196.

80. Ibid., 207. Also, McCormick, 173-175.

81. Jonsen, "Do no harm," 209.

82. Fletcher, "Four Indicators of Humanhood," 377. Ref., Tooley, 37-65.

83. Dickens, 24.

84. Beauchamp, *Philosophic Ethics,* Ch. 9. See *Oxford American Dictionary,* Herald Colleges Edition (New York: Avon, 1980), 295.

85. Daniel Eleazar, *Covenant and Commonwealth* (New Brunswick: Rutgers University Press, 1995), 323ff.

86. John Rawls, "Justice, Utilitarianism, Deontology," in *Philosophic Ethics: An Introduction of Moral Philosophy,* Ed. Tom L. Beauchamp (Washington, DC: Georgetown University, 1982), 113-14. See Ruth Benedict, "Relativism and Patterns of culture," in *Value and Obligation,* Ed. Richard B. Brandt (New York: Harcourt, Brace, and World, 1961), 457. Also, Robert M. Sade, "Medical Care as a Right, a Refutation," in *Cross-Cultural Perspectives in Medical Ethics: Readings,* Ed. Robert Veatch (Boston: Jones and Bartlett Publishers, 1989), 300. Ref. Kennedy-Griffith Bill.

87. Gen. 1:26-27. Jean-Marc Chouraqui, "Des Devoirs Aux Droits de l'homme une perspective juive," in *Les dimensions universelles des Droits de l'homme,* Eds. A. Lapeyre, F. de Tinguy, K. Vasak (Brussels: UNESCO, 1990), 1:81.

88. *Mishnah,* Sanhedrin IV.5.

89. *Mishnah,* IV.4.

90. Chouraqui, 1:81. See Eleazar, 323ff. Ref., Ex. 20:1-17; 23:3, 6, 9; *Mishnah,* 38a.

91. Robert Morgan, *Romans: New Testament Guide* (Sheffield: Sheffield Academic Press, 1995), 19ff.

92. John Witte and Johann D. van der Vyver, eds., "Introduction," in *Human Rights in Global Perspective: Religious Perspectives* (Boston: Martinus Nijhoff Publishers, 1996), xxvii. See James E. Wood, Jr., "An Apologia for Religious Human Rights," in *Human Rights in Global Perspective: Religious Perspectives* (Boston: Martinus Nijhoff Publishers, 1996), 475.

93. Jean Imbert, "Conférence internationale sur la tolérance et loi (Sienne, Italy 8-10 April 1995): Tolérence et loi: aperçu historique," *Conscience et liberté* 2:2 (1995): 93-96, 98-103. See A. Lapeyre, F. de Tinguy, and K. Vasak, eds., *Les dimensions universelles des Droits de l'homme,* 2 Vols. (Brussels: UNESCO, 1990), introduction, 1:5-8, 77-78.

94. Pascale Boucard, *Laïcité, libertés de conscience and religion* (Lyon, France: Catholique de Lyon, 1995), 96-101.

95. Anne David, "Freedom of Association and Civil Society: Freedom of Association and Freedoms of Associations," *Freedom of Association Seminar* (in Reykjavik, Iceland) (Leiden, Netherlands: Center for Human Rights Studies, University of Leiden, 26-28 August 1993). Refs. Right of Association: Germany, Art. 30, Prussian Constitution (1850), Art. 9 Basic Law, 5 Apr. 1964; Italy, Art. 2 Const. Charter, 1942 Civil Code, 11 Aug. 1991; Luxembourg, Art. 26, Const. 17 Oct. 1868-clubs and assoc. 21 Apr. 1928; Belgium, Art. 20 Const.; Netherlands, 1848 Const.; Denmark, Art. 78-1 Const. Act; Switzerland, Art. 56, Fed. Const. 29 May 1974; Spain, Act of 24 Dec. 1964 (Sec. 3, para. 1) amended 1987 Const.; Portugal, Sec. 41 Const. Act amended 25 Apr. 1976; Greece, Art. 12-1, 1975 Constitution.

96. Council of Europe Press, *Human Rights in International Law* (Haaksbergen, Netherlands: In Or publikaties, 1995), 449. Refer to Charter of Paris for a New Europe, Paris, 21 November 1990.

97. GWF Hegel, *Philosophy of Right* (1821), translation by T. M. Knox (London: Oxford University Press, 1952), preface. Also refer to Keith Ward, *God: A Guide for the Perplexed* (Oxford: Oneworld, 2002).

98. Stuart Hampshire, *Public and Private Morality* (Cambridge: Cambridge University Press, 1978), 23ff.

99. Ronald Dworkin, "Taking Rights Seriously," in *Philosophic Ethics: An Introduction of Moral Philosophy,* Ed. Tom L. Beauchamp (Washington DC: Georgetown University, 1982), 192. See Hampshire, 23-50. Also, T. M. Scanlon, "Rights, Goals and Fairness," in *Public and Private Morality,* Ed. Stuart Hampshire (Cambridge: Cambridge University Press, 1978), 93-113.

100. R. Dworkin, 195.

101. Joel Feinberg, "The Nature of Rights," in *Philosophic Ethics,* 197-98. See R. Sade, "Is Health Care a Right?" *Image* 7 (1974). Also ref., R. Sade, "Medical Care as a Right, a Refutation," in *Cross-Cultural Perspectives in Medical Ethics: Readings,* Ed. Robert Veatch (Boston: Jones and Bartlett Publishers, 1989). 299-301. See also, Allen Buchanan, "Justice: A Philosophical Review," in *Cross-Cultural Perspectives in Medical Ethics: Readings,* Ed. Robert Veatch (Boston: Jones and Bartlett Publishers, 1989), 287ff. Ref., Robert Nozick, *Anarchy, State and Utopia* (New York: Basic Books, 1977).

102. Harold J. Berman, *Faith and Order: The Reconciliation of Law and Religion* (Atlanta: Scholars Press, 1993), 5-6.

103. J. Ian H. McDonald, *Christian Values: Theory and Practice in Christian Ethics Today* (Edinburgh: T & T Clark, 1995), 45.

104. Gene Outka, "Social Justice and Equal Access to Health Care," in *On Moral Medicine: Theological Perspectives in Medical Ethics*, Eds. Stephen E. Lammers and Allen Verney, 2nd ed. (Grand Rapids: Wm. B. Eerdmans Publishing Company, 1998), 956. See Beauchamp, *Philosophical Ethics: An Introduction of Moral Philosophy*, Ed. Tom L. Beauchamp (Washington DC: Georgetown University, 1982), 223-25. Ref., Stanley I. Bean, "Justice," in *The Encyclopedia of Philosophy*, Ed. Paul Edwards (New York: Macmillan, 1963) 3:299.

105. Wood et al., *Church and State in Scripture, History, and Constitutional Law*, introduction. Also, David C. Thomasma, "The Basis of Medicine and Religion: Respect for Persons," in *On Moral Medicine*, 424. Ref., Derek Davis, "Preserving the Moral Integrity of the Constitution: An Examination of Deconstruction and Other Hermeneutical Theories," in *Law and Morality*, Eds. James Wood, Jr. and Derek Davis (Waco, TX: J.M. Dawson Institute, Baylor University Press, 1995).

106. Berman, 67, 76-77, 82.

107. Andrew Williams, "Egalitarian Justice and Personal Responsibility," Lecture (Oxford: All Soul's College, 1999), 1-4.

108. John Rawls, "Justice, Utilitarian, Deontology," in *Philosophic Ethics: An Introduction of Moral Philosophy*, Ed. Tom L. Beauchamp (Washington DC: Georgetown University, 1982), 113-14. Also ref., John Rawls, *A Theory of Justice* (Cambridge, Mass: Harvard University Press, 1971).

109. Walzer, 5.

110. Beauchamp, 278.

111. Buchanan, 287ff. Ref. Nozick, *Anarchy, State and Utopia* (New York: Basic Books, 1977).

112. Gerald Dworkin, "Moral Autonomy," in *Morals, Science, and Sociality*, Eds. G. Dworkin, H. Tristram Engelhardt Jr., and David Callahan (Hastings-On-Hudson, NY: The Hastings Center, 1978).

113. G.A. Cohen, *Ethics* (Oxford: Oxford University Press, 1989), 920.

114. A. Williams, "Egalitarian Justice and Personal Responsibility," Lecture (Oxford: University of Oxford, 2000), 2.

115. Ibid., 4.

116. T. M. Scanlon, *What We Owe Each Other* (Oxford: Oxford University Press, 1999), 254.

117. K. Danner Clouser, "Models: A Critical review and a New View," in *Cross-Cultural Perspectives in Medical Ethics: Readings*, Ed. Robert Veatch (Boston: Jones and Bartlett Publishers, 1989), 182-185.

118. "President's Commission for the Study of Ethical Problems in Medicine and Biomedical and Behavioral Research. Securing Access to Health Care," in *Cross-Cultural Perspectives: Readings*, Ed. Robert Veatch (Boston: Jones and Bartlett Publishers, 1989), 303-309.

119. Immanuel Kant, "On the Supposed Right to Tell Lies From Benevolent Motives," in *Cross-Cultural Perspectives*, 216-219.

120. Beauchamp, 281f.

121. Carol Gilligan, *In a Different Voice: Psychological Theory and Women's Development* (Cambridge: Harvard University Press, 1982), 7, 17.

122. Sidgwick, introduction.

123. Gilligan, 62.

124. Lois K. Daly, "Ecofeminism, Reverence for Life, Feminist Theological Ethics," in *Feminist Theological Ethics: A Reader,* Ed. Lois K. Daly (Louisville, KY: John Knox Press, 1994), 299-300. See Eleanor Humes Haney, "What is Feminist Ethics?: A Proposal for continuing Discussion," in *Feminist Theological Ethics: A Reader,* Ed. Lois K. Daly (Louisville, KY: John Knox Press, 1994), 4-5. Also, Carol S. Rob, "Framework for Feminine Ethics," in *Feminist Theological Ethics: A Reader,* Ed. Lois K. Daly (Louisville, KY: John Knox Press, 1994), 17. See also, Gilligan, 7. Ref., Susan Frank Parsons, *Feminism and Christian Ethics* (Cambridge: Cambridge University Press, 1996), 139-140. See ref., Nell Nodding, *Caring: A Feminist Approach to Ethics and Moral Education* (Los Angeles: University of California Press, 1984, 27.

125. Mary Midgley, "Putting Ourselves Together Again," in *Consciousness and Human Identity,* Ed. John Cornwall (Oxford: Oxford University Press, 1998), 160-162, 168. See Habgood, 68f, 137. See also, Gilligan, *In a Different Voice,* 8, 135.

126. Mary Daly, "The Spiritual Revolution: Women's Liberation as Theological Re-education," in *Feminist Theological Ethics: A Reader,* Ed. Lois K. Daly (Louisville, KY: John Knox Press, 1994), 122.

127. Haney, 12.

128. Gilligan, 148.

129. Parsons, 138-140. Nodding, 14, 56.

130. Gilligan, 165.

131. Haney, 12. See Margaret A. Farley, "Feminist Theology and Bioethics," in *Feminist Theological Ethics: A Reader,* Ed. Lois K. Daly (Louisville, KY: John Knox Press, 1994), 202.

132. Gilligan, 19.

133. Haney, 9. See Anne McGrew Bennett, "Overcoming the Biblical and Traditional Subordination of Women," in *Feminist Theological Ethics: A Reader,* Ed. Lois K. Daly (Louisville, KY: John Knox Press, 1994), 140. Also, Farley, 199-200. See also, Rosemary Ruether, *Sexism and God-Talk: Toward a Feminine Theology* (Boston: Beacon Press, 1983), 82. Ref., Daly, Lois, 297, 305, 312. Ref., Albert Schweitzer, *Philosophy of Civilization,* translation by CT Campion (New York: Macmillan, 1949, reprinted. Tallahassee, FL: University Press of Florida, 1981).

134. Haney, 7. See Lois Daly, 312. Ref., Martin Kheel, "The Liberation of Nature: A Circular Affair," *Environmental Ethics* 7 (Summer 1985), 144.

135. Gilligan, 5-24, 17.

136. Parsons, 140.

137. Lois Daly, 132.

138. Janice C. Raymond, "Reproductive Gifts and Gift-giving: The Altruistic Woman," in *Feminist Theological Ethics: A Reader,* Ed. Lois K. Daly (Louisville, KY: John Knox Press, 1994), 237-238.

139. Ibid., 237, 241.

140. Ibid., 238.

141. Lawrence Kohlberg, *The Philosophy of Moral Development* (San Francisco: Harper and Row, 1981). See Kohlberg and R. Kramer, "Continuities and Discontinuities in Child and Adult Moral Development," *Human Development* 12 (1969): 93-120.

142. Gilligan, 174.

143. Lisa Sowle Cahill, "'Embodiment' and Moral Critique: A Christian Social Perspective," in *On Moral Medicine: Theological Perspectives on Moral Medicine,* Eds. Stephen E. Lammers and Allen Verhey, 2nd ed. (Grand Rapids: William B. Eerdmans Publishing Co., 1998), 404.

144. Gen. 1:26 (NSRV). Farley, 196. Ref., George Herbert Mead, *Philosophy of the Present* (Promethius Books, 2002). Also ref., Martin Buber, *Two Types of Faith* (Prentice Hall, 1986). See Haney, 10.

145. Elizabeth E. Green, "The Transmutation of Theology: Ecofeminist Alchemy and the Christian Tradition," in *Ecofeminism and Theology: Yearbook of the European Society of Women in Theological Research* (Netherlands: Kok Pharos Publishing House, 1994), 49-53. See Jürgen Moltmann, *Gott in der Schöpfung: Oekolgische Schöpfungs lehre* (München: Christian Kaiser, 1985), 1985, Ch. 1, sec.5. Also, Mary Grey, *Redeeming the Dream: Feminism, Redemption and Christian Tradition* (London: SPCH, 1989), 34. See also, Farley, 203. Ref., I Cor. 15: 35-37, 38, 42-49; Lk. 8:8; 20:36 (NRSV).

146. Gilligan, 174.

147. Cahill, 401.

148. Ibid., 406. Ref., Mary Douglas, *Natural Symbols: Explorations I Cosmology* (Lon: Barrie & Jenkins, 1973).

Chapter 3

1. Gen 1:26-27 (NRSV).

2. Geoffrey Sawer, "Structures and divisions of the law," in *International Encyclopedia of Comparative Law: The Legal Systems of the World, Their Comparison and Unification,* Eds. K. Z. Zweigert, et al., Vol. II (The Hague: Mouton, 1975), 37-38. Ref., Max Lerner, ed., *The Mind and Faith of Justice Holmes* (Boston: Transaction Publisher, 1988), 74-75. (Reprint.)

3. Ref., Mircea Eliade, *From Medicine Men to Mohammed* (New York: Harper and Row, 1974).

4. B. M. Dickens, "Law, Ethics, and Justice in Human Reproduction," in *Aspects éthiques de la reproduction humaine—Ethical aspects of human reproduction,* Eds. Claude Sureau and Françoise Shenfield (Paris: John Libbey Eurotext, 1995), 21.

5. James B. Prichard, *Ancient Near Eastern Texts* (Princeton: Princeton University Press, 1969 (reprinted from 1939).

6. Ex. 20:1-2 (NRSV).

7. Acts 7:38 (NRSV).

8. Ex. 20:1-7 (NRSV).

9. Ex. 20:8-17 (NRSV).

10. Num. 11:16-17, 24-29 (NRSV).

11. Is. 61:1-3 and Mt. 5:1-17 (NRSV). Ref. Gen. 17:1, blamelessness.

12. Lk. 12:27, Mk. 12:29, Rom. 13:8b, Gal 5:14, Jas 2:8, Dt. 6:4-5, Lev. 19:18 (NRSV).

13. Ref. Keith Ward, *Religion and Community* (Oxford: Clarendon Press, 2000).

14. John Habgood, *Being a Person: Where Faith and Science Meet* (London: Hodder and Stoughton, 1998), 153-155.

15. Gal. 3:28. For Paul's Christology, see Robert Morgan, *Romans: New Testament Guide* (Sheffield: Sheffield Academic Press, 1995), 98f.

16. Morgan, 18. Rom. 1:17 (NRSV).

17. Morgan, 19ff. Rights, Gen 15:6, Rom. 4, Gal 3; the adjective, Hab. 2:4, Rom. 1:17, Gal. 3:11; the verb, Ps. 143:2, Rom. 3:20, Gal. 2:16 and Rom. 3:20 (NRSV).

18. Acts 9:3-22, 22:4-16; 26:9-18; compare Gal. 1:13 (NRSV).

19. A. Hyman and J.J. Walsh, eds., *Philosophy of the Middle Ages: The Christian, Jewish and Islamic Tradition* (Indianapolis: Hackett Publishing Co., 1973), 438-449. Deut. 10:15, Psalms 113-118 (NRSV).

20. Thomas Gilby, "Conscience," *Encyclopedia of Religion* (Farmington Hills, MI: MacMillan Reference Books, 1951), 1:884.

21. 1 Cor. 1:9; 10:13 (NRSV).

22. Rom. 10:4. See Tom Wright, *Climax of the Covenant* (London, 1998). Ward, *Religion and Community* (Oxford: Clarendon, 2000), 210.

23. Morgan, 86.

24. Jn. 1:17 (NRSV).

25. Morgan, 24-26, 28. Rom. 8:3 (NRSV).

26. Rom. 4:1, 4:11-12(NRSV).

27. Morgan, 21. See AJ Huktgren, "The *Pisitis Christou* Formulation in Paul," *NovT* 22 (1980): 253. Also, BW Longenecker, *The Triumph of Abraham's God: The Transformation of Identity in Galatians* (Edinburgh: T & T Clark, 1998), 96f. See also, EE Johnson and DM Hay, eds., *Pauline Theology, Volume IV, Looking Back, Pressing On* (Sydney Biblical Association [SBA] Symposium Series, 1997), 35-81.

28. Ex. 5:1, 6:6, 8:1 and the Psalter (NRSV).

29. Morgan, 86. Rom. 9:5; antithetical to salvation, Phil. 3:9 (NRSV).

30. Charles Conti, *Metaphysical Personalism—An Analysis of Austin Farrar's Theistic Metaphysics* (Oxford: Clarendon, 1995), xx. See, P. D. Bookstaber, *The Idea of the Development of the Soul in Jewish Medieval Philosophy* (Phil.: Maurice Jacobs, Inc., 1950/5711), 36.

31. Morgan, 82-83, 87. Cites Rom. 4:8, 13-14; 9:13 (c.f., Joel 2:32).

32. Morgan, 86-87.

33. Ibid., 91.

34. David Réne, "Comparative Function," in *International Encyclopedia of Comparative Law: The Legal Systems of the World, Their Comparison and Unification,* Eds. K. Z. Zweigert, et al., Vol. II (The Hague: Mouton, 1975), 4.

35. Mt. 5:17; Mt. 23:23. Also, Ex. 25:17, 1 Ch.21:13, Ps. 40, Dan. 9:9, Hab. 3:2, Zech. 1:12, Mt. 9:13, Rom. 9:15, Eph. 2:4, 1 Tim. 1:13, Tit. 3:5, Heb. 4:16, Jas. 2:13, Sir. 2:17 (NRSV).

36. Geoffrey Sawer, "Structures and divisions of the law," in *International Encyclopedia of Comparative Law: The Legal Systems of the World, Their Comparison*

and Unification, Eds. K. Z. Zweigert, et al., Vol. II (The Hague: Mouton, 1975), 17, 46.

37. Ibid.

38. *Kingdom... on earth:* Mt. 6:10, Lk. 11:2 (NRSV).

39. Ref. Kallistos Ware, *The Orthodox Church* (London: Penguin, 1993).

40. G. Sawer, 17, 46.

41. Dickens, 21.

42. Réne, 16.

43. James E. Wood, Bruce Thompson, and Robert T. Miller *Church and State in Scripture, History, and Constitutional Law* (Waco, TX: Baylor University Press, 1958), 57ff.

44. Sawer, 18.

45. Ibid., 19.

46. Ibid.

47. Ibid., 21f.

48. Charles Szadits, "Structures and Divisions of Law," in *International Encyclopedia of Comparative Law: The Legal Systems of the World, Their Comparison and Unification,* Eds. K. Z. Zweigert, et al., Vol. II (The Hague: Mouton, 1975), ch. 3, 21.

49. Berman, *Faith and Order: The Reconciliation of Law and Religion* (Atlanta, Georgia: Scholars Press, 1993), 35ff.

50. Wood, et al., *Church and State in Scripture, History, and Constitutional Law,* 57ff.

51. Dickens, 21.

52. Réne, 100-101.

53. Sawer, 23.

54. Berman, 60f.

55. Ibid., 23-24.

56. *Quinn v. Leatham* (1901) AC 495, 506 (H.L.). See Sawer, 25-27.

57. Ibid., 25-27.

58. Ibid., 25.

59. Berman, 102ff.

60. John Emerich Edward Dalberg Acton, *Lectures on the French Revolution,* Eds. J.N. Figgis and R.V. Lawrence (New York: Noonday Press, 1959), 115.

61. Berman, 135.

62. Ibid., 33, 86f.

63. Sawer, 34-35.

64. See Christopher Columbus Langdell, *The Development of Equity Leading from Canon Law Procedures* (Cambridge: Cambridge University Press, 1905).

65. Alasdair MacIntyre, *After Virtue* (Notre Dame: University of Notre Dame, 1981), 1-6.

66. Jean-Jacques Rousseau, *On the Social Contract (1762) or Principles of Political Right,* translated and edited by Donald A. Cress (Indianapolis: Hackett, 1983), 52f.

67. Calvin Woodard, "Morality as a Perennial Source of Indeterminacy in the Life of the Law," in *Law and Morality in a Free Society,* Eds. James E. Wood, Jr. and Derek Davis (Waco, TX: JM Dawson Institute of Church-State Studies, 1994), 29f.

68. Berman, 289, 292f.

69. Derek Davis, "Preserving the Moral Integrity of the Constitution: An Examination of Deconstruction and Other Hermeneutical Theories," in *Law and Morality,* Eds. James E. Wood, Jr. and Derek Davis (Waco, TX: JM Dawson Institute of Church-State Studies, 1994), 215.

70. Berman, 278f.

71. Sawer, 37-38. N.n. Lerner, 74-75.

72. Sawer, 39. Ref., H.L.A. Hart, *The Concept of Law* (Oxford: Oxford University Press, 1961).

73. Sawer, 46, 48.

74. Roger B. Dworkin, *The Role of the Law in Bioethical Decision-Making* (Indianapolis, Indiana University Press, 1996), 2-7, 108.

75. Ibid., 162.

76. Ibid., 87-88.

77. Ibid., 84, 90.

78. Dickens, 27.

79. R. Dworkin, 82-84. George P. Smith II, "Australia Frozen Orphan Embryos: A Medical, Legal and Ethical Dilemma," 24 *J. Family L.* 27 (1985-86), 82. Also, David Mangolick, "15 Vials of Sperm: the Unusual Bequest of an even More Unusual Man," *New York Times* (29 April 1994): B18.

80. Sheila Jasonoff, *Science at the Bar: Law, Science, Technology in America* (Cambridge: Harvard University Press, 1995), 139-40. See also, Dickens, 84, 88, 90. Daniel E. Koshland, "Judicial Impact Statements," *Science* 239 (1988): 1225.

81. Jasonoff, 140, 144-145.

82. Genetic Forum, *The Case Against Patients in Genetic Engineering* (London: Genetic Forum, April, 1996), 4-6, 14-15.

83. Los Angeles Times Editorial, "Gene Patent Reform Vital," *Los Angeles Times* (February 2000, n/d), n/p.

84. Ruth Deech, HFEA Chair, *Blood* decision ref. *Kass v. Kass,* NJ, Case No. 7808640.

85. Réne, 113-115.

86. James E. Wood, Jr., "Religion, Morality and the Law," in *Law and Morality,* Eds. James E. Wood, Jr. and Derek Davis (Waco, TX: JM Dawson Institute of Church–State Studies, 1994), 15.

87. Berman, 300.

88. Réne, 17, 19, 20, 23, 100.

89. G.W.F. Hegel, *Philosophy of Right* (1821), translation by T.M. Knox (London: Oxford University Press, 1952), 14f., 25, 79f (§117), 86f. (§128-129).

90. Berman, 309f.

91. Ibid. See Réne, 24.

92. Wood, "Religion, Morality and the Law," 12f.

93. Michael Perry, "Is the Idea of Human Rights Ineliminably Religious?" in *Law and Morality,* Eds. James E. Wood, Jr. and Derek Davis (Waco, TX: JM Dawson Institute of Church-State Studies, 1994), 70.

94. Perry, 84.
95. Alasdair MacIntyre, *After Virtue* (Notre Dame: University of Notre Dame Press,˚1981), 3.
96. UNESCO Bioethics Committee, "Universal Declaration on the Human Genome and Human Rights" (November 1997), 1. Recalling, "Universal Declaration of Human Rights" (10 December 1948); "UN Covenant on Economic, Social, and Cultural Rights" (16 December 1966); "UN Civil and Political Rights" (16 December 1966); "UN Convention on the Prevention and Punishment of the Crime of Genocide" (9 December 1948); "UN Convention on the Elimination of All Forms of Racial Discrimination" (21 December 1965); "UN Declaration on the Rights of Mentally Retarded Persons" (20 December 1971); "UN Declaration on the Rights of Disabled Persons" (9 December 1975); "UN Declaration on the Elimination of All Forms of Discrimination against Women" (18 December 1979); "UN Declaration on Basic Principles of Justice on Victims of Crimes and Abuse of Power" (29 November 1985); "UN Convention on the Rights of the Child" (20 November 1985); "UN Standard Rules on the Equalization of Opportunities for Persons with Disabilities" (20 December 1993); "UN Convention on Biological Diversity" (5 June 1992); "Convention on the Prohibition of the Development, Production and Stockpiling of Bacteriological (Biological) and Toxin Weapons and on their Destruction" (16 December 1971); "UNESCO Convention against Discrimination in Education" (14 December 1960); "UNESCO Declaration of the Principles of International Cultural Co-operation" (4 November 1966); "UNESCO Recommendation on the Status of Scientific Researchers" (20 November 1974); "UNESCO Declaration on Race and Racial Prejudice" (27 November 1978); "ILO Convention (No. 111) concerning Discrimination in Respect of Employment and Occupation" (25 June 1958); and, "ILO Convention (No. 169) Concerning Indigenous and tribal Peoples in Independent Countries" (27 June 1989). Instruments applicable to intellectual property, *inter alia* "Bern Convention for the Protection of Literary and Artistic Works" (9 September 1886); "UNESCO Universal Copyright Convention" (6 September 1952, revision 24 July 1971); "Paris Convention for the Protection of Industrial Property" (20 March 1883, revised 14 July 1967); "Budapest Treaty of the WIPO on International Recognition of the Deposit of Micro-organisms for the Purposes of Patent Procedures" (28 April 1977); and, "Trade Related Aspects of Intellectual Property Rights Agreement (TRIPs) annexed to the Agreement establishing the World Trade Organization" (1 January 1995). Resolutions in accordance with the "Preamble to the Universal Declaration of Human Rights" 22 C/Resolution 13.1, 23 C/Resolution 13.1, 24 C/Resolution 13.1, 25 C/Resolutions 5.2 and 7.3, 27 C/Resolution 5.15 and 28 C/Resolutions 1.12, 2.1 and 2.2.
97. UNESCO Bioethics Committee, Universal Declaration on the Human Genome and Human Rights (November 1997), 3-8.
98. Jean Michaud, "The Internationalization of a framework for Genetic Diagnosis," lecture at the International Conference on Genetic Diagnosis (Rennes, France, 1998), ref. Art. 11, 12, and 13 of the *Convention*.

Chapter 4

1. Henrik Wulff, Stig Andur Pedersen, Raben Rosenberg, *Philosophy of Medicine: Introduction* (London: Blackwell Scientific Publications, 1986), ix. See also, Robert B. Baker, Arthur L. Caplan, Linda L. Emanuel, and Stephen R. Latham, eds, *The American Medical Ethics Revolution: How the AMAs Code of Ethics Has Transformed Physicians Relationships to Patients, Professionals, and Society* (Baltimore: The Johns Hopkins University Press, 2001).

2. Wulff, Pedersen, Rosenberg, 3.

3. Leon Kass, "Regarding the End of Medicine and the Pursuit of Health," *The Public Interest* 40 (Summer 1975): 27-29.

4. Christopher Boorse, "Health is a Theoretical Concept," *Philosophy of Science* 44 (1977): 542-573.

5. James M. Gustafson, *Intersections: Science, Theology, and Ethics* (Cleveland: The Pilgrim Press, 1996), 95-96.

6. William F. May, *The Physician's Covenant* (Philadelphia: The Westminster Press, 1983), 109.

7. E.H. Ackerknect, *A Short History of Medicine* (Baltimore: Johns Hopkins University Press, 1982), chapters 1-4.

8. Michel Foucault, *The Birth of the Clinic: An Archeology of Medical Perception*, translation of *Naissance de la Clinic* by A.M. Sheridan Smith (New York: Pantheon Books, 1973), 59, 168, 190-195.

9. John H. Brooke, *Science and Religion* (Cambridge: Cambridge University Press, 1998), 254-55, 293, 323, 336. Ref. Darwin, *Origin of Species* (1859). Also, John Brooke and Geoffrey Cantor, *Reconstructing Nature: The Engagement of Science and Religion* (Edinburgh: T & T Clark, 1998), 160, 164-66. See Holmes Rolston, *Genes, Genesis and God: Values and Their Origins in Natural and Human History* (Cambridge: Cambridge University Press, 1999), 1-21. Also see John Maynard Smith, *On Evolution* (Edinburgh: University of Edinburgh, 1972), 89, 93-98.

10. Wulff, Pedersen, Rosenberg, 42. See Ackerkneckt, chapters 5 to end.

11. Ref. Daniel Jonah Goldhagen, *Hitler's Willing Executioners* (New York: Vintage Books, 1997).

12. Hans Guater Zmärzlik, *"Der Sozialdarwinismus im Deutschland als geschichtliches Problem," Vierteljahrshefte für Zeitgeschichte* 11 (1963): 246-273. See R. Proctor, *Racial Hygiene: Medicine Under the Nazis* (Cambridge: Harvard University Press, 1988): 29, 46-47. Also, Donald J. Dietrich, "Catholic Eugenics in Germany, 1920-1945: Hermann Muckermann, S.J. and Joseph Mayer," *Journal of Church and State* 34 (Summer 1992), 3:575. Ref., Michael H. Kater, *Under Hitler* (Chapel Hill: University of North Carolina Press, Inc., 1989).

13. Yehuda Bauer, "Euthanasia, Nazism and Psychiatry," *Holocaust Conference* (Oxford, England, July 1988): 2. See William Brennan, *Medical Holocaust I: Exterminative Medicine in Nazi Germany and Contemporary America* (Boston: Nordland Publishing International, Inc., 1980), 20. Also, E. BenGershôm, "From Haeckel to Hackethal: Lessons from Nazi Medicine for Students and Practitioners

of Medicine," *Holocaust and Genocidal Studies* 5, No.1 (Oxford: Pergamon Press, Winter 1990): 78.

14. BenGershôm, 78.

15. Dietrich, 3:591.

16. Robert Jay Lifton, *The Nazi Doctors: Medical Killing and the Psychology of Genocide* (New York: Basic Books, Inc. Publications, 1986), 31.

17. BenGershôm, 79f. See Lifton, 31.

18. Dietrich, 577-78, 582-583.

19. National Archives, RG 238 CI-FIR/123, 9 January 1947 Annex V; *Süddeutsche Zeitung,* 15 February 1967. See Dietrich, 584, 590, 591, 593. For origin and content of sin: Clement, Origin, J. Chrysostum and Gratian.

20. George J. Annas and Michael Grodin, eds., *The Nazi Doctors and the Nuremberg Code* (Oxford: Oxford University Press, 1992), 23.

21. Dietrich, 584, 591. Aly Götz, Peter Chroust and Christian Pross, *Cleansing the Fatherland, Nazi Medicine and Racial Hygiene* (Baltimore: Johns Hopkins University Press, 1994), 14. See also, Hans-Heimrich Wilhelm, "Euthanasia Program," in *Encyclopedia of the Holocaust,* Vol. 2, Ed., Israel Gutman (New York: Macmillan Publishing Co., 1990), 2:451, 593-594.

22. Dietrich, 576-77. Also, Lifton, 30f. See "The 'Euthanasia' Programme 1939-1945," in *Nazism 1919-1945, Vol. 3 Foreign Policy, War and Racial Extermination, Exeter Studies in History* 13, eds., J. Noakes and G. Pridham (University of Exeter, n.d.), 998. Ref. Annas and Grodin, ix.

23. "The Programme," 1001; Annas, 23.

24. Bauer, 3-4, 53. Also, "The Programme, 998. See Wilhelm, 2:451. Also see Götz, 3.

25. KdF was an government organization; the acronym stands for "kraft durch freud" (Eng., strength through joy). Annas, 25. See, Götz, 190-91. Bauer, 5-7. "The Programme," 1001, 1005f

26. "The Programme," 1001.

27. Annas, 23. See Bauer, 7.

28. "The Programme," 997. See Lifton, 93, 480. Also, Wilhelm, 2:453. See also, Annas, 23, 33.

29. BenGershôm, 24-25.

30. Götz, 24.

31. Ibid., 3, 208. See, "The Programme," 1000. Also, Dietrich, 595. See also, Lifton, 31.

32. Bauer, 11.

33. "The Programme," 1019. Bauer, 7, 11, 15-16, 19. See Leni Yahil, "Kristallnach," in *Encyclopedia of the Holocaust,* 4 Vols., Ed., Israel Gutman (New York: MacMillan Co., Inc.), 2:836. Ref., F. Kapp wrote "On sterilization of Hereditary Mental Deficit's and Its meaning in the Fight Against Crime," in *Monthly Journal for Criminal Biology and Criminal Law Reference* (1930). Also, Annas, Eli Wiesel's introduction, vii, 24-25. See also, BenGershôm, 10. See Wladyslaw T. Bartoszewski, *Surviving Treblinka* (Oxford: Basil Blackwell, 1989), 3. Also, Wilhelm, 2:452-453. Ref., M.H. Pappworth, *Human Guinea Pigs* (London: Rutledge and Kegan Paul, 1967), 61, 83.

34. Annas, 28.

35. Ibid., 71. Götz, 69, 70, 72, 257.

36. Götz, 47-49, 169, 176, 217-128, 205, 220-225.

37. Annas, *Doctors,* 83. Götz, 16, 99f., 105.

38. BenGershôm, 80, 82-83. Götz, 12-13, 32f. Annas, vii, 47, 266.

39. BenGershôm, 80-81. Bauer, 12. Götz, 5, 7-8.

40. BenGershôm, 82.

41. Ibid., 46.

42. Ibid., xii. See, Bauer, 2.

43. Annas, 272. See also, G.J. Annas, "Nancy Cruzan and the Right to Die," *New England Journal of Medicine* 323 (1990): 670-73. See also, D. Andrusko, ed., *A Passion for Justice* (Washington D.C.: National Right to Life, 1998). Also, N. Hentoff, "Nazi Bioethics and a Doctor's Defense," *Human Life Review* 8 (1982): 55-69. See F. Wertham, *A Sign for Cain* (New York: Warner, 1973); *The German Euthanasia Program* (Cinn.: Hayes, 1988). Post-war advocates: Dr. Erhardt, *Euthanasia and Destruction of Life Devoid of Value,* Forum of Psychology Series (Marburg: F. Encke Publishers, 1965).

44. Steve Jones, "Genetics in Medicine: Real Promises, Unreal Expectations— One Scientist's Advice to Policymakers in the United Kingdom and the United States," from the Millbank Memorial Fund Prospectus (New York: Millbank Memorial Fund, 2000), 3.

45. Rolston, 35. See Ronald Cole-Turner, *The New Genesis: Theology and the Genetic Revolution* (Louisville: Westminster/John Knox Press, 1993), 13-14. Also, Rom Harre, *The Philosophy of Science: An Introductory Survey* (Oxford: Oxford University Press, 1985), 255. Ref. text: Lubert Stryer, *Biochemistry,* 4th ed. (New York: W.H. Freeman, 1999). Ref. text: Bruce Alberts et al., *Molecular Biology of the Cell,* 3rd ed. (N/c: Garland Publishing Co., 1994).

46. Stephen Rose, "The Rise of Neurogenic Determinism," in *Consciousness and Human Identity,* Ed., John Cornwall (Oxford: Oxford University Press, 1998), 98. Ref. text: James Watson et al., *Recombinant DNA,* 2nd ed. (New York: Scientific American Books/ W.H. Freeman, 1992).

47. T. D. McKnight, "Transcription and elongation," *Genes and Development* 10 (1996): 367. Also see, A. Wolff, "Gene repression by targeted deacetylation," *Nature* 387 (1997): 16-17.

48. Peter Cook, "99rep" (replication info.) or "nuc99" (transcription) Peter. Cook@path.ox.ac.uk. Immobile *replication:* P. Hozak, D.A. Jackson, and P.R. Cook, "The Role of nuclear structure in DNA Replication," in *Eukaryotic DNA Replication: Frontiers in Molecular Biology,* Ed. J.J. Blow (Oxford University Press, 1996), 124-42. See K. P. Lemon and A.D. Grossman, "Localization of bacterial DNA polymerase: evidence for a factory model of replication," *Science* 282 (1998): 1516-19. Immobile *transcription:* P.R. Cook and I.A. Brazell, "Supercoils in Human DNA," *Journal Cellular Science* 19 (1975): 261-79. See A. Wolff, *Chromatin: Structure and Function,* 3rd ed. (London: Academic Press, 1998). Also, S.M. Gasser and U.K. Laemmli, "Cohabitation of scaffold binding regions with upstream/enhancer elements of 3 developmentally regulated genes of D. melanogaster," *Cell* 46 (1986): 521-30. Ref. P. Schediand F. Grosveld, "Domaines and

Boundaries," in *Chromatin Structure and Gene Expression*, Ed. S.C.R. Elgin (Oxford: Oxford University Press, 1996). Transient attachment: D.A. Jackson and P.R. Cook, "Transcriptionally active minichromosomes are attached transiently in nuclei through transcription units," *Journal Cellular Science* 105 (1993): 1143-1150. Ref. Text: Thomas Strachen and Andrew Read, *Human Molecular Genetics Bios.*, 2nd ed. (London: Wiley John and Sons and Co., 1999), chaps. 4, 5, 6, 19, 20.

49. Cole-Turner, *The New Genesis*, 20. Jones, 5. Ref. text: Strachan and Read.

50. Ref., Rolston, chapter 2.

51. Edmund Samturri, "Prenatal Diagnosis: Some Moral Considerations," in *Questions about the Beginning of Life: Christian Appraisals of Seven Bioethical Issues* (Minneapolis, Minn.: Augsburg, 1985): 120, 122-123, 125-126, 130. See Andrew Simons, "Brave New Harvest," *Christianity Today* (19 November 1990): 25-28. Also, André Boué, "The Evolution of Genetic Diagnosis Before Birth: Past, Present, and Future," at the *International Conference on Genetic Diagnosis: From Prenatal to Preimplantation, Ethical, Legal and Social Issues* (Rennes, FR, 1998).

52. Allan Sekine et al., "Fgf10 is essential for limb and lung formation," *Nature Genetics* 21 (1999): 138-41. Also, Gerald Neubüser et al., "The role of FGF signaling in positioning the tooth germs in the mandible," *Cell* 90 (1997): 247-255.

53. Gary Taubes, "Ontogeny Recapitulated," *Discover* (May 1998): 66, 68-71. Ref. Text, Lewis Wolpert, *Principles of Development* (Oxford: Oxford University Press, 1995).

54. Wolpert, 304-19. See Scott Gilbert, *Developmental Biology*, 5th ed. (London: Sinuar, 1995), 701-26. Also, W.J. Larsen, *Human Embryology* (London: Churchill Livingston, 1996), 300-05. See also, C. Tickel, "The Number of polarizing regions cells required to specify additional digits in the chick wing," *Nature* 289 (1981): 295-298.

55. S.J. Goss, "Differentiation," Lecture, Oxford: University of Oxford (1999).

56. J.R. Hinchliffe and T.J. Horder, "Testing the theoretical models for limb patterning," in *Experimental and Theoretical Advances in Biological Pattern Formation*, Ed. H.G. Othmer, et al. (London: Plenum, 1993).

57. Robin Marantz Henig, "Tempting," *Discover* (May 1998): 62.

58. Jones, 12,15.

59. Ibid., 8f. See Robert C. Stern, "The Diagnosis of Cystic Fibrosis," *New England Journal of Medicine* 336, no. 7 (13 February 1997): 487, 490. See also, Biesecker, "Genetic Counseling: Practice of Genetic Counseling" in *Encyclopedia of Bioethics*, Vol. 2 (New York: Macmillan Library, 1995): 2:926.

60. Jones, 12.

61. Ibid., 6f.

62. Andrew Simons, "Brave New Harvest," *Christianity Today* (19 November 1990): 24f. See Jones, 9.

63. Kay Davis, "Identification of Disease," Lecture, Oxford: University of Oxford (1999).

64. Simons, 6f.

65. Taubes, 68, 71-72.

66. Simons, 25-28. See Samturri, 125-126, 130.

67. Richard D. Devine, *Good Care, Painful Choices: Medical Ethics for Ordinary People* (New York: Paulist Press, 1996), 127. See Burtness, 71, 83-84, 86. Also, Eric Juengst and LeRoy Walters, "Gene Therapy: Ethical and Social Issues," in the *Encyclopedia of Bioethics,* 5 Vols. (New York: Macmillan Library, 1995): 2:917-918.

68. D. Nakada, B. Magasanik. "The Roles of Inducer and Catabolite Repressor in the Synthesis of Beta-Galactosidase by Escherichia Coli". *Journal of Molecular Biology* 8 (1964): 105-127. See Gros et al., *Cold Spring Harbor Symposium* (1961): 26, 111.

69. Robert Pool, "Saviors," *Discover* (May 1998): 54-56.

70. Ibid., 56. See www.abcnews.go.com/sections/living/daileynews/pigorgans 991103.htm.

71. David Morley, *The Sensitive Scientist: Report of a British Associated Study Group* (London: SCM, 1978), 122. See Paul M. McNeil, *Ethics and the Politics of Human Experimentation* (Cambridge: Cambridge University Press, 1993): 165-66. Also, P.S. Appelbaum, C.W. Lutz, A. Morsel, *Informed Consent: Legal Theory and Clinical Practice* (New York: Oxford University Press, 1987), 238. Also see, Alex Capron, "Human Experiment," in *Biological Law: A Legal Reporter on Medicine, Health Care and Bioengineering,* Eds. J.F. Childress, et al. (Frederick, MD: University Publication of America, 199), 1:217-252.

72. Morley, 119, 122-123, 125-129. See H.J. Eysenck, "The Ethics of Science and the Duties of Scientists," *The Advancement of Science,* no. 1 (1975): 23-25. Also, Jacques Monad, *"Leçon inaugurale au college de France,"* College de France, Paris (3 Nov. 1967), published in *Chance and Necessity* (Collins).

73. Morley, 32, 119, 122.

74. Robert Twycross, "Palliative Care," in *Encyclopedia of Applied Ethics,* Vol. 3 (Oxford: Oxford University Press, 1998), 419.

75. Twycross, 420. See May, 131.

76. Twycross, 421-423. Ref., R. Sims and V.A. Moss, *Palliative Care for People with AIDS,* 2nd ed. (London: Edward Arnold, 1995). See ref., A. Armstrong-Dailey and S.Z. Goltzer, eds., *Hospice Care for Children* (Oxford: Oxford University Press, 1993). Also ref., S. DuBoulay, *Cicely Saunders: The Founder of the Modern Hospice Movement* (London: Hodder and Stroughton, 1997).

77. Ref. Text: V. Mor, *Hospice Care Systems: Structure, Process, Costs and Outcome* (New York: Springer, 1987).

78. Twycross, 423f. See *Cancer Pain Relief* (Geneva: World Health Organization, 1986).

79. Twycross, 424, 426.

80. Ibid., 427f. See N. Dickey, "Council on Ethical and Judicial Affairs, American Medical Association, Statement on Withholding or Withdrawing Life-Prolonging Medical Treatment," *Journal of the American Medical Association* 256 (1986): 471.

81. Twycross, 427.

82. Ibid, 431.

83. Ibid, 429.

84. David Jones, "On Death," Lecture, Oxford: University of Oxford (2000).

85. Twycross, 431.

86. Gen. 1:26-31. Murphy and Ellis, *On the Moral Nature of the Universe,* 116 (c.f. MacIntyre, *After Virtue* [Notre Dame: University of Notre Dame Press, 1981], 23).

87. Jyoti Thottam, "Hope in a Test Tube," *Time Special Issue* (5 March 2001): 38-39.

88. *State Initiatives in End-of-Life Care: Policy Leaders* 9 (January 2001): 1-6. Ref., California Department of Health Services, Public Law 101-508. See UCI Medical Center *Patients' Rights* (Irvine: University of California, 2000). Also ref., UCIMC, *Patient's Responsibilities* (Irvine: University of California, 2000). Reference: www.ucihealth.com.

Chapter 5

1. David Morley, *The Sensitive Scientist: Report of a British Associated Study Group* (London: SCM, 1978), 121. See Herbert J. Eysenck, "The Ethics of Science and the Duty of Scientists," *The Advancement of Science* 1 (1975), 23-25.

2. Carol S. Robb, "Framework for Feminine Ethics," in *Feminist Theological Ethics,* Ed. Lois. K. Daly (Louisville: John Knox Press, 1994), 15.

3. Gen. 3; 16:2ff.; Gen. 21:12. Robb, 15.

4. Carol Gilligan, *In a Different Voice: Psychological Theory and Women's Development* (Cambridge: Harvard, 1982), 128, 148f.

5. Gen. 1:27 (NRSV).

6. Cahill, " 'Embodiment' and Moral Critique: A Christian Social Perspective," in *On Moral Medicine: Theological Perspectives in Medical Ethics,* Eds. Stephen E. Lammers and Allen Verney, 2nd ed. (Grand Rapids: Wm. D. Eerdmans Publishing Company, 1998), 406-407.

7. Lois K. Daly, "Ecofeminosm, Reverence for Life, Feminist Theological Ethics," in *Feminist Theological Ethics: A Reader,* Ed. Lois Daly (Louisville, KY: John Knox Press, 1994), 311. See H. Richard Niebuhr, *The Responsible Self* (San Francisco: Harper Row, 1963), 143.

8. Elizabeth E. Green, "The Transmutation of Theology: Ecofeminist Alchemy and the Christian Tradition," in *Ecofeminism and Theology: Yearbook of the European Society of Women in Theological Research* (Netherlands: Kok Pharos Publishing House, 1994), 49. Also see Cahill, 406.

9. Susan Frank Parson, *Feminism and Christian Ethics* (Cambridge: Cambridge University Press, 1996), 140. See Nell Nodding, *Caring: A Feminist Approach to Ethics and Moral Education* (Los Angeles: University of California Press, 1984), 56. Also, Gilligan, 8, 17, 148. Also see, Robb, 22.

10. Margaret A. Farley, "Feminist Theology and Bioethics," in *Feminist Theological Ethics: A Reader,* Ed. Lois K. Daly (Louisville, KY: John Knox Press, 1994), 202. See Janice G. Raymond, "Reproductive Gifts and Gift Giving: The Altruistic Woman," in *Feminist Theological Ethics: A Reader,* Ed. Lois K. Daly (Louisville, KY: John Knox Press, 1994), 237. See also, Gilligan, 148. Eleanor Humes Hancy, "What is Feminist Ethics?" in *Feminist Theological Ethics: A Reader,* Ed. Lois K. Daly (Louisville, KY: John Knox Press, 1994), 5. See Robb, 17. Also, Anne

McGrew Bennett, "Overcoming the Biblical and Traditional Subordination of Women," in *Feminist Theological Ethics: A Reader,* Ed. Lois K. Daly (Louisville, KY: John Knox Press, 1994), 144. See also, Barbara Hilkert Andolsen, "Agape in Feminist Ethics," in *Feminist Theological Ethics: A Reader,* Ed. Lois K. Daly (Louisville, KY: John Knox Press, 1994), 156.

11. Dt. 6:5; Mt. 22:37; Mk. 12:28, Lk. 9:48.

12. Jn. 15:13 (NRSV).

13. Cahill, 406. For virtues see Mary Daly, "The Spiritual Revolution: Women's Liberation as Theological Re-education," in *Feminist Theological Ethics: A Reader,* Ed. Lois K. Daly (Louisville, KY: John Knox Press, 1994), 122. See L. K. Daly, 304ff. References Albert Schweitzer, *Philosophy of Civilization,* translated by C. T. Campion (New York: Macmillan, 1949, reprint Tallahassee, FL: Univ. Press of Florida, 1981). See also, Gilligan, 62f., 129.

14. Sophie Boukhari and Amy Otchet, "Uncharted terrain on tomorrow's genetic map," *The UNESCO Courier* (September 1999): 19. See L. K. Daly, 295f. Also, Hancy, 10, 12. See also, Robb, 15. Ref., Gilligan, 19, 22. Antithetical ref., Lawrence Kohlberg, *The Philosophy of Moral Development* (San Francisco: Harper and Row, 1981).

15. M. Daly, 132. See Paul Tillich, *Systematic Theology.*

16. McNeil, 175. See P.S. Appelbaum, C.W. Lutz, A. Meisel, *Informed Consent: Legal Theory and Clinical Practice* (New York: Oxford University Press, 1987), 239, 246-247.

17. Morley, 127. See Jean-Marie Mpendawatu, *"Questions Generales Sur le Conseil Genetic,"* at http:www.unesco/ethics.

18. Ruth S Downie and Elizabeth Telfer, "Respect for Persons," in *Philosophic Ethics: An Introduction of Moral Philosophy,* Ed. Tom L. Beauchamp (Georgetown Univ., 1982), 131-34 (c.f., Telfer Downie, *Respect for Persons* [New York: Schoken Books, Inc., 1970], 23-29. See also, Tom L. Beauchamp, ed., *Philosophic Ethics: An Introduction of Moral Philosophy* (Washington DC: Georgetown University, 1982), 4f.

19. Ibid., 72, 88.

20. Hancy, 12. See H.R. Niebuhr, *The Responsible Self* (San Francisco: Harper Row, 1963), 31.

21. H.R. Niebuhr, 47f.

22. Gilligan, 129.

23. Cahill, "'Embodiment' and Moral Critique," 405. See Gilligan, 69. Also, Feinberg, 229-230, 257-261. See also, Cole-Turner, 40, 42, 45. Ref., John A. Robertson, "Genetic Selection of Offspring Characteristics," *Boston University Law Review* 76 (June 1996): 470, 473, 481. Legal cases, *Custody of Minor,* 393 N.E. 2d 836, 837-838 (Mass. 1979) and *Skinner v. Oklahoma,* 316 US 535, 541. See Thomas H. Murray and Jeffrey R. Botkin, "Genetic Testing and Screening: Ethical Issues," in the *Encyclopedia of Bioethics,* 5 Vols. (New York: Macmillan Library, 1995), 2:1008-1009. Also, Eric Juengst and LeRoy Walters, "Gene Therapy: Ethical and Social Issues," in *Encyclopedia of Bioethics,* Vol. 2 (New York: Macmillan Library, 1995), 920.

24. John Fletcher, "Moral Problems in Genetic Counseling," in *Ethical Issues in Moral Medicine,* Eds. Robert J. Hunt and John Arras (Palo Alto, CA: Mayfield Publishing Co., 1977), 108ff.

25. Counsel of Europe, "Written Declaration No. 247," *Parliamentary Assembly* (Strasbourg, France 26 April 1996), 1.

26. Farley, 206-7. See S. Riddick, "Maternal thinking," *Signs* 6 (1980): 342-367.

27. *Personal Origins,* 2nd ed. (London: Church House Publishing, 1996), 64ff. See Barbara Biesecker, "Genetic Counseling: Practice of Genetic Counseling," in the *Encyclopedia of Bioethics,* Vol. 2 (New York: Macmillan Library, 1995), 2: 923. See Andrew Simons, "Brave New Harvest," *Christianity Today* (19 November 1990): 25-28. See also, Edmund Samturri, "Prenatal Diagnosis: Some Moral Considerations," in *Questions about the Beginning of Life* (Minneapolis: Augsburg, 1985): 125-126, 130.

28. R. H. Niebuhr, *The Responsible Self,* 132ff.

29. Farley, 199.

30. James F. Drane, *Becoming a Doctor: The Place of Virtue and Character in Medical Ethics* (Kansas City, MO: Sheed and Ward, 1988), 33, 122, 125. See Cole–Turner, *Pastoral Genetics,* 41, 43.

31. Drane, 33, 122, 125.

32. James F. Drane, *Clinical Bioethics: Theory and Practice of Medical–Ethical Decision-Making* (Kansas City, MO: Sheed and Ward, 1994), 5-9.

33. Glenn McGee, *The Prefect Baby: The Pragmatic Approach to Genetics* (Lanham, Maryland: Rowman and Littlefield Publishers, 1977), 75, 80, 92. See Niebuhr, 100. Also, Ronald Cole-Turner and Brent Waters, *Pastoral Genetics: Theology and Care at the Beginning of Life* (Cleveland: Pilgrims Press, 1996), 41.

34. McGee, 73.

35. Cole-Turner, *Pastoral Genetics,* 35-36, 39-40. See also, Robert Murray, "Genetic Counseling: Ethical Issues," in the *Encyclopedia of Bioethics,* Vol. 2 (New York: Macmillan Library, 1995), 927-928. Also see, Biesecker, 2:924-925.

36. Cahill, "'Embodiment' and Moral Critique," 403, 406. Drane, *Clinical Bioethics,* xv-xvii. Raymond, 241.

37. Biesecker, 2:924.

38. John S. Feinberg and Paul D. Feinberg, *Ethics for a Brave New World* (Wheaton, Ill.: Crossways Books, 1993), 257-261. See Biesecker, 2:925-926. For dysgenics, R.E. Murray, 2:928. Also, Richard D. Devine, *Good Care, Painful Choices: Medical Ethics for Ordinary People* (New York: Paulist Press, 1996), 129. Also see, R. Murray, 2:929-930. Cole-Turner, *Pastoral Genetics,* 41, 43. James M. Childress, "Genetic Screening and Counseling," in *Questions about the Beginning of Life: Christian Appraisals of Seven Bioethical Issues* (Minneapolis, Minn.: Augsburg, 1985): 114-117. Case, *Howard v. Lecher,* 42 NY 2d 109; NYS 2d 363; 366 NE 2d 64.

39. McGee, 41, 47.

40. McGee, 80. Barbara Rothman, *The Tentative Pregnancy: Amniocentesis and Sexual Politics of Motherhood* (London: Pandora, 1986), 263.

41. Samturri, 120, 122-123.

42. Bernard Steinbock, "Maternal–fetal conflict and *in utero* fetal Therapy," in *Aspects éthicques de la reproduction humaine—Ethical aspects of human reproduction*, Eds. Claude Sureau and Françoise Shenfield (Pars: Libby Eurotext, 1995), 6-68. See Childs, 114-117. Case ref., *Custody of a Minor*, 393 N.E. 2d 836, 837-838 (Mass 1979).

43. Rothman, 167, 183, 221-263.

44. Lappé, Marc and James E. Bowman, "Genetics and Racial Minorities: Genetic Testing," in *Encyclopedia of Bioethics*, Vol. 2 (New York: Macmillan Library, 1995), 982. See Biesecker, 2:925. Also, Marc Lappé, "Eugenics: Ethical Issues," in the *Encyclopedia of Bioethics*, Vol. 2 (New York: Macmillan Library, 1995): 773-775. See also, R. Murray, 930.

45. Rothman, 119ff., 195. See Joseph G. Schenker, "Transplantation of Fetal Tissue, Gametes, and Organs," in *Aspects éthiques de la reproduction humanine*, ed. Claude Sureau and Françoise Shenfield (Paris: John Libby Eurotext, 1995), 155, 157. Also, Patricia Baird, "Research on Pre-embryos, zygotes," in *Aspects éthiques de la reproduction humanine*, Ed: Claude Sureau (Paris: John Libby Eurotext, 1995), 333-34. Also see John A. Robertson, "Embryo and Fetal Research," in *Aspects éthiques de la reproduction humanine*, Ed. Claude Sureau (Paris: John Libby Eurotext, 1995), 352-54. Women's dignity, Cahill, 404-05. Surgical aspects, B. Steinbock, "Maternal Fetal Conflict in *in utero Fetal Therapy*," in *Aspects éthiques de la reproduction humanine*, Ed. Claude Sureau and Françoise Shenfield (Paris: John Libby Eurotext, 1995), 70, 77.

46. Jean-Marie Mpendawatu, *"Questions Generales Sue Le Conseil Genetique,"* www.UNESCO/ethic. See Alan Meisel, "Informed Consent: Where is it going?" *Health Law News*, Vol. XV, (June 2001): 6. Case ref., *Salgo v. Leland Stanford Jr. University* Board of Trustees (1957).

47. Steinbeck, 75, 77. Case ref., *In re* President and Directors of Georgetown College, 331 F. 2d 1010, 1017 (D.C.Cir), certificate denied, 377 US 978, 1964.

48. Thomas H. Murray and Jeffrey R. Botkin, "Genetic Testing and Screening: Ethical Issues," in the *Encyclopedia of Bioethics*, 5 Vols. (New York: Macmillan Library, 1995), 2:1008-09. See Cole-Turner, 32-34, 40. Also, Biesecker, 2:924. See also, Cahill, "'Embodiment' and Moral Critique," 404.

49. McNeil, *Ethics and the Politics of Human Experimentation*, 175. Ref. Student-volunteer case: *Halushka v. University of Sashkatchewan* (1965) 53 DLR 2d: 436. See Hans Jonas, "Report on the National Commission: Good as Gold," *Medical Legal News* 8 (Dec. 1980): 4-7.

50. Lisa A. Cahill, "Within Shouting Distance: Paul Ramsey and Richard McCormick on Method," in *Cross-Cultural Perspectives in Medical Ethics: Readings*, Ed. Robert Veatch (Boston: Jones and Bartlett Publishers, 1989), 70-81. Ref., Paul Ramsey, *Ethics at the Edges of Life* (New Haven: Yale University Press, 1978).

51. *Roe v. Wade*, 410 U.S. 113 (1973).

52. Leonard Glantz, "Is the Fetus a Person? A Lawyers View," in *Abortion and the Status of the Fetus*, Eds. William B. Bandeson, H. Tristan Engelhardt, Jr., Stuart I. Spickler, and Daniel H. Winship, (Dordreet: D. Reidel Publishing Company, 1983), 108. See Anita L Allen, "The Proposed Equal Protection Fix for the Abortion Law: Reflections on Citizenship, Gender and the Constitution," *Harvard Journal of*

Law and Public Policy 18 (Spring 1995): 419-55. Also Michael Tooley, "Abortion and Infanticide, In the Rights and Wrongs of Abortion," 52 (1974): 77. Ref., Richard H. Feen, "Abortion and Exposure in Ancient Greece: Assessing the Status of the Fetus and 'New Born' from Classical Sources," in *Abortion and the Status of the Fetus,* Ed., William B. Bandeson; H. Tristan Engelhardt, Jr.; Stuart I. Spickler, and Daniel H. Winship (New York: D. Reidel Publishing Company, 1983), 285-287.

53. Feen, 292.

54. Ibid., 289. Plato, *Politics,* 7.16.15.

55. Stephen M. Krason, *Abortion, Politics, Morality and the Constitution* (New York: University Press of America, 1984), 255.

56. *State v. Winthrop,* 43 Iowa 519 (1876).

57. Glantz, 109; 116.

58. *Doe v. Bolton,* 319 F. Supp. 1048 (1973). See Krason, APMC, 81.

59. *Roe v. Wade,* 410 U.S. 113 (1973).

60. *Griswold v. Connecticut,* 381 U.S. 479 (1965). Allen, 429.

61. Krason, APMC, 81.

62. Tara K. Kelly, "Silencing the Lambs: Restricting First Amendment Rights of Abortion Clinic Protesters," *Southern California Law Review* 68 (January 1995): 453.

63. David M. Smolin, "The Jurisprudence of Privacy in a Splintered Supreme Court," *75 Marquardt 2 Review* 975 (1992): 1020. See Allen, 423.

64. *Roe v. Wade,* 410 U.S. 113 (1973). See Allen, 424-25, 429. Ref., Leo Pfeffer, "An Autobiographical Sketch," in *Church, State, and Freedom,* Rev. Ed. (Boston: Beacon Press, 1967), 510.

65. *Planned Parenthood v. Casey,* 112 S. Ct. 2791 (1992). Janice C. Biskin, "The Hyde Amendment: An Infringement Upon the Free Exercise Clause?" *Rutgers Law Review* 33 (Summer 1981): 1058. Allen, 446.

66. *Beal v. Doe,* 432 U.S. 438 (1977); *Maher v. Doe,* 432 U.S. 519 (1977); *Poelker v. Doe,* 432 U.S. 519 (1977).

67. Biskin, 1058-1059.

68. Allen, 446, 453.

69. Biskin, 1065-1067, 1069. Pfeffer, "An Autobiographical Sketch," 511.

70. Robert L. Maddox and Blaine Bortnick, "Webster v. Reproductive Health Services: Do Legislative Declarations that Life Begins at Conception Violate the Establishment Clause?" *Campbell Law Review* 12 (Winter 1989): 3-5.

71. *McRae v. Califano,* 491 F. Supp. 630 (E.D. N.Y. 1980). *Harris v. McRae,* 448 U.S. 297 (1980). Samuel Krislov, "Alternatives to Separation of Church and State in Countries Outside the United States," in *Religion and the State,* Ed. James E. Wood (Waco: Baylor University Press, 1985), 422.

72. *Epperson v. Arkansas,* 393 U.S. 97 (1968). *Lemon v. Kurtzman,* 403 U.S. 602 (1971). Jan D. Feldman, "The Establishment Clause and Religious Influences on Legislation," *Northwestern University Law Review* 75 (December 1980): 974-975.

73. Legal cases, *McGowan v. Maryland,* 366 U.S. 420 (1961); *McDaniel v. Paty,* 435 U.S. 618 (1978); *Everson v. Board of Education,* 330 U.S. 1 (1947). See, Maddox, Bortnick, Legislative Declarations, 7-8. Also, Feldman, 963-965. See also, Biskin, 1054. Ref., John Martin Cummings, "The State, the Stork, and the Wall: The

Establishment Clause and Statutory Abortion Regulation," *Catholic University Law Review* 34 (Summer 1990): 1192, 1218, 1230-33. In favor of McRae, *Commission for Public Education and Religious Liberty v. Nyquist,* 413 U.S. (1973).

74. *Harris v. McRae,* 448 U.S. 297 (1980) at 297.

75. Feldman, 994-995.

76. "Embryos are out there, but not for Research," News 6-7.

77. Robert T. Miller and Ronald B. Flowers, *Toward Benevolent Neutrality: Church, State and the Supreme Court* (Waco: Markham Press Fund of Baylor University Press, 1992), 471. *Bradfield v. Roberts,* 175 U.S. 291 (1899). Sectarian cases, *Roemer v. Maryland Board of Public Works, Tilton v. Richardson, Hunt v. Mc Nair, Bradfield v. Roberts.* Indirect, *Witters v. Washington, Mueller v. Allen, Everson v. Board of Education,* and *Walz v. Tax Commission,* 397 U.S. 602 (1971).

78. *Bowen v. Kendrick,* 487 U. S. 589 (1988).

79. Miller, Flowers, 392; 485; 487; 490-491. *Walz v. Tax Commission,* 397 U.S. 602 (1971). See also, Dean M. Kelly, "Tax Exemption and the Free Exercise of Religion," in *Religion and the State,* Ed. James E. Wood, Jr. (Waco: Baylor University Press, 1985), 271.

80. Miller, Flowers, 479. Neutrality, *Grand Rapids v. Ball,* 473 U.S. 373 (1985) and *Grand Rapids School District v. Ball. Committee for Public Education v. Regan,* 444 U.S. 646 (1980).

81. Kent Greenawalt, "Conscientious Objection and the Liberal State," in *Religion and the State,* Ed. James E. Wood, Jr. (Waco: Baylor University Press, 1985), 271-72. *Chrisman v. Sisters of St. Joseph of Peace,* 506 F. 2d 308 (9th Cir. 1974).

82. Angela Marie Hubbell, "FACE'ing the First Amendment: Application of RICO and the Clinic Entrances Act to Abortion Posters," *Ohio Northern University Law Review* 21(Spring 1995): 1080-1081.

83. G. Benagiano, "Debate," in *Aspects éthiques de la reproduction humaine,* Eds. Claude Sureau and Françoise Shenfield (Paris, France: John Libbey Eurotext, 1995), 176.

84. Wulff et al., 54-59. See Boorse, 542-573. Also, A. Ross, *Det psychopatologiske sysdomsbegrab* (Netherlands: Bibliotek *Laeger,* 1980), 172:1-23.

85. Rothman, 214-216.

86. Bryan K. Larsen, "RICOs Application to Non-Economic Actors: A Serious Threat to First Amendment Freedoms," *Review of Litigation* 14 (Summer 1995): 708, 712, 715. Also see, Joel A. Youngblood, "The First Amendment Falls Victim to RICO," *Tulsa Law Journal* 30 (Fall 1994): 203-204, 210-212. *Madsen v. Women's Health Center,* 114 S. Ct. 2516 (1994). *National Organization for Women v. Scheidler,* 114 S. Ct. 798 (1994).

87. Larsen, 733.

88. *Thornburgh v. American College of Obstetricians and Pediatricians,* 106 S. Ct. 2169 (1986). Dennis J. Horan, et al., *Abortion and the Constitution: Reversing Roe v. Wade Through the Courts* (Washington, DC: Georgetown University Press, 1987), 245.

89. Kelly, 431-432, 487.

90. *Employment Division v. Smith,* 494 U.S. 872 (1990).

91. *Church of Lukumi Babalu Aye v. Hialeah,* 113 S. Ct. 2217 (1993).

92. Hubbell, FACE'ing, 1079-1080.

93. *Cantwell v. Connecticut,* 310 U.S. 296 (1940). *Schneider v. New Jersey,* 308 U.S. 147 (1939). (*Shelton v Tucker,* 364 U.S. 479 [1960] used *Cantwell* and *Schneider.*) *Califano v. Yamasaki,* 442 U.S. 682 (1979). See Richard A. Griggs, "First Amendment Facelift: Renquist Court Crafts New Scrutiny Level for Content-Neutral Speech Restricting Injunctions," *Mercer Law Review* 46 (Spring 1995): 1197-1210. Also see, Kelly, 449. *NAACP v. Clairbourne Hardware,* 458 U.S. 886 (1982).

94. Griggs, 1197-2010. Ref. *Reynolds v. U.S.,* 98 U.S. 145 (1878).

95. Kelly, 450, 475. *Heffron v. International Society of Krishna Consciousness,* 452 U.S. 640 (1981) at 647; and *U.S. v. Grace,* 461 U.S. 171 (1983) at 177-178.

96. Kelly, 489.

97. Larsen, 737. In *Madsen v. Women's Health Center,* 114 S. Ct. 2516 (1994). Kelly, 457. Scalia cited *Ward v. Rock Against Racism,* 491 U.S. 781 (1989); *United States v. O'Brien,* 391 U.S. 367 (1968).

98. Larsen, 722, 725-726. *Northeastern Women's Center Inc. v. McMonagle,* 665 F. Supp. 1147 (1987).

99. Kelly, 487-488.

100. Hubbell, 1073-1078. *Riely,* 860. F. Supp. at 693 and *Brock,* 863 F. Supp. at 851; *American Life League,* 855 F. Supp @ 137; *Council for Life Coalition,* 856 F. Supp. at 1922.

101. Larsen, 708, 712, 715, 726. See Joel A. Youngblood, "The First Amendment Falls Victim to RICO," *Tulsa Law Journal* 30 (Fall 1994): 203-204, 212. See Kelly, 460. *National Organization for Women v. Scheidler,* 114 S. Ct. 798 (1994). RICO § 1961 (1) 18 U.S.C., (1988).

102. Hubbell, 1068-69. Also, Larsen, RICOs Application, 729; 733. *NAACP v. Clairbourne Hardware,* 458 U.S. 886 (1982).

103. *National Organization for Women v. Scheidler,* 114 S. Ct. 798 (1994).

104. Evelyn Schuster, "Progress in Embryology and Diagnosis," Symposium on *Bioethics and The Rights of the Child* (Monaco: UNESCO/AMADE, 2000). Ref., Universal Declaration of Human Rights: Art. 1, 4; UN Rights of the Child: 8, 29. See Farley, 208ff.

105. "Embryos are out there, but not for Research," *Orange County Register* (26 August 2001): News 6-7. Originally printed in the *New York Times* (24 August 2001).

106. Ibid.

107. James H. Burtness, "Genetic Manipulation," in *Questions about the Beginning of Life: Christian Appraisals of Seven Biological Issues,* Ed. James M. Childs (Minneapolis, MN: Augsburg, 1985), 81.

108. Morley, 31.

109. Ibid., 30, 125. Edward Slater, "Severely Malformed Children. Wanted—A New Basic Approach," *British Medial Journal,* II (73): 285-86. Jacque Monad, "Leçon inaugurale au College de France," College of France, Paris (3 November 1967); also Monad, *Chance and Necessity* (n/c: Collins, 1967).

110. Morley, 119-29. See Eysenck, 80. Also, B. Glass, *Science and Ethical Values* (Oxford: Oxford University Press, 1966), 47-48.

111. Morley, 126-129.

112. Baruch Brody, "Protecting Scientific Integrity Through Disclosure of Conflicts of Interest" (Houston: Baylor College of Medicine, 2000), 1-4.

113. Lappé, "Eugenics: Ethical Issues," 2:775-776.

114. O. Guillod, "Genetics, the Family and Human Rights," lecture at the International Society of Family Law Symposium on *Biomedicine, the Family and Human Rights* (Oxford: St. Anne's College, August 1999).

115. Madame Professor B. Feuillet-Le Mintier, "Genetics, the Family and Human Rights," lecture at the International Society of Family Law Symposium on *Biomedicine, the Family and Human Rights* (Oxford: St. Anne's College, August 1999).

116. Claude Sureau, "Conclusion: A Narrow Path," in *Aspects éthiques de la reproduction humaine*, Eds. Claude Sureau and Françoise Shenfield (Paris: John Libbey Eurotext, 1995), 377.

Chapter 6

1. B. Steinbock, "Maternal–fetal Conflict and *in utero* Fetal Therapy," in *Aspects éthiques de la reproduction humaine*, Eds. Claude Sureau and Françoise Shenfield (Paris, France: John Libbey Eurotext, 1995), 68. See S. Blacklee, "Fetus returned to womb, following surgery," *New York Times* (7 October 1987): C1-3.

2. Steinbock, 67. Also, M.R. Harrison and Adzick N. Scott, "Fetus as a Patient: Surgical Considerations," in *Ann Surg*, 213 (1991): 279-290.

3. M. Brower, et al., "Saving Lives not yet begun," *People* (18 June 1990): 38.

4. M.R. Harrison, "Congenital diaphragmatic hernia; an unsolved problem," *Seminal Pediatric Surgery*, 2 (1993): 109-111.

5. Steinbock, 69. See K.J.S. Analand and P.R. Hickey, "Pain and its effects in the human neonate and the fetus," *New England Journal of Medicine* 317 (1987): 1231-1232.

6. H. Edgar, "Discussion: Fetal Cell Transplantation," in *Aspects éthiques de la reproduction humaine*, Eds. Claude Sureau and Françoise Shenfield (Paris, France: John Libbey Eurotext, 1995), 169-173.

7. Alexander McCall Smith and Michel Revel, "The Use of Embryonic Stem Cells in Therapeutic Research," 7th Session, Proceedings (Paris, FR: UNESCO, 2000), 38.

8. Steinbock, 71.

9. McCall Smith and Revel, 39. See Caroline Whitbeck, "The Moral Implications of Regarding Women as People: New Perspectives on Pregnancy and Personhood," Eds. William Bondeson, H. Tristan Engelhardt, Stuart F. Spinker, Daniel H. Winship, *Abortion and the Status of the Fetus* (Boston: Kluwer, 1984), 254-256.

10. Patricia Baird, "Research on Preembryos (zygotes)," in *Aspects éthiques de la reproduction humaine*, Eds. Claude Sureau and Françoise Shenfield (Paris, France: John Libbey Eurotext, 1995), 328.

11. McCall Smith and Revel, 39-40.

12. Steinbock, 70.

13. Baird, 328.

14. Robert C. Solomon, "Reflections on the Meaning of Fetal Life," in *Abortion and the Status of the Fetus,* Eds. William Bondeson, H. Tristan Englehardt, Stuart F. Spinker, Daniel H. Winship, (Boston: Kluwer, 1984), 208.

15. McCall Smith and Revel, 39-40.

16. Joseph H. Schenker, "Transplantation of Fetal Tissue, Gametes, and Organs," in *Aspects éthiques de la reproduction humaine,* Eds. Claude Sureau and Françoise Shenfield (Paris, France: John Libbey Eurotext, 1995), 155ff.

17. George J. Boer, "Discussion: The key issues of embryonic and fetal tissue transplantation, a response for discussion," in *Aspects éthiques de la reproduction humaine,* Eds. Claude Sureau and Françoise Shenfield (Paris, France: John Libbey Eurotext, 1995), 165ff. See John A. Robertson, "The Embryo and Fetal Research," in *Aspects éthiques de la reproduction humaine,* Eds. Claude Sureau and Françoise Shenfield (Paris, France: John Libbey Eurotext, 1995), 352ff.

18. Schenker, 154.

19. Ibid., 155ff.

20. George J. Annas, "Pregnant Women as Fetal Containers," *Hastings Center Report* (December 1986): 13-14.

21. Annas, 13-14. See Schenker, 155-157.

22. Justice Michel Kirby, "Economic Aspects of Genome Research," 7th Session, Quito, Ecuador (Paris, FR: UNESCO IBC, 2000), 17-18. Also, Huanming Yang, "Economic Aspects of Genome Research," 7th Session, Proceedings (Paris, FR: UNESCO IBC, 2000), 18.

23. Boer, 165,167.

24. Ibid., 167. See Schenker, 157.

25. Boer, 167

26. Schenker, 159, 162.

27. Michel Revel, "Discussion: Ethical Aspects of Embryonic Stem Cell Research," 7th Session (Paris, FR: UNESCO IBS, 2000), 11. See A. Baguisi, E. Behoodi, D.T. Melican, J.S. Pollock, M.M. Destrempes, C. Cammuso, J.L. Williams, S.D. Nims, C.A. Porter, P. Midura, M.J. Palacios, S.L. Ayres, R.S. Dennison, M.L. Hayes, C.A. Ziomek, H.M. Meade, R.A. Godke, W.G. Gavin, E.W. Overstom, and Y. Echelard, "Production of goats by somatic cell transfer," *Natural Biotechnology* 17 (1999): 456-461. Also, K.H. Cambell, J.McWhir, W.A. Ritchie, and I. Wilmut, "Sheep cloned by nuclear transfer from cultured cell line," *Nature* 380 (1996): 64-66. See also, J.B. Cebelli, S.L. Slice, P.J. Golueke, J.J. Kane, J. Jerry C. Blackwell, F.A. Ponce de Leon, and J.M. Robl, "Cloned transgenic calves produced from non-quiescent fetal fibroblasts," *Science* 280 (1998): 1256-1258 and by the same authors, "Transgenic bovine chimeric offspring produced somatic cell–derived stem-like cells," *Natural biotechnology* 16 (1998): 642-646.

28. Patricia Baird, 330. See G.J. Annas, A. Caplan, and S. Elias, "Stem Cell Politics, Ethics, and Medical Progress," *Natural Medicine* 5 (1999): 1339-1341. Also, M.B. Frielle, ed., *Embryo Experimentation in Europe: Biomedical, Legal, and Philosophical Aspects* (Bad Neuenahr-Ahrweiler: Europäische Akademie, 2001).

29. Alexander McCall Smith and Michel Revel, "The Use of Embryonic Stem Cells in Therapeutic Research," 7th Session, Proceedings (Paris, FR: UNESCO, 2000), 30.

30. James Pickel, "State of the Art of Neuroscience," 7th Session, Acts and Proceedings (Paris: UNESCO IBC, 2000): 89.

31. Baird, 330. See McCall Smith and Revel, 30.

32. Baird, 331-322. See Pickel, 89.

33. S. Geber and M. Sampaio, "Blastomere development after embryo biopsy: a new model to predict embryo development and to select for transfer," *Human Reproduction* 14 (1999): 782-786. See R. Revel, "Ongoing Research on mammalian cloning and embryo stem cell technologies: Bioethics of their potential medical applications," *Israel Medical Association Journal* (IMAJ) 2, *Supplement* (July 2000): 8-14. Also see, Baird, 328-329.

34. G. Serour, "Debate," in *Aspects éthiques de la reproduction humaine,* Eds. Claude Sureau and Françoise Shenfield (Paris, France: John Libbey Eurotext, 1995), 359-363.

35. Baird, 332. See McCall Smith and Revel, 31-32. Also, Pickel, 9. See also, O. Brustle, K.N. Jones, R.D. Learish, K. Karram, K. Choudhary, O.D. Wiestler, I.D. Duncan, and R.D. McKay, "Embryonic stem cell-derived glial precursors: a source of myelinating transplants," *Science* 285 (1999): 754-756. Refer to O. Brustle, A.C. Spiro, K. Karram, K. Choudhary, S. Okabe, and R.D. McKay, "In vitro-generated neural precursors participate in mammalian brain development," *Proceedings, National Academy of Science U.S.A.* 94 (1997): 14809-14814. See T. Deacon, J. Dinsmore, L.C. Costantini, J. Ratliff, and O. Isacson, "Blastula-stage stem cells can differentiate into dopaminergic and serotonergic neurons after transplantation," *Exp Neurology*149 (1998): 28-41.

36. McCall Smith and Revel, 51. See N. Hole, G.J. Grapham, U. Menzel, J.D. Nasell, "A limited temporal window for the deviation of multilineage repopulating hematopoietic progenitors during embroyonal stem cell differentiation," *Blood* 88 (1996): 1266-76. Also, G. Hottois, "Is cloning the absolute evil?," *Human Reproductive Update* 4 (1999): 787-790. See also, N. Kikyo and A.P. Wolffe, "Reprogramming nuclei: insights from cloning, nuclear transfer and heterokaryons," *Journal of Cell Science* 113 (2000): 11-20. Reference, D. Kipling and R.G. Faragher, "Telomeres. Aging hard or hardly ageing?" *Nature* 398 (1999): 191, 193. Additionally, R.P. Lanza, J.B. Cibelli, M.D. West, "Prospect for the use of nuclear transfer in human transplantation," *Nature Biotechnology* 17 (1999): 1171-1174.

37. McCall Smith and Revel, 42.

38. Serour, 359-363.

39. McCall Smith and Revel, 49. Refer to 1948 Universal Declaration on Human Rights (1948), International Covenant on Civil and Political Rights (1996); Universal Declaration on the Human Genome and Human Rights (1997), Convention for the Protection of Human Rights and the Dignity of the Human Being with Regard to the Application of Biology and Medicine (1997), Additional Protocol to the Convention for the Protection of Human Rights and Dignity of the Human Being with Regard to the Application of Biology and Medicine, on the Prohibition of Cloning Human Beings (1998), European Union Charter of Fundamental Rights of the European Union (2000), European Resolution on Human Cloning (2000), African Charter on Human and People's Rights (1981), American Convention on Human Rights (1969).

40. Christine Gosden, "Progress and Achievements of Biotechnology," at the International Society of Family Law, Biomedicine, The Family and Human Rights, (Oxford: St. Anne's College, 1999).

41. Claude Sureau and Françoise Shenfield, "A Narrow Path," in *Aspects éthiques de la reproduction humaine,* Eds. Claude Sureau and Françoise Shenfield (Paris, France: John Libbey Eurotext, 1995), 376. See Ellen K. Wondra, "How do we Judge? Theological Assessment of Scientific Developments," *Anglican Theological Review* 18, 4 (Fall 1999), 593.

42. Rom 1:6.

43. McCall Smith and Revel, 40.

44. Ibid., 47-48. Refer to: National Legal Sources, Constitutions, Ecuador's Constitution of 5 June 1998, Ireland's Constitution of 1 July 1937 (amended 7 October 1983), and Switzerland's Constitution of 18 April 1999. Legislation, Australia, Gene Technology Act 2000 (enactment 2001); Austria, Law no. 275 of 1992 on reproductive medicine; Brazil, Law no. 8974/95 of 5 January 1995 on genetic engineering; Costa Rica, Law no. 7739 of 1998, Code of Childhood and Adolescence; Finland, Statute no. 488/1999 of 9 April 1999, Medical Research Act; France, Law no. 94-654 of 29 July 1994 on the donation and use of elements and products of the human body, medically assisted procreation and prenatal diagnosis; Germany, Law of 13 December 1990, the Federal Embryo Protection Law; Hungary, Law no. LXXIX of 17 December 1992 on protection of the life of the embryo; Japan, Law of 30 November 2000 concerning regulation relating to the techniques of human cloning and on the similar techniques; Norway, Law no. 56 of 5 August 1994 on the medical use of biotechnology (amended by Law no. 29 of 16 May 1997); Peru, Law no. 26.842 General Law of Public Health/Law no. 27.337 Code of Childhood and Adolescence; Poland, Law of 7 January 1993 on family planning, protection of the human fetus and the admissibility conditions for the artificial termination of pregnancy (as amended on 30 August 1996); Spain, Law no. 35 of 1988 on assisted reproduction procedures; Sweden, Law no. 115 of 14 March 1991 on measures relating to the use of human fertilized ovocytes for research or therapeutic purposes; United Kingdom, Law of 1 November 1990, Human Fertilization and Embryology Act/Law of 232 January 2001, amending the Human Fertilization and Embryology Act of 1 November 1990. Bills, Belgium, Bills on the protection of embryos, Senate; France, Draft of the revised "Bioethics Law," presented by the Prime Minister on 28 November 2000; Italy, Bill no. 4048 on the discipline of medically assisted procreation; Netherlands, Bill containing rules relating to the use of gametes and embryos (Embryos Bill). Pontificia Academia Pro Vita, Declaration on the Production and the Scientific and Therapeutic Use of Human Embryonic Stem Cells, August 2000. U.S.A. National Bioethics Advisory Commission, "Ethical Issues in Human Stem Cell Research," September 1999/National Institutes of Health, "Guidelines for Research Using Human Pluripotent Stem Cells," 25 August 2000.

45. Patrick Robinson, "Proposals of the IBC Working Group with a view to the follow-up on the International Symposium on 'Ethics, Intellectual Property, and Genomics'," 8th session, Proceedings (Paris, FR: UNESCO IBC, 2001).

46. McCall Smith and Revel, 41-44.

272   COUNSELING PREGNANCY, POLITICS, AND BIOMEDICINE

47. Ibid., 41-47. Also, Baird, 332-333. George Radwanski (Canada), "Hearings of Commissioners for the Protection of Personal Data," 8th session, Proceedings (Paris, FR: UNESCO, 2001).

48. Radwanski (Canada), "Hearings of Commissioners for the Protection of Personal Data," 8th Session, Proceedings (Paris, FR: UNESCO IBC, 2001).

49. Sylvia Rumball (New Zealand) and Alexander McCall Smith (U.K.), "Draft Report on Collection, Treatment, Storage and Use of Genetic Data," Draft Report (Paris, FR: UNESCO IBC 2001): 9-17.

50. Troylyn Ball, "The Mystery of Marshall," *Guideposts* Vol. LV, No. 11 (January 2001), 56-60. Marshall Ball, *Kiss of God: The Wisdom of a Silent Child* (Austin, n/p, n/d).

Sources Consulted

Ackernecht, E.H. *A Short History of Medicine.* Baltimore: Johns Hopkins University Press, 1982.
Acton, John Emerich Edward Dalberg. *Essays on Church and State.* New York: Crowell, 1968.
———. *Lectures on the French Revolution.* J.N. Figgis and R.V. Lawrence Eds. New York: Noonday Press, 1959.
Aertsen, A. and G.L. Gerstein. "Dynamic Aspects of Neuronal Cooperativity: Fast Stimulus-Locked Modulation of Effective Cooperativity." In *Neuronal Cooperativity,* Ed. J. Kruger. New York: Springer-Verlag (1991): 52-67.
Aghajanian, G.K., J.S. Sprouse, and K. Rasmussen. "Physiology of the Midbrain Serotonin System." In *Psychopharmacy.* H.Y. Meltzer Ed. New York: Raven Press (1987): 141-150.
Aland, Kurt, et al., eds. *The Greek New Testament.*4th ed. Münster/Westphalia: Deutsche Bibelgesellschaft, 1993.
Alberts, Bruce, et al. *Molecular Biology of the Cell,* 3rd ed. N/c: Garland Publishing Co., 1994.
Allen, Anita L. "The Proposed Equal Protection Fix for the Abortion Law: Reflections on Citizenship, Gender and the Constitution." *Harvard Journal of Law and Public Policy* 18 (Spring 1995): 419-455.
Alschuler, Albert W. "Part Six: Should We Have Public Policy?" In *Active Euthanasia, Religion, and the Public Debate.* Ron Hamel Ed. Chicago: The Park Ridge Center (1991): 105-109.
Aly, Götz, Peter Chroust, and Christian Pross. *Cleansing the Fatherland, Nazi Medicine and Racial Hygiene.* Baltimore: Johns Hopkins University Press, 1994.
Amen, Daniel G. *Images Into Human Behavior: A Brain SPEC Atlas.* Los Angeles: Mindworks Press, 1998. CD-ROM, http://brain.com/atlas and http://amenclinics. com/bp/atlas.
———. *Healing the Hardware of the Soul.* Los Angles: Mindworks Press, 2002.
Analand, K.J.S., and P.R. Hickey. "Pain and its effects in the human neonate and the fetus." *New England Journal of Medicine* 317 (1987): 1231-1232.
Andrusko, D. ed. *A Passion for Justice.* Washington DC: National Right to Life, 1998.
Annas, George J. "Nancy Cruzan and the Right to Die." *New England Journal of Medicine* 323 (1990): 670-673.

Counseling Pregnancy, Politics, and Biomedicine
© 2007 by The Haworth Press, Inc. All rights reserved.
doi:10.1300/5697_10

————. "Pregnant Women as Fetal Containers." *Hastings Center Report* (December 1986): 13-14.

Annas, George J. and Michael Grodin, eds. *The Nazi Doctors and the Nuremberg Code.* Oxford: Oxford University Press, 1992.

Annas, G.J., A. Caplan, and S. Elias. "Stem Cell Politics, Ethics, and Medical Progress." *Natural Medicine* 5 (1999): 1339-1341.

Applebaum, P.S., C.W. Lutz and A. Morsel. *Informed Consent: Legal Theory and Clinical Practice.* New York: Oxford University Press, 1987.

Appenzellar, Tim. "Someplace Like Earth." In *National Geographic: Searching the Stars for New Earths* (December 2004): 68, 82-84.

Aquinas, T. *Summa Theologica.* Translation by the Fathers of the English Dominican Province. New York: Benziger Bros., 1947.

————. *Commentary on Politics.* Translation by C.I. Litzinger. Chicago: Regnery, 1964.

Aristotle. *Nichomachean Ethics and Politics.* CRW Publishing Limited Book Blocks, 2004.

Armstrong-Dailey, A. and S.Z. Goltzer, eds. *Hospice Care for Children.* Oxford: Oxford University Press, 1993.

Athanasius. *Four Discourses Against the Arians.* St. Vladimir's Seminary Press, 1989.

Augustine. *City of God.* New York: Penguin Classics, 1975.

————. *On the Trinity.* Translated and Edited by Desmond M. Matthews, Gareth B. Clarke. Cambridge: Cambridge University Press, 2002.

Baguisi, A., E. Behoodi, D.T. Melican, J.S. Pollock, M.M. Destrempes, C. Cammuso, J.L. Williams, S.D. Nims, C.A. Porter, P. Midura, M.J. Palacios, S.L. Ayres, R.S. Dennison, M.L. Hayes, C.A. Ziomek, H.M. Meade, R.A. Godke, W.G. Gavin, E.W. Overstom, and Y. Echelard. "Production of goats by somatic cell transfer." *Natural Biotechnology* 17 (1999): 456-461.

Baird, D.C. *Experimentation.* Englewood Cliffs, NJ: Prentice Hall, 1995.

Baker, Robert B., Arthur L. Caplan, Linda L. Emanuel, and Stephen R. Latham, Eds. *The American Medical Ethics Revolution: How the AMAs Code of Ethics Has Transformed Physicians' Relationships to Patients, Professionals, and Society.* Baltimore: The Johns Hopkins University Press, 2001.

Ball, Marshall. *Kiss of God: The Wisdom of a Silent Child* (Austin, n/p, n/d).

Ball, Troylyn. "The Mystery of Marshall." *Guideposts.* Vol. LV, No. 11 (January 2001): 56-60.

Ballentine, Bernard, Anthony Dickenson. "Consciousness—The Interface Between Effect and Cognition." In *Consciousness and Human Identity.* John Cornwell Ed. Oxford: Oxford University Press, 1998.

Barbour, Ian. *Religion and Science—Historical and Contemporary Issues.* London: SCM, 1998.

————. *Ethics in an Age of Technology.* London: SCM, 1992.

Barrett, C.K. *New Testament Documents.* 2nd ed. London: SPCK, 1978.

Barth, Karl. *Church Dogmatics.* 2 Vols. Trans. G.W. Bromiley. Edinburgh: T&T Clark, 1975.

Bartoszewski, Wladyslaw T. *Surviving Treblinka.* Oxford: Basil Blackwell, 1989.

Basil of Caesarea. *On the Holy Spirit.* Translated by David Taylor. Lovanii: Peeter Press.

Bauer, Yehuda. "Euthanasia, Nazism and Psychiatry." *Holocaust Conference.* Oxford, England, July 1988.

Bauer, Yehuda. *A History of the Holocaust.* New York: Franklin Watts, 1982.

Baylor, Michael. *Action and Person: Conscience in Late Scholasticism and the Young Luther.* Leiden: Brill, 1977.

Bean, Stanley I. "Justice." In *The Encyclopedia of Philosophy.* Vol. 3. Paul Edwards Ed. New York: Macmillan, 1963.

Beauchamp, Tom L. "Introduction." In *Ethics and Public Policy.* Englewood Cliffs, NJ: Prentice Hall (1975): 361-370.

Beauchamp, Tom L., ed. *Philosophic Ethics: An Introduction of Moral Philosophy.* Washington DC: Georgetown University, 1982.

Benagiano, G. "Debate." In *Aspects éthicques de la reproduction humaine.* Claude Sureau and Françoise Shenfield Eds. Paris, France: John Libbey Eurotext, 1995.

Benedict, Ruth. "Relativism and Patterns of culture." In *Value and Obligation.* Richard B. Brandt Ed. New York: Harcourt, Brace, and World, 1961.

BenGershôm, E. "From Haeckel to Hackethal: Lessons From Nazi Medicine For Students and Practitioners of Medicine." In *Holocaust and Genocide Studies 5,* No. 1. Oxford: Pergamon Press (Winter 1990): 73-87.

Bennett, Anne McGrew. "Overcoming the Biblical and Traditional Subordination of Women." In *Feminist Theological Ethics: A Reader.* Lois K. Daly Ed. Louisville, KY: John Knox Press, 1994.

Bentham, , Jeremy. *The Works of Jeremy Bentham.* Vol X. Continuum International Publishing Group Ltd., 1994.

Berman, Harold J. *Faith and Order: The Reconciliation of Law and Religion.* Atlanta, Georgia: Scholars Press, 1993.

Berry, A. Caroline. "Genetic Counseling: A Medical Perspective." In *Genetic Counseling: Practice and Principles.* London: Rutledge, 1994.

Bettoni, Efrem. *Duns Scotus: The Basic Principles of His Philosophy.* Trans. Bonansea. Washington DC: Catholic University of America Press, 1961.

Biblia Hebraica: Stuttgartensia. Stuttgart: Deutsche Bibelgesellschaft, 1990.

Biesecker, Barbara Bowles. "Genetic Counseling: Practice of Genetic Counseling." In *Encyclopedia of Bioethics.* Vol. 2. New York: Macmillan Library, 1995.

Biskin, Janice C. "The Hyde Amendment: An Infringement Upon the Free Exercise Clause?" *Rutgers Law Review* 33 (Summer 1981): 1054-1075.

Blacklee, S. "Fetus returned to womb, following surgery." *New York Times* (7 October 1987): C1-3.

Boden, M. "Consciousness and Human Identity: An Interdisciplinary Perspective." In *Consciousness and Human Identity.* John Cornwell Ed. Oxford: Oxford University Press, 1998.

Boer, George J. "Discussion: The key issues of embryonic and fetal tissue transplantation, a response for discussion." In *Aspects éthiques de la reproduction humaine.* Claude Sureau and Françoise Shenfield Eds. Paris, France: John Libbey Eurotext, 1995.

Bohr, Neils. *Atomic Theory and the Description of Nature*. Cambridge: Cambridge University Press, 1934.

———. *Atomic Physics and Human Knowledge*. New York: Science Editions, 1958.

———. *The Theory of Spectra and Atomic Constitution*. Cambridge: Cambridge University Press, 1922.

Bonaventure. *The Mind's Journey to God*. Translated by Lawrence S. Cunningham. Chicago: Franciscan Herald Press, 1979.

Bondeson, William, H. Tristan Engelhardt, Stuart F. Spicker, and Daniel H. Winship, eds. *Abortion and the Status of the Fetus*. Boston: Kluwer, 1984.

Bonniksen, Andrea. *What Kind of Policy Formation Do We Need for Preimplantation Diagnosis?* Lecture. International Conference on Genetic Diagnosis. Rennes, FR: University of Rennes, 1998.

Bookstaber, Philip David. *The Idea of the Development of the Soul in Jewish Medieval Philosophy*. Philadelphia: Maurice Jacobs, Inc., 1950/5711.

Boorse, Christopher. "Health is a Theoretical Concept." *Philosophy of Science* 44 (1977): 542-573.

Borowitz, Eugene B. "Rethinking our Holocaust Consciousness." *Judaism* 40 (Fall, 1991): 389-390.

Bosk, Charles L. *All God's Mistakes: Genetic Counseling in a Pediatric Hospital*. Chicago: University of Chicago Press, 1992.

Boucard, Pascale. *Laïcité, libertés de conscience and religion*. Lyon, France: Catholique de Lyon, 1995.

Boué, André. *The Evolution of Genetic Diagnosis Before Birth: Past, Present, and Future*. Lecture. International Conference on Genetic Diagnosis. Rennes, FR: University of Rennes, 1998.

Boukhari, Sophie and Amy Otchet. "Uncharted terrain on tomorrow's genetic map." *The UNESCO Courier* (September 1999): 19.

Bowman, James E. "Genetics and Racial Minorities: Genetic Testing. In *Encyclopedia of Bioethics*. Vol. 2. New York: Macmillan Library, 1995.

Braham, Randolph L., ed. *The Origins of the Holocaust: Christian Anti-Semitism*. New York: Columbia University Press, 1986.

Brennen, William. *Medical Holocaust 1: Exterminative Medicine in Nazi Germany and Contemporary America*. Boston: Nordland Publishing International, Inc., 1980.

Broad, Charles D. *Five Types of Ethical Theory*. London: Routledge & Kegan Paul, 1967.

Brody, Baruch A. *Life and Death Decision Making*. Oxford: Oxford University Press, 1988.

———. *Protecting Scientific Integrity through Disclosure of Conflicts of Interest*. Houston: Baylor College of Medicine Survey Form (2000).

Brooke, John Hedley. *Science and Religion – Some Historical Perspectives*. Cambridge: Cambridge University Press, 1998. (Reprint of 1991 edition.)

Brooke, John H and Geoffrey Cantor. *Reconstructing Nature: The Engagement of Science and Religion*. Edinburgh: T & T Clark, 1998.

Brower, M. et al. "Saving Lives not yet begun." *People* (18 June 1990): 38.

Brown, Harold O.J., C. Everett Koop. A. D. *Restatement of the Oath of Hippocrates (Circa 400 B.C.).* Bingham, Mass.: Value of Life Committee, Inc., 1995.

Brown, Jennifer. "Vertebrate Limb Development: Chick Insights." Lecture. University of Oxford, 1999.

Brunner, Emil. *The Mediator.* London: Lutterworth Press, 1947.

Brustle, O., A.C. Spiro, K. Karram, K. Choudhary, S. Okabe, and R.D. McKay. "In vitro-generated neural precursors participate in mammalian brain development." *Proceedings, National Academy of Science U.S.A.* 94 (1997): 14809-14814.

Brustle, O., K.N. Jones, R.D. Learish, K. Karram, K. Choudhary, O.D. Wiestler, I.D. Duncan, and R.D. McKay. "Embryonic stem cell-derived glial precursors: a source of myelinating transplants." *Science* 285 (1999): 754-756.

Buber, Martin. *I and Thou.* Translation by Ronald Gregor Smith. Edinburgh: T and T Clark, 1939.

Buchanan, Allen. "Justice: A Philosophical Review." In *Cross-Cultural Perspectives in Medical Ethics: Readings.* Robert Veatch Ed. Boston: Jones and Bartlett Publishers, 1989.

Bultmann, Rudolph. "New Testament and Mythology." Vol. I. London: SCM, 1985.

Burtness, James H. "Genetic Manipulation." In *Questions about the Beginning of Life: Christian Appraisals of Seven Bioethical Issues.* Minneapolis, MN: Augsburg, 1985.

Cahill, Lisa Sowle. "'Embodiment'" and Moral Critique: A Christian Social Perspective." In *On Moral Medicine: Theological Perspectives in Medical Ethics.* Stephen E. Lammers and Allen Verney Eds. 2nd ed. Grand Rapids: Wm. B. Eerdmans Publishing Company, 1998.

———. "Within Shouting Distance: Paul Ramsey and Richard McCormick on Method." In *Cross-Cultural Perspectives in Medical Ethics: Readings.* Robert M. Veatch Ed. Boston: Jones and Bartlett Publishers, 1989.

Cambell, K.H., J.McWhir, W.A. Ritchie, and I. Wilmut. Sheep cloned by nuclear transfer from cultured cell line. *Nature* 380 (1996): 64-66.

Capron, Alex. "Human Experiment." In *Biological Law: A Legal Reporter on Medicine, Health Care and Bioengineering.* J.F. Childress, et al. Frederick, Eds. MD: University Publication of America, 1999.

Cebelli, J.B, S.L. Slice, P.J. Golueke, J.J. Kane, J. Jerry. C. Blackwell, F.A. Ponce de Leon, and J.M. Robl. "Cloned transgenic calves produced from nonquiescent fetal fibroblasts." *Science* 280 (1998): 1256-1258.

———. "Transgenic bovine chimeric offspring produced somatic cell–derived stem-like cells." *Natural biotechnology* 16 (1998): 642-646.

"Celebrating the Medieval Heritage: a Colloquy on the Thought of Aquinas and Bonaventure." Edited by Tracey, D. *The Journal of Religion* 58, suppl. (1978).

Childress, James F. *Practical Reasoning in Bioethics.* Indianapolis: Indiana University Press, 1997.

Childs, James M. "Genetic Screening and Counseling." In *Questions about the Beginning of Life: Christian Appraisals of Seven Bioethical Issues.* Ed. James Childs. Minneapolis, Minn.: Augsburg, 1985.

Chouraqui, Jean-Marc. "Des Devoirs Aux Droits de l'homme une perspective juive." In *Les dimensions universelles des Droits de l'homme,* Eds. A. Lapeyre, F. de Tinguy, K. Vasak. Brussells: UNESCO (1990): 1:81-1:112.

Churchland, Patricia S., T.J. Sejnowski. "Perspectives on Cognitive Neuroscience." *Science* 242 (1988): 741-745.

Clarke, Angus. "Is non-directive genetic counseling possible?" *The Lancet* 338 (19 Oct. 1991) : 741-745.

Clouser, K. Danner. "Models: A Critical review and a New View." In *Cross-Cultural Perspectives in Medical Ethics: Readings.* Robert Veatch Ed. Boston: Jones and Bartlett Publishers, 1989.

Coakley, S. *Christ Without Absolutes.* Oxford: Clarendon, 1988.

Coakley, S. and Palin D., eds. *The Making and Remaking of Christian Doctrine.* Oxford: Clarendon, 1993.

Cohen, GA. *Ethics.* Oxford: Oxford University Press, 1989.

Cole-Turner, Ronald. *The New Genesis: Theology and the Genetic Revolution.* Louisville: Westminster/John Knox Press, 1993.

Cole-Turner, Ronald and Brent Waters. *Pastoral Genetics: Theology and Care at the Beginning of Life.* Cleveland: Pilgrims Press, 1996.

Conti, Charles. *Metaphysical Personalism—An Analysis of Austin Farrer's Theistic Metaphysics.* Oxford: Clarendon, 1995.

Cook, Peter. "99rep" (replication info.). Peter.Cook@path.ox.ac.uk.

———. "nuc99" (transcription). Peter.Cook@path.ox.ac.uk.

Cook, Peter, I.A. Brazell. "Supercoils in Human DNA." *Journal Cellular Science* 19 (1975): 261-279.

Cullman, O. *Immortality of the Soul or Resurrection of the Dead.* London: Epworth Press, 1958.

Cummings, John Martin. "The State, the Stork, and the Wall: the Establishment Clause and Statutory Abortion Regulation." *Catholic University Law Review* 34 (Summer 1990): 1191-1238.

Conti, Charles. *Metaphysical Personalism – An Analysis of Austin Farrer's Theistic Metaphysics.* Oxford: Clarendon, 1995.

Cornwell, John. *Consciousness and Human Identity.* Oxford: Oxford University Press, 1998.

Council of Europe Press. *Human Rights in International Law.* Haaksbergen, Netherlands: In Or Publikaties, 1995.

Council of Europe Bioethics Committee (CDBI). *Texts of the Council of Europe on Bioethical Matters.* Strasbourg: Council of Europe, April 2000.

Crisp, Roger. "Medical Ethics." Lecture. Oxford: University of Oxford, 1999.

Daly, Mary. "The Spiritual Revolution: Women's Liberation as Theological Re-education." In *Feminist Theological Ethics: A Reader.* Lois K. Daly Ed. Louisville, KY: John Knox Press, 1994.

Daly, Lois K., ed. *Feminist Theological Ethics: A Reader.* Louisville, KY: John Knox Press, 1994.

Darwin, Charles. *Origin of Species.* 1859.

David, Anne. "Freedom of Association and Civil Society: Freedom of Association and Freedoms of Associations." Lecture. Leiden, Netherlands: University of Leiden (1993): 91-94.

Davies, Carolyn Franks. *The Evidential Force of Religious Experience*. Oxford: Clarendon, 1981.

Davis, Derek. "Preserving the Moral Integrity of the Constitution: An Examination of Deconstruction and Other Hermeneutical Theories." In *Law and Morality in a Free Society*. James E. Wood, Jr. and Derek Davis Eds. Waco, TX: JM Dawson Institute of Church–State Studies, 1994.

Davis, Kay. *Duchemes Muscular Dystrophy*. Lecture. Oxford: University of Oxford, 1999.

Dawkins, Richard. *The Selfish Gene*. Oxford: Oxford University Press, 1989.

Deacon, T., J. Dinsmore, L.C. Costantini, J. Ratliff, and O. Isacson. "Blastula-stage stem cells can differentiate into dopaminergic and serotonergic neurons after transplantation." *Exp Neurology*149 (1998): 28-41.

de Cataranzaro, C. J. *Sources chrétiennes*. New York: The Classics of W. Spirituality, 1980.

de Chardin, Teilhard. *Man's Place in Nature*. Translated by Rene Hague. New York: Harper and Row, 1966.

———. *The Phenomenon of Man*. Translated by Rene Hague. New York: Harper, 1959.

———. *Science and Christ*. Translated by Rene Hague. New York: Harper and Row, 1968.

Deech, Ruth. "British Blood Case." Lecture. International Society of Family Law. Oxford: University of Oxford, 1999.

Delitzsche, Franz. *New Commentary on Genesis*. Translated by Sophia Taylor. Minneapolis: Klock and Klock Christian Publishers, 1978. (Original by T & T Clarke, 1888).

Devine, Richard D. *Good Care, Painful Choices: Medical Ethics for Ordinary People*. New York: Paulist Press, 1996.

Dickens, B. M. "Law, Ethics, and Justice in Human Reproduction." In *Aspects éthiques de la reproduction humaine – Ethical aspects of human reproduction*, Eds. Claude Sureau and Françoise Shenfield. Paris: John Libbey Eurotext, 1995.

Dickey, N. "Council on Ethical and Judicial Affairs, American Medical Association, Statement on Withholding or Withdrawing Life-Prolonging Medical Treatment." *Journal of the American Medical Association* 256 (1986): 471.

Dietrich, Donald J. "Catholic Eugenics in Germany, 1920-1945: Hermann Muckermann, S.J. and Joseph Mayer." *Journal of Church and State* 34 (Summer 1992): 575-600.

Douglas, Mary. *Natural Symbols: Explorations in Cosmology*. London: Barrie & Jenkins, 1973.

Downie, R.S., Elizabeth Telfer. *Respect for Persons*. New York: Schoken Books, Inc., 1970. In *Philosophic Ethics: An Introduction of Moral Philosophy*. Washington DC: Georgetown University, 1982.

Drane, James F. *Becoming a Good Doctor: The Place of Virtue and Character in Medical Ethics*. Kansas City, MO: Sheed & Ward, 1988.

————. *Clinical Bioethics: Theory and Practice in Medical–Ethical Decision Making*. Kansas City, MO: Sheed & Ward, 1994.

Driver, Samuel. *The Book of Genesis*. London: Methuen and Co., 1904.

DuBoulay, S. *Cicely Saunders: The Founder of the Modern Hospice Movement*. London: Hodder and Stroughton, 1997.

Dworkin, Gerald. "Moral Autonomy." In *Morals, Science, and Sociality*, Eds. G. Dworkin, H. Tristram Engelhardt Jr., and David Callahan. Hastings-On-Hudson, NY: The Hastings Center, 1978. In *Philosophic Ethics: An Introduction of Moral Philosophy*. Washington DC: Georgetown University, 1982.

Dworkin, Roger B. *The Role of Law in Bioethical Decision-Making*. Indianapolis: Indiana UP, 1996.

Dworkin, Ronald. "Taking Rights Seriously." In *Philosophic Ethics: An Introduction of Moral Philosophy*. Tom L. Beauchamp Ed. Washington DC: Georgetown University, 1982.

Doherty, Peter, ed. *Man-Made Man: Ethical and Legal Issues in Genetics*. Dublin: Open Air, 1997.

Edgar, H. "Discussion: Fetal Cell Transplantation." In *Aspects éthiques de la reproduction humaine*. Claude Sureau and Françoise Shenfield Eds. Paris, France: John Libbey Eurotext, 1995.

Edwards, Ruth. *Gospel of John*. London: SPCH, 2004.

Eleazar, Daniel. *Covenant and Commonwealth*. New Brunswick: Rutgers University Press, 1995.

Eliade, Mircea Eliade. *From Medicine Men to Mohammed*. New York: Harper and Row, 1974.

"Embryos are out there, but not for Research." *Orange County Register* (26 August 2001): News 6-7. Originally printed in the *New York Times* (24 August 2001).

Erhardt, N.n. *Euthanasia and Destruction of Life Devoid of Value*. Forum of Psychology Series. Marburg: F. Encke Publishers, 1965.

"The 'Euthanasia' Programme 1939-1945." In *Nazism 1919-1945 Vol. 3 Foreign Policy, War and Racial Extermination*. Exeter Studies in History No. 13. J. Noakes, and G. Pridham Eds. Exeter: University of Exeter, n.d.

"Evangelical Doctrine of Theosis." *Journal of the Evangelical Society* (June 1997).

Eysenck, H.J. "The Ethics of Science and the Duties of Scientists." *The Advancement of Science*, no. 1 (1975): 23-25.

Farley, Margaret A. "Feminist Theology and Bioethics." In *Feminist Theological Ethics: A Reader*. Lois K. Daly Ed. Louisville, KY: John Knox Press, 1994.

Farrar, Austin. *The Freedom of the Will*. London: A & C Black, 1958.

————. *The Glass Vision*. Westminster: Dacre, 1948.

————. *A Science of God?* London: Geoffrey Bles, 1966.

Feen, Richard H. "Abortion and Exposure in Ancient Greece: Assessing the Status of the Fetus and 'New Born' from Classical Sources." In *Abortion and the Status of the Fetus*. William B. Bandeson, H. Tristan Engelhardt, Jr., Stuart I. Spickler, and Daniel H. Winship Eds. New York: D. Reidel Publishing Company, 1983.

Feinberg, Joel. "Obligations and Supererogation." From "Supererogation and Rules." *Ethics* 71 (1961). Reprinted in Feinberg, J. *Doing and Deserving*. Princeton, New Jersey: Princeton University Press, 1970. In *Philosophic Ethics: An Intro-*

duction of Moral Philosophy, Ed. Tom L. Beauchamp. Washington DC: George-town University, 1982.

Feinberg, John S., and Paul D. Feinberg. *Ethics for a Brave New World.* Wheaton, Ill.: Crossways Books, 1993.

Feldman, Jan D. "The Establishment Clause and Religious Influences on Legislation." *Northwestern University Law Review* 75 (December 1980): 944-976.

Feuillet-Le Mintier, B. *Genetics, the Family and Human Rights.* Lecture. International Society of Family Law Symposium. Oxford: University of Oxford (1999).

Fiddes, Paul. *The Creative Suffering of God.* Oxford: Clarendon, 1988.

Fine, Beth A. "The Evolution of Nondirectiveness in Genetic Counseling and Implications of the Human Genome Project." In *Prescribing Our Future.* New York: Aldine de Gruyter, 1993.

Fleming, Gerald. *Hitler and the Final Solution.* Berkeley: University of California Press, 1984.

Fletcher, Joseph F. "Four Indicators of Humanhood—The Enquiry Matures." In *On Moral Medicine: Theological Perspectives on Moral Medicine.* Stephen E. Lammers and Allen Verney Ed. 2nd ed. Grand Rapids: William B. Eerdmans Publishing Co, 1998.

Fletcher, Joseph. *Situation Ethics.* Philadelphia: The Westminster Press, 1966.

Fowler, Gregory, Eric T. Juengst, and Burke K. Zimmerman, eds. "Germline Gene Therapy and the Clinical Ethos of Medical Genetics." *Theoretical Medicine* 10 (1989): 151-165.

Foucault, Michel. *The Birth of the Clinic: An Archeology of Medical Perception.* Translation of *Naissance de la Clinic.* Translated by A.M. Sheridan Smith. New York: Pantheon Books, 1973.

Frankel, Victor E. *Man's Search for Meaning.* New York: Beacon Press, 1984.

Friedlander, Henry. *The Origins of the Nazis Genocide: From Euthanasia to Final Solution.* Chapel Hill: The University of North Carolina Press, 1995.

Frielle, M.B. ed. *Embryo Experimentation in Europe: Biomedical, Legal, and Philosophical Aspects.* Bad Neuenahr-Ahrweiler: Europäische Akademie, 2001.

Fuller, M. *Atoms and Icons – A Discussion of the Relationships Between Science and Theology.* London: Mowbray, 1995.

Gasser, S.M., U.K. Laemmli. "Cohabitation of scaffold binding regions with upstream/enhancer elements of 3 developmentally regulated genes of *D. melanogaster*." *Cell* 46 (1986): 521-530.

Geber. S., M. Sampaio. "Blastomere development after embryo biopsy: A new model to predict embryo development and to select for transfer." *Human Reproduction* 14 (1999): 782-786.

Genetic Forum. *The Case Against Patients in Genetic Engineering.* London: Genetic Forum, 1996.

Gilbert, Scott. *Developmental Biology,* 5th ed. London: Sinuar, 1995.

Gilby, Thomas. "Conscience." In the *Encyclopedia of Religion.* Vol. 1. Farmington Hills, MI: MacMillan Reference Books, 1985.

Gilligan, Carol. *In a Different Voice: Psychological Theory and Women's Development.* Cambridge: Harvard University Press, 1982.

Gilson, Etienne. *The Spirit of Medieval Philosophy*. Trans. By A.H.C. Downes. New York: Charles Schribner's Sons, 1936.

————. History of Christian Philosophy in the Middle Ages. New York: Random House, 1955.

Glantz, Leonard. "Is the Fetus a Person? A Lawyers View." In *Abortion and the Status of the Fetus*. William B. Bandeson, H. Tristan Engelhardt, Jr., Stuart I. Spickler, and Daniel H. Winship Eds. 283-293. Dordreet: D. Reidel Publishing Company, 1983.

Glass, B. *Science and Ethical Values*. Oxford: Oxford University Press, 1966.

Goldhagen, Daniel Jonah. *Hitler's Willing Executioners*. New York: Vintage Books, 1997.

Golding, Martin P. "Ethical Issues in Biological Engineering." In *Ethics and Public Policy,* Ed. Tom L. Beauchamp. Englewood Cliffs, NJ: Prentice Hall, 1975.

Gosden, Christine. *Progress and Achievements of Biotechnology*. Lecture. International Society of Family Law. Oxford: University of Oxford, 1999.

Goss, Steve J. *Differentiation*. Lecture. Oxford: University of Oxford, 1999.

Götz, Aly, Peter Chroust, and Christian Pross. *Cleansing the Fatherland, Nazi Medicine and Racial Hygiene*. Baltimore: Johns Hopkins University Press, 1994.

Green, Elizabeth E. "The Transmutation of Theology: Ecofeminist Alchemy and the Christian Tradition." In *Ecofeminism and Theology: Yearbook of the European Society of Women in Theological Research*. Netherlands: Kok Pharos Publishing House, 1994.

Greenawalt, Kent. *Religiously Based Premises and Laws Restrictive of Liberty*. Lexington, VA: n.n. 1984.

————. *Private Consciences and Public Reasons*. Oxford: Oxford University Press, 1995.

————. *Religious Convictions and Political Choice*. New York: Oxford University Press, 1988.

Greenfield, Susan. *Journey to the Center of the Mind: Toward a Science of Consciousness*. New York: W.H. Freeman and Co., 1995.

Gregory of Nazianzus. *Ep. Cled.* St. Vladimir's Seminary Press, 1986.

————. *Funeral Oration for Basil*. SLG Press Fairacres Publications, 1986.

Grey, Mary. *Redeeming the Dream: Feminism, Redemption and Christian Tradition*. London: SPCH, 1989.

Griggs, Richard A. "First Amendment Facelift: Renquist Court Crafts New Scrutiny Level for Content-Neutral Speech Restricting Injunctions." *Mercer Law Review* 46 (Spring 1995): 1197-1210.

Gross, Richard. *Psychology: Science of Mind and Behavior.* London: Hodder and Stroughton, 1996.

Gruman, Gerald J. "Death and Dying: Euthanasia and Sustaining Life, I. Historical Perspectives." In *Encyclopedia of Bioethics,* Ed. Warren T. Reich. London, Collier Macmillan Publishers, 1978.

Guillod, Oliver. *Genetics, the Family and Human Rights*. Lecture. International Society of Family Law. Oxford: University of Oxford, 1999.

Gustafson, James M. *Ethics from a Theocentric Perspective*. 2 Vols. *Ethics and Theology*. Chicago: University of Chicago, 1984.

————. *Intersections: Science, Theology, and Ethics.* Cleveland: The Pilgrim Press, 1996.

Habgood, John. *Being a Person—Where Faith and Science Meet.* London: Hodder & Stoughton, 1998.

Hallowell, John. "The Liberal Expression of Individualism." In *Cross Cultural Perspectives in Medical Ethics: Readings.* Robert Veatch Ed. Boston: Jones and Bartlett Publishers, 1989.

Hampshire, Stuart, ed. *Public and Private Morality.* Cambridge: Cambridge University Press, 1978.

————. *Two Theories of Morality.* Oxford: Oxford University Press, 1977.

Haney, Eleanor Humes. "What is Feminist Ethics?: A Proposal for continuing Discussion." In *Feminist Theological Ethics: A Reader,* Ed. Lois K. Daly. Louisville, KY: John Knox Press, 1994.

Harre, Rom. *Language of Morals.* Oxford: Oxford University Press, 1952.

————. *The Philosophies of Science – An Introductory Survey.* Oxford: Oxford University Press, 1985.

————. *Varieties of Realism.* Oxford: Basil Blackwell, 1986.

Harrison, M.R., and Adzick N. Scott. "Fetus As a Patient: Surgical Considerations." In *Ann Surg* 213 (1991): 279-90.

Haren, Michael. *Medieval Thought,* 2nd ed. Toronto: University of Toronto Press, 1992.

Hart, H.L.A. *The Concept of Law.* Oxford: Oxford University Press, 1961.

Hartland-Swann, John. *An Analysis of Morals.* London: George Allen and Unwin Ltd., 1960.

Hauerwas, Stanley. *The Peaceable Kingdom: A Primer in Christian Ethics.* Notre Dame, IN.: University of Notre Dame Press, 1983.

Hefner, Philip. *The Human Factor: Evolution, Culture, and Religion.* Minneapolis: Fortress Press, 1993.

Hegel, G.W.F. *Philosophy of Right* (1821). Translated by T.M. Knox. London: Oxford University Press, 1952.

Henig, Robin Marantz. "Tempting." *Discover* (May 1998): 62.

Hensley, Scott. "In Odd Pairing, Celera, University to Map Rat DNA." *Wall Street Journal* (1 March 2001), B1, B6.

Hentoff, N. "Nazi Bioethics and a Doctor's Defense." *Human Life Review* 8 (1982): 55-69.

Heschel, Abraham. *Who is Man?* Stanford: Stanford University Press, 1965.

Heyd, David. *Genethics: Moral Issues in the Creation of People.* Berkeley: University of California Press, 1992.

Hick, John. *Death and Eternal Life.* New York: Harper and Row.

Hilberg, Raul. *The Destruction of the European Jews.* Chicago: Quadrangle Books, 1961.

Hildegard of Bingen. *Scivias.* Translation by Bruce Hozeski. Santa Fe, NM: Bear, 1986.

Himmelfarb, Gertrude. *The De-Moralization of Society.* New York: Alfred A. Knopf, 1995.

Hitler, Adolf. *My Battle (Mein Kampf)*. Translation by E.T.S. Dugdale. Boston, Mass.: Houghton Mifflin Co., 1937. (Complete, unabridged version: New York: Reynal and Hitchcock, 1939).

Hinchliffe, J.R., T.J. Horder. "Testing the theoretical models for limb patterning." In *Experimental and Theoretical Advances in Biological Pattern Formation*. H.G. Othmer, et al. Ed. London: Plenum, 1993.

Hobsley, M. *Pathways in Surgical Management*. 2nd ed. London: Edward Arnold, 1986.

Hoedeman, Paul. *Hitler or Hippocrates*. Translation by Ralph de Rijke. Sussex, Eng.: The Book Guild, Ltd., 1991.

Hoffman, B. *The Strange Story of the Quantum*. 2nd ed. Mass.: Harmonsworth and Glouchester, 1963.

Hole, N., G.J. Grapham, U. Menzel, J.D. Nasell. "A limited temporal window for the deviation of multilineage repopulating hematopoietic progenitors during embroyonal stem cell differentiation." *Blood* 88 (1996): 1266-1276.

Horan, Dennis J., et al. *Abortion and the Constitution: Reversing Roe v. Wade Through the Courts*. Washington DC: Georgetown University Press, 1987.

Hottois, G. "Is cloning the absolute evil?" *Human Reproductive Update* 4 (199).

Hozak, P., D.A. Jackson, and P.R. Cook. "The Role of nuclear structure in DNA Replication." In *Eukaryotic DNA Replication: Frontiers in Molecular Biology*, Ed. J.J. Blow. Oxford: Oxford University Press, 1996.

Hubbell, Angela Marie. "FACE'ing the First Amendment: Application of RICO and the Clinic Entrances Act to Abortion Protesters." *Ohio Northern University Law Review* 21 (Spring 1995): 1061-1083.

Huktgren, A.J. "The *Pisitis Christou* Formulation in Paul." *NovTestamentum* 22 (1980).

Hunt, Robert and John Arras, eds. *Ethical Issues in Modern Medicine*. Palo Alto, CA: Mayfield Publishing Company, 1977.

Hyman, A. and J.J. Walsh, eds. *Philosophy of the Middle Ages. The Christian, Islamic and Jewish Tradition*. Indianapolis: Hackett Publishing Co., 1973.

Imbert, Jean. "Conférence internationale sur la tolérance et loi (Sienne, Italy 8-10 April 1995): Tolérence et loi: aperçu historique." *Conscience et liberté* 2:2 (1995): 93-104.

Jackson, D.A., and P.R. Cook. "Transcriptionally active minichromosomes are attached transiently in nuclei through transcription units." *Journal Cellular Science* 105 (1993): 1143-1150.

Johannes, Laura. "Protein Clears Alzheimer's Plaque on Brains of Mice, Study Shows." *Wall Street Journal* (1 March 2001), B1, B11.

James, William. *Varieties of Religious Experience*. New York: Modern Library, 1936.

Jasonoff, Sheila. *Science at the Bar: Law Science and Technology in America*. Cambridge: Harvard Univ. Press, 1995.

Jasper, H.H., J. Tessier, "Acetylcholine Liberation from Cerebral Cortex during Paradoxical (REM) Sleep." *Science* 172 (1971): 601-602.

John of the Cross. *Dark Night of the Soul*. Halcyon Backhouse Ed. London: Hodder and Stroughton, 1988.

Johnson, Alan G. *Pathways in Medical Ethics.* London: Edward Arnold, 1990.

Johnson, E.E., and D.M. Hay, eds. *Pauline Theology, Volume IV, Looking Back, Pressing On.* Sydney Biblical Association [SBA] Symposium Series, 1997.

Jonas, Hans. "Report on the National Commission: Good as Gold." *Medical Legal News* 8 (Dec. 1980): 4-7.

Jones, David. *On Death.* Lecture. Oxford: University of Oxford, 2000.

Jones, Steve. "Genetics in Medicine: Real Promises, Unreal Expectations—One Scientist's Advice to Policymakers in the United Kingdom and the United States." *Millbank Memorial Fund Prospectus.* New York: Millbank Memorial Fund, 2000.

Jonsen, Albert R. "Part Six: Should We Have Public Policy?" In *Active Euthanasia, Religion, and the Public Debate,* Ed. Ron Hamel. Chicago: The Park Ridge Center (1991): 100-105.

Jonsson, John N. *Creation, Law, Gospel.* Pretoria, South Africa: University of Natal, 1965. Reprint, Charlottesville, S. Carolina: Nilses Publications, 1998.

———. *Mythologem and High God in Ancient Mythology.* Charlotte, So. Carolina: Nilses Publications, 1979.

———. *Mythology: The Entmythologisierung Controversy.* Charlotte, So. Carolina: Nilses Publications, 1979.

———. *Religion Within World Phenomena: A Phenomenological Approach to the Study of Religion—Praesis ut Prosis.* Charleston: Nilses Publications, 1996.

———. *The Transfiguration of Jesus.* Pietermaritzburg, S. Africa: Universtiy of Natal, 1979.

Juengst, Eric, and LeRoy Walters. "Gene Therapy: Ethical and Social Issues." In the *Encyclopedia of Bioethics.* Vol. 2. New York: Macmillan Library, 1995.

Kant, Immanuel. *Kant: Political Writings.* Edited by Hans Reiss. Cambridge: Cambridge University Press, 1970.

———. *Groundwork of the Metaphysics of Morals* (1785). Translated by H.J. Paton. New York: Harper and Row, 1956.

Kapp, F. "On sterilization of Hereditary Mental Deficit's and Its meaning in the Fight Against Crime." *Monthly Journal for Criminal Biology and Criminal Law Reference* (1930).

Kass, Leon R. "The New Biology: What Price Relieving Man's Estate?" In *Ethics and Public Policy.* Tom L. Beauchamp ed. Englewood Cliffs, NJ: Prentice Hall, 1975.

———. "Regarding the End of Medicine and the Pursuit of Health." *The Public Interest* 40 (Summer 1975): 27-29.

Kater, Michael H. *Under Hitler.* Chapel Hill: University of North Carolina Press, Inc., 1989.

Katz, Wilbur G. *Religion and the American Constitution.* Evanston, IL: Northwestern University Press, 1964.

Kaufman, Walter and Forrest E. Baird, Ed. *Medieval Philosophy.* 2 Vols. Englewood Cliffs, NJ: Prentice Hall, 1994.

Kelly, Tara K. "Silencing the Lambs: Restricting First Amendment Rights of Abortion Clinic Protesters." *Southern California Law Review* 68 (January 1995): 427-492.

Kendrew, J.C. *The Thread of Life: An Introduction to Molecular Biology.* London: Bell and Sons, 1966.

Kheel, Martin. "The Liberation of Nature: A Circular Affair." *Environmental Ethics* 7 (Summer 1985): 144.

Kikyo N., and A.P. Wolffe. "Reprogramming nuclei: insights from cloning, nuclear transfer and heterokaryons." *Journal of Cell Science* 113 (2000): 11-20.

Kipling D., and R.G. Faragher. "Telomeres. Aging hard or hardly ageing?" *Nature* 398 (1999): 191-193.

Kirby, Justice Michel. "Economic Aspects of Genome Research." In the *International Bioethics Committee of UNESCO (IBC),* 7th Session: Proceedings. Vol. 1. Paris, France: UNESCO, 2003.

Knoppers, Bartha Marie. *The Internationalization of Norms in Genetic Medicine.* Lecture. International Conference on Genetic Diagnosis. Rennes, FR: University of Rennes, 1998.

Kohlberg, Lawrence. *The Philosophy of Moral Development.* San Francisco: Harper and Row, 1981.

Kohlberg, Lawrence and R. Kramer. "Continuities and Discontinuities in Child and Adult Moral Development." *Human Development* 12 (1969): 93-120.

Konner, Melvin. *The Tangled Wing: Biological Constraints on the Human Spirit.* New York: Harper Colophon Books, 1982.

Koshland, , Daniel E. "Judicial Impact Statements." *Science* 239 (1988): 1225.

Krason, Stephen M. *Abortion, Politics, Morality and the Constitution.* New York: University Press of America, 1984.

Krislov, Samuel. "Alternatives to Separation of Church and State in Countries Outside the United States." In *Religion and the State.* James E. Wood Ed. Waco: Baylor University Press, 1985.

Küng, Hans. "A Global Ethic: A Challenge for the New Millennium." *Gresham Special Lecture.* London: St. Paul's Cathedral, 2000.

Küng, Hans and Helmut Schmidt. *A Global Ethic and Global Responsibilities: Two Declarations.* London: SCM Press Ltd., 1998.

Ladd, George Eldon. *A Theology for the New Testament.* Eerdmans, 1987.

Langdell, Christopher Columbus. *The Development of Equity Leading from Canon Law Procedures.* Cambridge: Cambridge University Press, 1905.

Lanza, R.P., J.B. Cibelli, M.D. West. "Prospect for the use of nuclear transfer in human transplantation." *Nature Biotechnology* 17 (1999): 1171-1174.

Lapeyre A., F. de Tinguy, and K. Vasak, Eds. *Les dimensions universelles des Droits de l'homme.* Vol. 1. Brussels: UNESCO, 1990.

Lappé, Marc. "Eugenics: Ethical Issues." In the *Encyclopedia of Bioethics,* 5 vols. 2:773-77. New York: Macmillan Library, 1995.

———. "Eugenics, II. Ethical Issues." In *Ethics and Public Policy.* Tom L. Beauchamp Ed. Englewood Cliffs, NJ: Prentice Hall (1975): 462-468.

Larsen, Bryn K. "RICOs Application to Non-Economic Actors: A Serious Threat to First Amendment Freedoms." *Review of Litigation* 14 (Summer 1995): 707-739.

Larsen, W.J. *Human Embryology.* London: Churchill Livingston, 1996.

Leaky, Richard, Roger Lewen. *The Sixth Extinction: Biodiversity and its Survival.* London: Orion Books, Ltd., 1996.

Lemkow, Louis. *Public Attitude to Genetic Engineering: Some European Perspectives*. Dublin: Loughlinstown House, Shankill Co., 1993.

Lemon, K.P., and A.D. Grossman. "Localization of bacterial DNA polymerase: evidence for a factory model of replication." *Science* 282 (1998): 1516-1519.

Lepin, J. "Introduction." In *Scientific Realism*. J. Leplin. Berkley Ed. University of California Press, 1984.

Lerner, R. and M. Mahdi, Eds. *Medieval Political Philosophy: A Sourcebook*. Ithaca, New York: Cornell University Press, 1963.

Lerner, Max. *Mind and Faith of Holmes*. Boston: Transactoin Publishers, 1988. (Reprint.)

Leslie, Stephen. *Science of Ethics* (1882).

Leuprecht, Peter. "Le Sous - Dévelopment des droits culturels, vu depuis le Conseil de L' Europe." In *Les droits culturels*. Fribourg, Suisse: Universitaires Fribourg Suise [St. Paul] (1993) : 73-88.

Lifton, Robert Jay. *The Nazi Doctors: Medicine, Killing and Psychology of Genocide*. New York: Basic Books, Inc. Publications, 1986.

Lindberg, David C. *The Beginnings of Western Science: The European Scientific Tradition of Philosophical, Religious, and Institutional Context, 600BC to AD 1450*. Chicago: University of Chicago Press, 1992.

Little, David. *Religion, Order and Law*. New York: Harper and Row, 1994.

Lockley, Harold. *Dietrich Bonhoeffer: His "Ethics" and its Value for Christian Ethics Today*. London: Phoenix Press (Swansea), 1993.

Longenecker, B.W. *The Triumph of Abraham's God: The Transformation of Identity in Galatians*. Edinburgh: T & T Clark, 1998.

Los Angeles Times Editorial. "Gene Patent Reform Vital." *Los Angeles Times*, February 2000, n/d.

Loskey, Vladamir. *The Mystical Theology of the Eastern Church*. Cambridge: James Clarke and Co., Ltd., 1957.

MacIntyre, Alaisdair. *After Virtue*. Notre Dame: University of Notre Dame, 1981.

Maclin, Ruth. "Moral Concerns and Appeals to Rights and Duties." *The Hastings Center Report* (October 1976).

Maddox, Robert L., and Blaine Bortnick. "Webster v. Reproductive Health Services: Do Legislative Declarations that Life Begins at Conception Violate the Establishment Clause?" *Campbell Law Review* 12 (Winter 1989): 1-21.

Maloney, George A. *Pseudo Marcarius*. Edited and translated by George Maloney. New York: Paulist Press, 1992.

Mangolick, David. "15 Vials of Sperm: the Unusual Bequest of an even More Unusual Man." *New York Time* (29 April 1994), B18.

Marineau, James. *Types of Ethical Theory* (1885).

Martin-Archard, , R. *From Death to Life*. Edinburgh: Oliver and Boyd, 1960.

Mauer, Armand A. *Medieval Philosophy*, 2nd ed. 2 Vols. Toronto, Ontario: Pontifical Institute of Medieval Studies, 1982.

May, William. "The Morality of Abortion." *Catholic Medical Quarterly* 26 (1974).

May, William F. *The Physician's Covenant*. Philadelphia: The Westminster Press, 1983.

Mayo, Bernard. "Ethics and The Moral Life." In *Ethics and the Moral Life*. New York: Macmillan and Co., 1958. In *Philosophic Ethics: An Introduction of Moral Philosophy*. Tom L. Beauchamp Ed. Washington, DC: Georgetown University, 1982.

McCall Smith, Alexander, and Michel Revel. "The Use of Embryonic Stem Cells in Therapeutic Research." In the *International Bioethics Committee of UNESCO (IBC)*, 7th Session, Proceedings. Vol. 1. Paris, France: UNESCO, 2003.

McCormick, Richard A. "To Save or Let Die, The Dilemma of Modern Medicine." *Journal of the American Medical Association* 299 (8 July 1974): 172-176.

McDonald, J. Ian H. *Christian Values: Theory and Practice in Christian Ethics Today*. Edinburgh: T & T Clark, 1995.

McGee, Daniel B. "Euthanasia and Physician-Assisted Suicide: A Believer's Church Perspective." In *Must We Suffer Our Way to Death?*, Eds. Ronald B. Hamel and Edwin R. DuBose. Dallas: Southern Methodist University Press, 1996.

McGee, Glenn. *The Perfect Baby: A Pragmatic Approach to Genetics*. Lanham, Maryland: Rowman & Littlefield Publishers, Inc., 1977.

McFayden, Alistair J. *The Call to Personhood: A Christian Theory of the Individual in Social Relationships*. Cambridge: Cambridge University Press, 1990.

McKay, Donald. *Behind the Eye*. Gifford Lectures, ed. Valerie MacKay. Oxford: Blackwell, 1991.

McKnight, T. D. "Transcription and elongation." *Genes and Development* 10 (1996): 367.

McNeil, Paul M. *Ethics and Politics of Human Experimentation*. Cambridge: Cambridge University Press, 1993.

Mead, Sydney E. *The Nation with the Soul of a Church*. New York: Harper and Row, 1975.

Meisel, Alan. "Informed Consent: Where is it going?" *Health Law News*. Vol. XV. (June 2001): 6.

Michaud, Jean. *The Internationalization of a Framework for Genetic Diagnosis*. Lecture. International Conference on Genetic Diagnosis. Rennes, FR: University of Rennes, 1998.

Midgley, Mary. "Putting Ourselves Together Again." In *Consciousness and Human Identity*, Ed. John Cornwall. Oxford: Oxford University Press, 1998.

Mills, John Stuart. *On Liberty and Considerations on Representative Government* (1859). Edited by R. B. McCallum. Oxford: Basil Blackwell, 1946.

Miller, Robert T. and Ronald B. Flowers. *Toward Benevolent Neutrality: Church, State and the Supreme Court*. Waco: Markham Press Fund of Baylor University Press, 1992.

Mitchell, Basil. *The Justification of Religious Belief*. London: Macmillan, 1973.

Moltmann, Jürgen. *The Crucified God: The Cross of Christ as the Foundation and Criticism of Christian Theology*. Translation by R.A. Wilson and John Bowder. New York: Harper and Row, 1974.

————. *Gott in der Schöpfung: Oekolgische Schöpfungs lehre*. München: Christian Kaiser, 1985.

————. *Way of Jesus Christ*. London: SCM, 1990.

Monad, Jacque Monad. *Leçon inaugurale au College de France.* Lecture. College of France, Paris, 3 November 1967. Published as *Chance and Necessity.* N/c: Collins, 1967.

Montgomery, John Warwick Ed. "Human Dignity in Birth and Death: A Question of Values." *Christian Legal Journal.* Christian Legal Fellowship (Spring 1993): 3:17-23.

————. "Law and Christian Theology: Some Foundational Principles." *Christian Legal Journal.* Ed. Christian Legal Fellowship (Spring 1993): 3:24-31.

Mor, V. *Hospice Care Systems: Structure, Process, Costs and Outcome.* New York: Springer, 1987.

Morgan, Robert. *Romans: New Testament Guides.* Sheffield: Sheffield Academic Press, 1995.

Morley, David. *The Sensitive Scientist: Report of a British Associated Study Group.* London: SCM, 1978.

Morris-Kay, Gillian M., et al. *Signaling Systems in Development.* Lecture. Oxford: University of Oxford, 1999.

Mount, Eric. *Conscience and Responsibility.* Richmond, VA: John Knox Press, 1969.

Mpedawatu, Jean-Marie. *Questions Generales Sur le Conseil Genetic* at http:www.unesco/ethics.

Murphy, Margaret. "Part Six: Should We Have Public Policy?" In *Active Euthanasia, Religion, and the Public Debate,* Ed. Ron Hamel. Chicago: The Park Ridge Center (1991): 94-95.

Murphy, Nancey. *Beyond Liberalism and Fundamentalism.* Valley Forge, PA: Trinity Press, 1996.

————. "Mental Causation." www.st-edmunds.cam.ac.uk/cis/murphy.

————. *Theology in an Age of Scientific Reasoning.* New York: Cornell, 1990.

Murphy, Nancy and George F. R. Ellis. *On the Moral Nature of the Universe–Theology, Cosmology and Ethics.* Minneapolis: Fortress, 1996.

Murray, Robert E. "Genetic Counseling: Ethical Issues." In the *Encyclopedia of Bioethics.* Vol. 2. New York: Macmillan Library, 1995.

Murray, Thomas H. and Jeffrey R. Botkin. "Genetic Testing and Screening: Ethical Issues." In the *Encyclopedia of Bioethics.* Vol. 2. New York: Macmillan Library, 1995.

Mursell, Gordon. *Out of the Deep: Prayers of Protest.* London: SCM, 1998.

Nakada, D., B. Magasanik. "The Roles of Inducer and Catabolite Repressor in the Synthesis of Beta-Galactosidase by Escherichia Coli."*Journal of Molecular Biology* 8 (1964): 105-127.

Nelson, James B. *Moral Nexus: Ethics of Christian Identity and Community.* Philadelphia: Fortress Press, 1984.

Nesteruk, Alexi. *Orthodox Perspective of Science and Theology.* Lecture. Oxford: University of Oxford, 1999.

Neubüser, Gerald, at al. "The role of FGF signaling in positioning the tooth germs in the mandible." *Cell* 90 (1997): 247-255.

Neuhaus, John Richard. *The Naked Public Square: Religion and Democracy in America.* Grand Rapids: William B. Eerdmans, 1984.

New American Bible. Nashville: Thomas Nelson Publishers, 1987.

New International Version Study Bible.

New Oxford Annotated Bible: Revised Standard Version. New York: Oxford University Press, 1994.

Newton, L.H. "The Patient As Responsible Adult: Derivations and Consequences of Revised Perspective." In *Proceedings of the Fifty-fifth Annual Meeting of the American Catholic Philosophical Association.* Vol. LV, Eds. D.O. Dahlstrom, D.T. Ozar, and L. Sweeney. Washington DC: American Catholic Philosophical Association, 1981.

Nickelsberg, G. *Resurrection, Immortality and Eternal Life.* Cambridge, Mass: Harvard University Press, 1972.

Niebuhr, Reinhold. *The Nature and Destiny of Man.* New York: Charles Schribner's Sons, 1941.

Niebuhr, H. Richard. *Christ and Culture.* New York: Harper & Bros., 1951.

———. *Moral Man and Immoral Society.* New York: Charles Schribner's Sons, 1932.

———. *The Responsible Self: An Essay in Christian Moral Philosophy.* San Francisco: Harper & Row, Publishers, 1978.

Nisand, Israel. *Reproduction and New Technologies: State-of-the-Art.* Lecture. Monaco, FR: UNESCO/AMADE, 2000.

Nodding, Nell. *Caring: A Feminist Approach to Ethics and Moral Education.* Los Angeles: University of California Press, 1984.

Nozick, Robert. *Anarchy, State, and Utopia.* New York: Basic Books, 1977.

Olafson, Frederick. *What is a Human Being?: A Heideggarian View.* Cambridge: Cambridge University Press, 1995.

Orr, Harry T. "The Impact of the Human Genome Project for Genetic Counseling Services." In *Prescribing Our Future.* New York: Aldine de Gruyter, 1993.

Outka, Gene. "Social Justice and Equal Access to Health Care." In *On Moral Medicine: Theological Perspectives in Medical Ethics.* Stephen E. Lammers and Allen Verney 2nd Eds. Grand Rapids: Wm. B. Eerdmans Publishing Company, 1998.

Otto, Rudolph. *The Idea of the Holy,* 2nd ed. London: Oxford Univ. Press, 1950.

Oxford American Dictionary. Herald Colleges Edition. New York: Avon, 1980.

Pailin, David. *Probing the Foundations – A Study of Theistic Reconstruction.* The Netherlands: Pharos Kampen, 1994.

Pannenberg, Wolfgang. *The Apostle's Creed: In the Light of Today's Question.* Philadelphia: Westminster Press, 1972.

———. *Jesus—God and Man.* London: Westminster, 1968.

Pappworth, Michael H. *Human Guinea Pigs.* Boston: Beacon Press, 1967.

Parsons, Susan Frank. *Feminism and Christian Ethics.* Cambridge: Cambridge University Press, 1996.

Peacocke, Arthur. *Creation and the World of Science.* Oxford: Oxford University Press, 1979.

———. *Paths From Science towards God: The End of All our Exploring.* Oxford: Oneworld, 2001.

———. *Theology for a Scientific Age.* London: SCM, 1996.

Pearlman, Robert A., Steven H. Miles, and Robert M. Arnold. "Contributors of Empirical Research to Medical Ethics." *Theoretical Medicine* 14 (1993): 197-210.

Pelligrino, Edmund D. and David C. Thomasma. *For the Patient's Good: The Restoration of Beneficence in Health Care.* Oxford: Oxford University Press, 1988.

Pentateuch with Targum Onkelos, Haphtaroth and Rashi's Commentary, trans. and annotated by M. Rosenbaum and A. Silbermann. New York: Hebrew Publishing Company, 1965.

Perry, Michael. "Is the Idea of Human Rights Ineliminably Religious?" In *Law and Morality,* Eds. James E. Wood, Jr. and Derek Davis. Waco, TX: JM Dawson Institute of Church–State Studies, 1994.

Perry, Patrick. "Craig Ventor: At the Helm of the Genetic Revolution." *The Saturday Evening Post* (Jan/Feb 2000).

Personal Origins, 2nd ed. London: Church House Publishing, 1996.

Petermann, Thomas. "Human Dignity and Genetic Tests." In *Sanctity of Life.* Kurt Bayertz Ed. Boston: Kluwer Academic Publishers, 1991.

Peters, Ted. *Playing God.* London: Rutledge and Kegan Paul, 1996.

Pfeffer, Leo. "An Autobiographical Sketch." In *Church, State, and Freedom.* Rev. Ed. Boston: Beacon Press, 1967.

Pfeffer, Leo. *Church, State, and Freedom.* Rev. Ed. Boston: Beacon Press, 1967.

Pickel, James. "State of the Art of Neuroscience." In the *International Bioethics Committee of UNESCO (IBC),* 7th Session: Proceedings. Vol. 1. Paris, France: UNESCO.

Pierce, Charles A. *Conscience and the New Testament.* London: SCM, 1955.

Pink, Arthur. *Gleanings in Genesis.* Chicago: Moody Press, 1922.

Polkinghorne, John. *Reason and Reality.* London: SPCK, 1991.

Pool, Robert. "Saviors." *Discover* (May 1998): 51 56.

Pope, Stephen J. *The Evolution of Altruism and the Ordering of Love.* Washington DC: Georgetown University Press, 1994.

Posner, Gerald L., John Ware. *Mengele.* New York: McGraw Hill Book Co., 1986.

Potter, Van Rensselaer. *Global Bioethics.* E. Lansing, Mich: Michigan State University Press, 1980.

Pritchard, James B. *The Ancient Near Eastern Texts.* Princeton: University of Princeton, 1950.

Proctor, Robert N. "Nazi Doctors, Racial Medicine, and Human Experimentation." In *The Nazi Doctors and the Nuremberg Code.* Oxford: Oxford University Press, 1975.

Proctor, R. *Racial Hygiene: Medicine Under the Nazis.* Cambridge: Harvard University Press, 1988.

Proudfoot, Nicholas J. *Modern Gene Technology.* Lecture. Oxford: University of Oxford, 1999.

————. *Regulated PolII Transcription.* Lecture. Oxford: University of Oxford, 1999.

————. *The Structure and Replication of DNA.* Lecture. Oxfrd: University of Oxford, 1999.

Radwanski, George. *Hearings of Commissioners for the Protection of Personal Data.* Lecture. 8th Session. Paris, FR: UNESCO, 2001.

Raff, R.A., T.C. Kauffman. *Embryos, Genes and Evolution.* New York: Macmillan, 1983.

Rahner, Karl. *Foundations of Christian Faith: An Introduction to the Idea of Christianity.* London: Darton, Longman, and Todd, 1976.

———. *Theological Investigations.* Vols. 1, 6, 9. New York: Herder and Herder, 1972.

Ramsey, Paul. *Ethics at the Edges of Life.* New Haven: Yale University Press, 1978.

Rawls, John. *A Theory of Justice.* Cambridge, Mass: Harvard University Press, 1971.

Raymond, Janice C. "Reproductive Gifts and Gift-giving: The Altruistic Woman." In *Feminist Theological Ethics: A Reader.* Lois K. Daly Ed. Louisville, KY: John Knox Press, 1994.

Rancourt, C., et al. "Genetic interaction between hoxb5 and Hoxb6 is revealed by nonallelic noncomplementation." *Genes Dev.* 9 (1995): 108-122.

Réne, David. "Comparative Function." In *International Encyclopedia of Comparative Law: The Legal Systems of the World, Their Comparison and Unification,* Eds. K. Z. Zweigert, et al., Vol. II. The Hague: Mouton, 1975).

Resher, Nicholas. "The Allocation of Exotic Medical Lifesaving Therapy." In *Ethics and Public Policy.* Tom L. Beauchamp Ed. Englewood Cliffs, NJ: Prentice Hall (1975): 425-441.

Revel, Michel. "Discussion: Ethical Aspects of Embryonic Stem Cell Research." 7th *Session, Proceedings.* Vol. 1. Paris, France: UNESCO, 2003.

———. "Ongoing Research on mammalian cloning and embryo stem cell technologies: Bioethics of their potential medical applications." *Israel Medical Association Journal* (IMAJ) 2, *Supplement* (July 2000): 8-14.

Riddick, S. "Maternal Thinking." *Signs* 6 (1980): 342-367.

Riley, Gregory J. *One Jesus, Many Christs.* San Francisco: Harper Collins, 1989.

Rob, Carol S. "Framework for Feminine Ethics." In *Feminist Theological Ethics: A Reader.* Lois K. Daly ed. Louisville, KY: John Knox Press, 1994.

Robertson, John A. "Genetic Selection of Offspring Characteristics." *Boston University Law Review* 76, no. 3 (June 1996):421-482.

Robinson, Patrick. *Proposals of the IBC Working Group with a view to the follow-up on the International Symposium on 'Ethics, Intellectual Property, and Genomics'.* Lecture. 8th Session. Paris, FR: UNESCO IBC, 2001.

Rolston, Holmes. *Genes, Genesis and God: Values and Their Origins in Natural and Human History.* Cambridge: Cambridge University Press, 1999.

Rooks, Alfred G. *Existence, Language, and Religion.* Pretoria: HSRC Publishers, 1991.

Rose, S. "The Rise of Neurogenic Determinism." In *Consciousness and Human Identity,* Ed. John Cornwell. Oxford: Oxford University Press, 1998.

Rosenbaum, M. and A. Silbermann. *Pentateuch with Targum Onkelos, Haphtaroth and Rashi's Commentary.* Translated and annotated by M. Rosenbaum and A. Silbermann. New York: Hebrew Publishing Company, 1965.

Ross, W.D. "What Makes Right Acts Right." In *Cross-Cultural Perspectives in Medical Ethics: Readings,* Robert Veatch Ed. Boston: Jones and Bartlett Publishers, 1989.

Rothman, Barbara. *The Tentative Pregnancy: Amniocentesis and Sexual Politics of Motherhood.* London: Pandora, 1986.

Rousseau, Jean-Jacques. *On the Social Contract* (1762). Translated and edited by Donald A. Cress. Indianapolis: Hackett, 1983.

Rowland, Christopher. "Gospel of John." Lectures. Oxford: University of Oxford, 1999.

———. "Resurrection." Lectures. Oxford: University of Oxford, 2001.

Ruether, Rosemary. *Sexism and God-Talk: Toward a Feminine Theology.* Boston: Beacon Press, 1983.

Rumball, Sylvia, and Alexander McCall Smith. *Draft Report on Collection, Treatment, Storage and Use of Genetic Data.* Draft report. 8th Session. Paris, FR: UNESCO IBC, 2001.

Sade, Robert M. "Medical Care as a Right, a Refutation." In *Cross-Cultural Perspectives in Medical Ethics: Readings.* Robert Veatch Ed. Boston: Jones and Bartlett Publishers, 1989.

Samturri, Edmund. "Prenatal Diagnosis: Some Moral Considerations." In *Questions about the Beginning of Life: Christian Appraisals of Seven Bioethical Issues.* Minneapolis, Minn.: Augsburg, 1985.

Sandel, Michael J. *Democracy's Discontent: America in Search of a Public Philosophy.* Cambridge, Mass: The Belknap Press of Harvard University Press, 1996.

Sawyer, Geoffrey. "Structures and divisions of the law" in *International Encyclopedia of Comparative Law: The Legal Systems of the World, Their Comparison and Unification.* K. Z. Zweigert, et al. Eds. Vol. II. The Hague: Mouton, 1975.

Scalding, J.G. "Diagnosis: The Clinician and the Computer." *Lancet* 11 (1967): 877-882.

Scanlon, Timothy M. *What We Owe Each Other.* Oxford: Oxford University Press, 1999.

Schediand, P., F. Grosveld, "Domaines and Boundaries." In *Chromatin Structure and Gene Expression.* S.C.R. Elgin Ed. Oxford: Oxford University Press, 1996.

Schenker, Joseph G. "Transplantation of Fetal Tissue, Gametes, and Organs." In *Aspects éthiques de la reproduction humaine.* Claude Sureau and Françoise Shenfield Eds. Paris: John Libby Eurotext, 1995.

Schuster, Evelyn. *Progress in embryology and in diagnosis.* Lecture. Monaco, FR: UNESCO/AMADE, 2000.

Schweitzer, Albert. *Philosophy of Civilization.* Translated by C. T. Campion. New York: Macmillan, 1949. Reprint Tallahassee, FL: University Press of Florida, 1981.

Scotus, John Duns. *God as First Principle.* Translated by Allan B. Wolter. Chicago: Franciscan Herald Press, 1969.

Searle, John. "How to Study Consciousness Scientifically." In *Consciousness and Human Identity.* John Cornwall Ed. Oxford: Oxford University Press, 1998.

Sekine, Allan, et al. "Fgf10 is essential for limb and lung formation." *Nature Genetics* 21 (1999): 138-141.

Serour, G. "Debate." In *Aspects éthiques de la reproduction humaine,* Eds. Claude Sureau and Françoise Shenfield. Paris, France: John Libbey Eurotext, 1995.

Seymour, Katy. "Chemical Boundaries of Psychopharmacology." In *Control of the Mind*, eds. Farber & Wilson. New York, 1961.

Sidgwick, Henry. *Outlines of the History of Ethics*. London: Macmillan and Co., Ltd., 1960.

Siegler, M. "Searching for Moral Certainty in Medicine: A Proposal for a New Model of the Doctor–Patient Encounter." *Bulletin of the New York Academy of Medicine*, 57(1): 56-69.

Simons, Andrew. "Brave New Harvest." *Christianity Today* (19 November 1990): 24-28.

Sims, R., and V.A. Moss. *Palliative Care for People with AIDS*, 2nd ed. London: Edward Arnold, 1995.

Skinner, John. *The International Critical and Exegetical Commentary on the Holy Scriptures of the Old and New Testaments: On Genesis*. Eds. Samuel Rolles Driver, Alfred Plummer, Charles Augustus Briggs. Edinburgh: T & T Clark, 1963.

Slater, Edward. "Severely Malformed Children. Wanted—A New Basic Approach." *British Medial Journal* II (1973): 285-286.

Smith, George P., II. "Australia Frozen Orphan Embryos: a Medical, Legal, and Ethical Dilemma." 24 *Journal of Family Law* 27 (1985-86): 82.

Smith, John Maynard. *On Evolution*. Edinburgh: University of Edinburgh, 1972.

Smolin, David M. "The Jurisprudence of Privacy in a Splintered Supreme Court." 75 *Marquardt 2 Review* 975 (1992): 1020.

Soloman, Robert C. "Reflections on the Meaning of Fetal Life." In *Abortion and the Status of the Fetus*. William Bondeson, H. Tristan Englehardt, Stuart F. Spinker, Daniel H. Winship Eds. Boston: Kluwer, 1984.

Sorenson, James R. "Genetic Counseling: Values That Have Mattered." In *Prescribing Our Future*. New York: Aldine de Gruyter, 1993.

Southgate, Christopher, et al. *God, Humanity and the Cosmos: A Textbook in Science and Religion*. Edinburgh: T & T Clark, 1999.

Snowden, R., G.D. Mitchell, and E.M. Snowden. *Artificial Reproduction: A Social Investigation*. London: George Allen & Unwin, 1983.

Stannard, Russell. *Science and Wonders*. London: Faber, 1996.

Steinbock, B. "Maternal–fetal Conflict and *in utero* Fetal Therapy." In *Aspects éthiques de la reproduction humaine*, Eds. Claude Sureau and Françoise Shenfield. Paris, France: John Libbey Eurotext, 1995.

Stern, Robert C. "The Diagnosis of Cystic Fibrosis." *New England Journal of Medicine* 336(7)(13 February 1997): 487-491.

Strachan, Thomas, and Andrew Read. *Human Molecular Genetics*, 2nd ed. London: Wiley John and Sons and Co., 1999.

Stryer, Lubert. *Biochemistry*, 4th ed. New York: W.H. Freeman, 1999.

Sureau, Claude and Françoise Shenfield, eds. *Aspects éthiques de la reproduction humaine–Ethical aspects of human reproduction*. Paris: John Libbey Eurotext, 1995.

Swinburne, Richard, Ed. *The Evolution of the Soul*. Oxford: Clarendon, 1997.

———. *Miracles*. New York: Macmillan, 1989.

Swinburne, Richard. "Resurrection." Lectures. Oxford: University of Oxford, 2001.

Sykes, Brian. *Origins of Man*. Lecture. Oxford: University of Oxford, 1999.

Szadits, Charles. "Structures and Divisions of Law." In *International Encyclopedia of Comparative Law: The Legal Systems of the World, Their Comparison and Unification*. K. Z. Zweigert, et al. Eds. Vol. II. The Hague: Mouton, 1975.

Taubes, Gary. "Ontogeny Recapitulated." *Discover* (May 1998): 66.

Taylor, Telford. "Opening Statement of the Prosecution December 9, 1946." In *The Nazi Doctors and the Nuremberg Code*. Oxford: Oxford University Press, 1992.

Teresa. *Interior Castle*, ed., Halcyon Backhouse. London: Hodder and Stroughton, 1988. "The 'Euthanasia' Programme 1939-1945." In *Nazism 1919-1945, Vol. 3 Foreign Policy, War and Racial Extermination, Exeter Studies in History 13*, Eds., J. Noakes and G. Pridham. University of Exeter, n.d.

Thomasma, David C. "The Basis of Medicine and Religion: Respect for Persons." In *On Moral Medicine: Theological Perspectives in Medical Ethics*. Stephen E. Lammers and Allen Verney, Eds. 2nd ed. Grand Rapids: Wm. B. Eerdmans Publishing Company, 1998.

Thottam, Jyoti. "Hope in a Test Tube." *Time Special Issue* (5 March 2001): 38-39.

Tickel, C. "The Number of polarizing regions cells required to specify additional digits in the chick wing." *Nature* 289 (1981): 295-298.

Tooley, Michael. "Abortion and Infanticide." *Philosophy and Public Affairs* 2 (Fall, 1972): 37-65.

Toulmin S. "The Tyranny of Principles." *Hastings Center Report*, Vol. 11, No. 6 (1981).

Twycross, Robert. "Palliative Care." In *Encyclopedia of Applied Ethics*. Vol. 3. Oxford: Oxford University Press, 1998.

———. "Hospice." Lecture. Oxford: University of Oxford, 2000.

van der Vyver, Johan D., and John Witte, eds. *Religious Human Rights in Global Perspective: Legal Perspectives*. Boston: Martinus Nijhoff Publishers, 1996.

———. *Religious Human Rights in Global Perspective: Religious Perspectives*. Boston: Martinus Nijhoff Publishers, 1996.

van Unnik, W. C. "The Newly Discovered Gnostic 'Epistle to Rheginos' on the Resurrection I," *JEH* 15 (1964), 141-144.

Veatch, Robert. *Cross-Cultural Perspectives in Medical Ethics: Readings*. Robert M. Veatch Ed. Boston: Jones and Bartlett Publishers 1989.

Veatch, Robert M. "Death and Dying: Euthanasia and Sustaining Life, III. Professional and Public Policies." In *Encyclopedia of Bioethics*. Warren T. Reich Ed. London, Collier Macmillan Publishers, 1978.

von Dillman, A. *Die Genesis*. Von der dritten Auflage an erklärt, 6th ed., 1892.

Voorst, R. *Jesus Outside the New Testament*. Grand Rapids: Eerdmans, 2000.

Walzer, Michael. *Spheres of Justice*. New York: Basic Books, 1983.

Ward, Keith. God: A Guide to the Perplexed. Oxford: Oneworld, 2004.

———. *God, Chance and Necessity*. Oxford: Oneworld, 1996.

———. *God Faith and the New Millennium*. Oxford: Oneworld, 1998.

———. *Religion and Creation*. Oxford: Oxford University Press, 1996.

———. *Religion and Community*. Oxford: Oxford University Press, 2000.

———. *Religion and Human Nature*. Oxford: Oxford University Press, 1998.

Ware, Kallistos. *The Orthodox Church*. London: Penguin, 1993.

Warnock, G.J. "The Object of Morality." In *Object of Morality.* London: Methusa and Co., 1971. In *Philosophic Ethics: An Introduction of Moral Philosophy.* Washington DC: Georgetown University, 1982.

Watson, James, et al. *Recombinant DNA.* New York: Scientific American Books/ W.H. Freeman, 1992.

Watts, Fraser. "Cognitive Neuroscience and Religious Consciousness." In *God, Humanity and the Cosmos: A Textbook in Science and Religion.* Christopher Southgate, et al Ed. Edinburgh: T & T Clark, 1999.

Watts, Fraser & M. Williams. *The Psychology of Knowing.* London: Geoffrey Chapman, 1988.

Weed, Laura. "The Amaydala and the Autonomic Nervous System in religious Ecstasy and Post Traumatic Stress Disorder Lecture." Philadelphia, PA: Villa Nova, 2002.

Wiesel, Elie. *Night.* New York: Hill and Wang, 1960.

———. *The Trial of God.* New York: Random House, 1964.

Wenz, Peter S. *Abortion Rights as Religious Freedom.* Phil.: Temple University Press, 1992.

Wertham, F. *A Sign for Cain.* New York: Warner, 1973.

Whitbeck, Caroline. "The Moral Implications of Regarding Women as People: New Perspectives on Pregnancy and Personhood," Eds. William Bondeson, H. Tristan Engelhardt, Stuart F. Spinker, Daniel H. Winship. In *Abortion and the Status of the Fetus.* Boston: Kluwer, 1984.

Wilhelm, Hans-Heinrich. "Euthanasia Program." In *Encyclopedia of the Holocaust.* Vol. 2. Ed., Israel Gutman. New York: Macmillan Publishing Co., 1990.

Williams, Andrew. *Egalitarian Justice and Personal Responsibility.* Paper. Oxford: University of Oxford, 1999.

Williams, Robert H. *To Live and To Die.* New York: Springer-Verlag, 1974.

Wilson, Edward O. *Consilience–The Unity of Knowledge.* London: Little, Brown, 1998.

Wingren, Gustaf. *Creation and Law.* Translated by Ross Mackenzie. London: Oliver and Boyd, 1961.

Witte, John, Johann D. van der Vyver, eds., "Introduction." In *Human Rights in Global Perspective: Religious Perspectives.* Boston: Martinus Nijhoff Publishers, 1996.

Wolff, A. "Gene repression by targeted deacetylation." *Nature* 387 (1997): 16-17.

Wolpert, Lewis. *Principles of Development.* Oxford: Oxford University Press, 1995.

Wondra, Ellen K. "How do we Judge? Theological Assessment of Scientific Developments." *Anglican Theological Review* 18(4)(Fall 1999): 593.

Wood, James E. "A Biblical View of Religious Liberty." *The Ecumenical Review* 30 (January 1978):32-41.

———. "Editorial: Religion and National Interest." *Journal of Church and State* 6 (1964): 7-16.

———. "Jewish–Christian Relations in Historical Perspective." In *Reflections of Church and State.* Waco: J.M. Dawson Institute of Church–State Studies, 1995.

Wood, James E., ed. *Religion and the State*. Waco, TX: Baylor University Press, 1985.

Wood, James E., Bruce Thompson, and Robert T. Miller. *Church and State in Scripture, History, and Constitutional Law*. Waco, TX: J.M. Dawson Institute, Baylor University Press, 1958.

Wood, James E., and Derek Davis, eds. *Law and Morality*. Waco, TX: J.M. Dawson Institute, Baylor University Press, 1995.

————. *Nationhood and the Kingdom*. Nashville, TN: Broadman Press, 1977.

————. *Religion and Politics*. Waco, TX: J.M. Dawson Institute, Baylor University Press, 1983.

————. *The Role of Religion in Making of Public Policy*. Waco, TX: J.M. Dawson Institute, Baylor University Press, 1991.

Woodard, Calvin. "Morality as a Perennial Source of Indeterminacy in the Life of the Law." In *Law and Morality in a Free Society,* Eds. James E. Wood, Jr. and Derek Davis. Waco, TX: JM Dawson Institute of Church–State Studies, 1994.

Wright, Thomas. *Climax of the Covenant*. London: SCM, 1998.

Wulff, Henrik, Stig Andur Pedersen, Raben Rosenberg. *Philosophy of Medicine: Introduction*. London: Blackwell Scientific Publications, 1986.

Xenotransplantation: http:www.abcnews.go.com/sections/living/DaileyNews/pigor gans991103.htm.

Xu, L. et al. "Fibroblast growth factors (FGFRs) and their roles in limb development." *Cell Tissue Research* 296 (1999): 33-43.

Yahil, Leni. *The Holocaust: The Fate of the European Jewry, 1932-1945*. New York: Oxford University Press, 1987.

————. "Kristallnach." In *Encyclopedia of the Holocaust*. Vol. 2. In *Encyclopedia of the Holocaust*. Israel Gutman Ed. New York: Macmillan Publishing Co., 1990.

Yang, Huanming. "Economic Aspects of Genome Research." 7th Session: Proceedings. Vol. 1. Paris, France: UNESCO IBC, 2003.

Youngblood, Joel A. "The First Amendment Falls Victim to RICO." *Tulsa Law Journal* 30 (Fall 1994): 195-212.

Zmärzlik, Hans Guater. *"Der Sozialdarwinismus im Deutschland als geschichtliches Problem."* Vierteljahrshefte *für Zeitgeschichte* 11 (1963): 246-73.

Zweigert, K. Z. et al., eds. *International Encyclopedia of Comparative Law: The Legal Systems of the World, Their Comparison and Unification*. Vol. II. The Hague: Mouton, 1975.

Index

Page numbers followed by the letter "f" indicate figures; those followed by the letter "t" indicate tables; and those followed by the letter "n" indicate endnote references.

T - #0476 - 101024 - C0 - 212/152/19 - PB - 9780789030450 - Gloss Lamination